Choledocholithiasis

AF793915

B. Fernando Santos • Nathaniel Soper
Editors

Choledocholithiasis

Comprehensive Surgical Management

Springer

Editors
B. Fernando Santos
Dartmouth College, Geisel School of Med
Hanover
NH
USA

Nathaniel Soper
Northwestern University
Chicago
IL
USA

ISBN 978-3-030-09007-4 ISBN 978-3-319-74503-9 (eBook)
https://doi.org/10.1007/978-3-319-74503-9

© Springer International Publishing AG, part of Springer Nature 2018
Softcover re-print of the Hardcover 1st edition 2018
This work is subject to copyright. All rights are reserved by the Publisher, whether the whole or part of the material is concerned, specifically the rights of translation, reprinting, reuse of illustrations, recitation, broadcasting, reproduction on microfilms or in any other physical way, and transmission or information storage and retrieval, electronic adaptation, computer software, or by similar or dissimilar methodology now known or hereafter developed.
The use of general descriptive names, registered names, trademarks, service marks, etc. in this publication does not imply, even in the absence of a specific statement, that such names are exempt from the relevant protective laws and regulations and therefore free for general use.
The publisher, the authors and the editors are safe to assume that the advice and information in this book are believed to be true and accurate at the date of publication. Neither the publisher nor the authors or the editors give a warranty, express or implied, with respect to the material contained herein or for any errors or omissions that may have been made. The publisher remains neutral with regard to jurisdictional claims in published maps and institutional affiliations.

Printed on acid-free paper

This Springer imprint is published by the registered company Springer International Publishing AG part of Springer Nature
The registered company address is: Gewerbestrasse 11, 6330 Cham, Switzerland

To my family, Amelia, Lucia, Oliver, and Corrina, Byron and Susy, Jim and Janice, for their endless love and support, and for believing in me.
To my mentors, Nat and Eric, and Bill and Ted, for encouraging my interest in biliary stone disease, and for their guidance over the years.
To George Berci for inspiring me.

—BFS

To my wife, Cindy, and the rest of my family, who have allowed me to pursue my academic passion.
Also, to the trainees who have allowed me to be part of their lives and, especially, to have taken on the responsibility of mastering the LCBDE curriculum and then push recalcitrant faculty to "do the right thing" for our patients.

—NJS

Preface

The management of choledocholithiasis is inherent to the practice of cholecystectomy. During the "open" era of surgery, general surgeons routinely managed this problem with a single-stage operation (open cholecystectomy plus common bile duct exploration), which remains the gold standard for choledocholithiasis. The laparoscopic revolution made cholecystectomy less invasive, but it made the management of choledocholithiasis more complicated. Laparoscopic cholangiography and common bile duct exploration were initially challenging for many surgeons, leading to the widespread and rapid adoption of two-stage management (endoscopic sphincterotomy plus laparoscopic cholecystectomy). While laparoscopic common bile duct exploration (LCBDE) was eventually shown to have equivalent efficacy and safety, two-stage management has become the norm in most institutions despite having several disadvantages for the patient: the need for additional procedures, longer hospital stays, higher costs, and typically the need for a different physician to perform the endoscopic procedure.

The loss of knowledge and technical skills for general surgeons in common duct exploration has been profound. As Dr. Jeffrey Ponsky pointed out in 2010:

> "A generation of surgeons has emerged from training with little experience in bile duct surgery… we must identify means to train our surgeons, residents, and those in practice in the techniques of bile duct exploration." [1]

The decline of bile duct exploration in the laparoscopic era has resulted in greater fragmentation of care, increased costs, and worse outcomes for the patient. A related and concerning recently reported trend is a decline in the use of intraoperative cholangiography and intraoperative imaging by surgeons. Recognition of this situation and a recent increased focus on improving the outcomes of laparoscopic cholecystectomy led a group of nationally recognized leaders in laparoscopic surgery in 2013 to call for the establishment of a national education project to train surgeons in LCBDE, calling this a "national priority." [2]

Ironically, it was in this age of decline in benign biliary surgery that my interest in surgical management of common duct stones began. As a resident in the research laboratory, one day I stumbled across a description of LCBDE and read about procedures that I had never seen but which made sense—both from a surgeon's perspective and from a patient perspective. I felt like a surgical archaeologist, rediscovering techniques that had been abandoned by most surgeons in the chaotic rush of the laparoscopic revolution. The traditional paradigm of the surgeon providing comprehensive care for both the gallbladder disease and biliary stone disease had obvious appeal to me, but in the current era it has largely been relegated to other consultants. I wondered how I could ever learn to perform LCBDE in the current environment, in which these cases were so rare? In my mind the answer eventually became clear: that unless we changed the way we teach surgeons LCBDE, this operation would continue to disappear. I set about trying to figure out how we could teach this operation in a better way in today's environment, by applying simulation as a tool. Development of an LCBDE simulator-based curriculum followed and continues to be an active area of work (see Chap. 16 for further details).

Since starting practice as an attending surgeon, I have developed a busy practice in gallbladder surgery that includes LCBDE. My driving vision continues to be to provide comprehensive management of gallbladder and CBD stones for my patients. Along the way I have learned many lessons and continue to refine my techniques of common duct exploration. Working with surgical residents, and teaching them LCBDE, I have been amazed at how enthusiastic today's residents are to learn these techniques. Many residents, after rotating on other services, would later tell me that they advocated for greater surgical involvement in CBD stone care on these services. As I endeavored to learn as much as I could about surgical management of CBD stones, it became clear to me that knowledge of this topic was scattered throughout the literature and that a comprehensive textbook on this subject was lacking. I felt that today's trainees and surgeons in practice who wanted to learn LCBDE and take on a more active role in the management of CBD stones needed a repository of information on this topic.

This volume has the goal of specifically addressing the current lack of knowledge of many general surgeons and trainees in the comprehensive management of patients with choledocholithiasis, with an emphasis on how the surgeon can provide single-stage management for the majority of patients. The book includes a discussion of historical perspectives on surgical techniques, preoperative evaluation, decision-making, economics, and simulation curricula and covers a range of surgical, endoscopic, and radiologic techniques available to care for CBD stone patients.

It is my hope that we, as surgeons, will once again embrace the management of common duct stones as a worthwhile cause and as the right thing to do for our patients.

References

1. Ponsky JL. Laparoscopic biliary surgery: will we ever learn? Surg Endosc. 2010;24(10):2367.
2. Berci G, Hunter J, Morgenstern L, Arregui M, Brunt M, Carroll B, Edye M, Fermelia D, Ferzli G, Greene F, Petelin J, Phillips E, Ponsky J, Sax H, Schwaitzberg S, Soper N, Swanstrom L, Traverso W. Laparoscopic cholecystectomy: first, do no harm; second, take care of bile duct stones. Surg Endosc. 2013;27(4):1051–4.

Hanover, NH, USA B. Fernando Santos
Chicago, IL, USA Nathaniel Soper

Contents

Contributors

Mazen R. Al-Mansour, MD Department of General and Gastrointestinal Surgery, The Ohio State University/Wexner Medical Center, Columbus, OH, USA

Horacio J. Asbun, MD, FACS Department of Surgery, Mayo Clinic Florida, Jacksonville, FL, USA

Todd H. Baron, MD, FASGE Department of Medicine, Division of Gastroenterology and Hepatology, University of North Carolina, Chapel Hill, NC, USA

George Berci, MD, FACS, FRCS ED Department of Surgery, Cedars-Sinai Medical Center, Los Angeles, CA, USA

Matthew B. Bloom, MD, MS Department of Surgery, Cedars-Sinai Medical Center, Los Angeles, CA, USA

Frank J. Brennan, MD Department of Radiology, Veteran Affairs Medical Center, White River Junction, VT, USA

Department of Radiology, Geisel School of Medicine, Dartmouth College, Hanover, NH, USA

Ryan Albert Campagna, MD Department of Surgery, Northwestern University Feinberg School of Medicine, Chicago, IL, USA

Robert D. Fanelli, MD, MHA, FACS, FASGE Department of Surgery, The Guthrie Clinic, Sayre, PA, USA

Morris E. Franklin Jr, MD, FACS Department of Minimally Invasive Surgery, Texas Endosurgery Institute, San Antonio, TX, USA

Miguel A. Hernández, MD Department of Minimally Invasive Surgery, Texas Endosurgery Institute, San Antonio, TX, USA

Eric S. Hungness, MD Department of Surgery, Northwestern Memorial Hospital, Chicago, IL, USA

Juaquito M. Jorge, MD Department of Surgery, University of South Florida, Tampa General Hospital, Tampa, FL, USA

Varun Kapur, MD Department of General Surgery, University Hospitals Case Medical Center, Cleveland, OH, USA

Jeffrey M. Marks, MD, FACS, FASGE Department of General Surgery, University Hospitals Cleveland Medical Center, Cleveland, OH, USA

H. Mason Hedberg, MD Department of Surgery, University of Chicago Medicine, Chicago, IL, USA

Timothy Mayfield, MD Department of General Surgery, UnityPoint Clinic Surgery, Des Moines, IA, USA

Ahmad Mirza, MD, FRCS Department of General Surgery, The Pennine Acute Hospitals NHS Trust, Manchester, UK

Vimal K. Narula, MD Department of General and Gastrointestinal Surgery, The Ohio State University/Wexner Medical Center, Columbus, OH, USA

Leslie K. Nathanson, FRACS, FRCS Ed(Hon) Wesley Hospital, Brisbane, QLD, Australia

Arslan Pannu, MBBS, MRCS Department of Colorectal/General Surgery, The Royal Oldham Hospital, Manchester, UK

Lucio Lucas Pereira, MD Department of General Surgery, Mayo Clinic Florida, Jacksonville, FL, USA

Joseph B. Petelin, MD, FACS Surgix™ Minimally Invasive Surgery Institute, Shawnee Mission, Kansas, USA

Department of Surgery, Shawnee Mission Medical Center, Shawnee, KS, USA

Edward H. Phillips, MD Department of Surgery, Cedars-Sinai Medical Center, Los Angeles, CA, USA

David W. Rattner, MD Department of Surgery, Division of General and Gastrointestinal Surgery, Massachusetts General Hospital, Harvard Medical School, Boston, MA, USA

Victor Sandoval, MD Department of General Surgery, University Hospitals of Cleveland, Cleveland, OH, USA

B. Fernando Santos, MD Department of Surgery, Geisel School of Medicine, Dartmouth College, Hanover, NH, USA

Veterans Affairs Medical Center, White River Junction, VT, USA

Harry C. Sax, MD Department of Surgery, Cedars-Sinai Medical Center, Los Angeles, CA, USA

Ben Schwab, MD Department of Surgery, Northwestern Memorial Hospital, Chicago, IL, USA

Nathaniel J. Soper, MD Department of Surgery, Northwestern University, Chicago, IL, USA

Thadeus L. Trus, MD Department of Surgery, Geisel School of Medicine, Dartmouth-Hitchcock Medical Center, Lebanon, NH, USA

Michael Ujiki, MD, FACS Department of Surgery, NorthShore University HealthSystems Evanston Hospital, Evanston, IL, USA

Brian Weinberg, BA, BS, MBA Department of Clinical Care Finance, Cedars-Sinai Health System, Los Angeles, CA, USA

Part I
Historical Perspective of Benign Gallbladder and Biliary Disease

Chapter 1
Historical Perspective on the Treatment of Choledocholithiasis: Lessons Learned and Techniques Prior to the Laparoscopic Era

George Berci

Selected Historical Data in Biliary Disease

- *Sir Granville Elliot Smith* in 1924 donated to the Royal College of Surgeons of England the mummy of a priestess from the twenty-first dynasty, 1500 BCE, whose gallbladder contained some 30 calculi. Unfortunately, this museum was destroyed during World War II.
- *Hippocrates* distinguished febrile from afebrile jaundice. There are many other historical stories, but it was not until the Renaissance when autopsy became legal and allowed for improved knowledge of the abdominal organs [1].
- *Andreas Vesalius* (1514–1564) made observations about gallstones [1].
- *Francis Glisson* (1597–1677) in his book *Anatomia Hepatis* described the sphincter and made detailed descriptions of biliary colic [1].
- In 1743, *John Petit*, a famous Parisian surgeon, described the first perforated gallbladder. He was also the first to identify obstructive cholecystitis [1].
- *Giovanni Morgagni* (1682–1771) removed three patient's calculi passed through a spontaneous biliary fistula [1].
- In 1878, *J. Marion Sims*, an American, and *Lawson Tait* in Scotland proposed cholecystostomy [1].
- *Emil Theodore Kocher* (1841–1917) in Switzerland proposed a surgery also on the gallbladder and introduced the right subcostal incision. (Kocher was the first to receive the Nobel Prize with his original outstanding work on the thyroid.)

G. Berci, MD, FACS, FRCS ED (Hon)
Department of Surgery, Cedars-Sinai Medical Center, Los Angeles, CA, USA
e-mail: George.Berci@cshs.org

© Springer International Publishing AG, part of Springer Nature 2018
B. F. Santos, N. Soper (eds.), *Choledocholithiasis*,
https://doi.org/10.1007/978-3-319-74503-9_1

- In 1867, *John Bobbs* operated on a woman on the third floor of a drugstore in Indianapolis, Indiana. He thought the patient had a tumor in the abdomen but found a distended gallbladder, which he drained and removed the gallstones. Bobbs thought it would be an ideal solution to create an opening to the abdominal wall and to create a cholecystostomy [2]. There were some followers who performed similar continuous drainage from the gallbladder with calculi in this time period [3].
- *Ludwig Courvoisier* published the first choledocholithotomy in 1890 [4]. He also introduced the eponym Courvoisier gallbladder in the diagnosis of cancer of the head of pancreas.
- *Carl Langenbuch* performed his first cholecystectomy in 1892. He prepared for the procedure by practicing on cadavers. He recommended careful removal of the gallbladder. In 1894 he published 26 successful operations dealing with liver and gallbladder disease [5].
- *Justice Ohage* of Saint Paul, Minnesota, performed the first cholecystectomy in America [6]. There was only one case reported [7].
- *Hans Kehr*, in my opinion, was the pioneer of systematically organized and well-recorded gallbladder surgery. His book or compendium was published in two volumes in 1913. He reported 2600 cholecystectomies and 400 common bile duct explorations. He mentioned complications of ductal injuries. He invented the T-tube, which is used for the drainage of the common bile duct (CBD). He was the first to recommend dilatation of the sphincter to facilitate removal of common duct stones. The American leaders in surgery at this time, William J. Mayo and William S. Halsted, visited Kehr [8].
- *William S. Halsted* the pioneer of American surgery is regarded as the founder of surgical schools and teaching systems. His first biliary surgery was performed in 1881 on his mother at her home in Albany, New York. She had jaundice, fever, and an abdominal mass. He incised and drained the gallbladder as well as removed several stones. She was never completely free from jaundice and died 2 years later. During the autopsy a large number of retained stones were found [9]. Halsted became a dominant figure in American surgery. Unfortunately, he developed acute cholecystitis and was operated on; however, 2 years later he became jaundiced and needed a re-exploration (retained stones). Our pioneer died from the complications of biliary surgery [10].
- *William J. Mayo* and his brother Charles performed 2147 procedures for cholecystitis and choledocholithiasis from 1893 to 1919 [11].

Early Cholangiography

In 1924, *Graham, Cole, and Copher* introduced a radiological examination of the gallbladder by intravenous injection of tetrabromophenolphthalein [12]. The hypothesis was that:

1. It will excrete slowly through the liver into the bile.
2. The cystic duct, if patent, will permit visualization of the gallbladder. There were 54 cases reported. After the injection some patients had side effects [13].

This experience began a new era of diagnostic examination in gallbladder disease. Films were taken 4, 8, 24, and 32 h after the injections.

In 1918, *Adolph Reich*, a radiologist, injected petroleum paste and bismuth into a female patient who presented with a fistula [14]. To his greatest surprise, the bile ducts were displayed. Other radiologists a few years later found the same phenomenon and injected through a cutaneous fistula a lipid solution and found retained stones or other anomalies after surgery [15].

A new era was introduced by injecting a safe contrast material directly into the biliary system.

In 1931, *Pablo Luis Mirizzi*, a surgeon from Argentina, recommended intraoperative cholangiography (IOC) [16] as a practical procedure by injecting contrast materials into the ductal system during surgery for the following reasons:

1. To recognize and remove CBD stones
2. To avoid unnecessary explorations of an empty or dilated CBD
3. To recognize the biliary anatomy and avoid ductal injuries

He published his experience in the American literature [17]. Lipiodol was used as a contrast material. He recommended intraoperative cholangiography (IOC) to be employed at the end of a choledocholithotomy. He reported 400 IOCs (including choledochotomies) without mortality. To quote Mirizzi about time-consuming events, "It must not be forgotten that in many cases the future welfare of the patient depends on the few minutes' delay."

N. Frederick Hicken reported his experience with IOC in the USA [18] and recommended also performing cholangiography in the postoperative period through the T-tube. A cholangiogram was performed using an X-ray machine. The personnel in the operating room (OR) had to be protected against radiation hazard. It had some disadvantages of being time-consuming; rapidly placing an X-ray plate under the patient and replacing it with two other plates in short time intervals were not easy. Despite a relatively short exposure, many films were not sharp, or the anatomy was missed. The anesthesiologist had to keep the patient apneic during the procedure, and on several occasions the procedure had to be repeated. There were only three films exposed using 5, 10, and 15 mL contrast material. It did not receive wide acceptance.

Early Choledocholithotomies

Frank Glenn reported a total of 907 patients' data from 1932 to 1938 for cholecystectomy. Out of those 907 cases, 120 had indications for choledocholithotomy. Calculi were found in 60 patients, but in 52 cases no stones were located. The mortality rate for all cases was 12.5% [19].

Duct exploration was indicated in acute and chronic cases and other conditions such as inflammatory strictures of the sphincter area. A stenotic part of the common bile duct was found in 12 cases. Cholangiography was not mentioned. There was an interesting description describing draining of the duct (T-tube) where the bile was collected in a sterile bag and transferred to an ice container. The bile was then filtered to remove debris and pus; however, it did not need to be treated with preservative. The bile output was between 800 and 1400 $cm^3/24$ h. The patient was instructed to ingest this filtered bile between meals in five or six equal increments.

A very detailed description was found about the closure of the CBD incision over a (Kehr) T-tube as well as a choledochoduodenostomy technique. Vitamin K was administered in the postoperative period and was recommended after checking the prothrombin time [20]. A high incidence of retained stones was noted despite careful palpation of the duct, irrigation, probing, etc. This report was the first time the use of the operative cholangiography by Hicken was mentioned.

In 1964, *Colcock and Perey* published their account of 1754 cholecystectomies out of which 29% of patients had choledochotomy [20]. Indications were similar to Glenn's: in 503 patients the CBD was explored and stones were found in 339 (67.4%), and 51 (4.2%) had stenosis of the sphincter. In three cases (0.6%), sclerosing cholangitis was found. In the series of 503 CBD explorations, the mortality was 1.8%. There were nine postoperative cases where patients developed jaundice. Cholangiography was not used routinely at the Lahey Clinic.

Retained Stone Removal Through a T-Tube

Many attempts were made to solve the problems of retained stones with less complication to the patient. Dissolving agents were attempted; however, the results were unsatisfactory [21].

If a stone was found in the postoperative cholangiogram, attempts were made to remove it through the T-tube tract.

H. Joachim Burhenne developed a remote-controlled catheter [22], introduced under continuous fluoroscopic guidance through the T-tube. The potential for higher radiation exposure was obvious. A specially trained radiologist was important to perform it.

Tatsuo Yamakawa converted Burhenne's technique to a direct endoscopic approach by introducing a flexible choledochofiberscope into the sinus tract to aid in the removal of retained stones under direct visual control [23]. The size of his instrument (6.5 mm O.D.) and relatively large turning radius caused some difficulty in negotiating the tract.

Our own institution employed a smaller, more pliable, flexible bronchoscope, which is only 4.8 mm in diameter [24]. The actual entrapment and retrieval maneuver was performed under direct visual control.

Following the procedure, a catheter was reintroduced into the extrahepatic biliary system and secured. Continuous bile drainage was maintained for a period of

3–4 days to allow for clearing of debris induced by manipulation, prior to final cholangiography. The catheter was then pulled after obtaining a negative cholangiogram.

We preferred a 5-week postoperative waiting period before scheduling the date of the manipulation through the T-tube tract. It was performed as an outpatient procedure. Patients received intravenous (IV) sedation and antibiotics. During the extraction procedure, first a guidewire was introduced through the T-tube controlled by fluoroscopy, and the T-tube was withdrawn.

Dilating (angioplasty balloon) was introduced sometimes to move a "wedged-in stone" or to dilate the sphincter. During fluoroscopic control, the scope was advanced over the guidewire so you could clearly visualize the anatomy. Manipulations were performed under direct visual rather than fluoroscopic guidance. Radiation dosage was reduced.

Results

Sixty-three patients were referred with a positive postoperative T-tube cholangiogram. Spontaneous passage had occurred in four patients. The filling defect in one case was found to be a fibrin thrombus. In the remaining 57 patients, we were able to completely clear the duct of calculi in 54 cases (94.6%). Twenty-eight patients required two sessions before we were able to declare the ductal system stone free. In another six patients, low fevers developed, which lasted 24–48 h. The success rate was predominately influenced by the size and position of the T-tube [24] (Fig. 1.1).

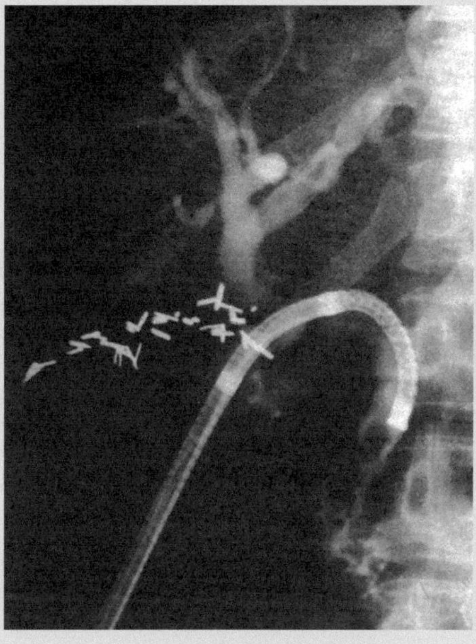

Fig. 1.1 In the postoperative period, a cholangiogram displayed the retained stone and a guidewire was introduced through the T-tube. The T-tube was pulled, the flexible bronchoscope introduced, and the stone entrapped in a basket, which was then removed. The drainage tube was reinserted and later, after a negative cholangiogram, was pulled. Reprinted with permission from Cuschieri A, Berci G, Hamlin JA, Paz-Partlow M. *Common Bile Duct Exploration: Intraoperative Investigations in Biliary Tract Surgery*. Boston, MA: Martinus Nijhoff Publishers (Springer). 1984

A drain tube was inserted at the completion of the procedure, which did not exceed 50 min. A final cholangiogram was performed 2 days later, before the tube was removed.

In our institution during the same time period, endoscopic retrograde cholangio-pancreatography (ERCP) was reported with a success rate of 80%, morbidity rate of 10%, and mortality rate of 0.5%.

Our success rate was 94.6% with minimal morbidity and no mortality.

Retained Stones

Ever since Kehr published his unique textbook of biliary surgery in 1913, the problem of retained CBD stones has plagued patients and surgeons alike [8]. The incidence of common bile duct stones in patients undergoing cholecystectomy is approximately 10–20%, depending on the age of the patient and the follow-up period. The real incidence of retained stone after duct exploration is not known but was reported as between 5 and 28% in the recent edition of *Blumgart's Surgery of the Liver, Biliary Tract and Pancreas*; Blumgart et al. produced a number of publications supporting the data that follows [25–32].

Early Operative Biliary Fluoroscopy

Lackner and *Volkel* introduced an image amplifier in conjunction with IOC [33]. The picture was seen through an optical viewer. A cassette was inserted for individual exposures. It became time-consuming, and radiation exposure was not insignificant. In general, this technique did not gain wide exposure.

Grace and Peckar in 1968 reported some successful cases [34].

Intraoperative Fluoro-cholangiography

The Introduction of the Mobile Video Amplifier

A new perspective was introduced by the image amplifier; invisible X-ray beams were converted to light by the fluorescent layer of the input screen. This is a very low-intensity light transmission that is transformed electronically to a bright optical image at the output screen. It can be seen through a viewer with a naked eye or with an altered television camera on a large screen. Its advantages are the reduction in radiation and immediate visibility without dark adaption, and multiple films can be exposed with lower radiation dosage (Fig. 1.2) [35].

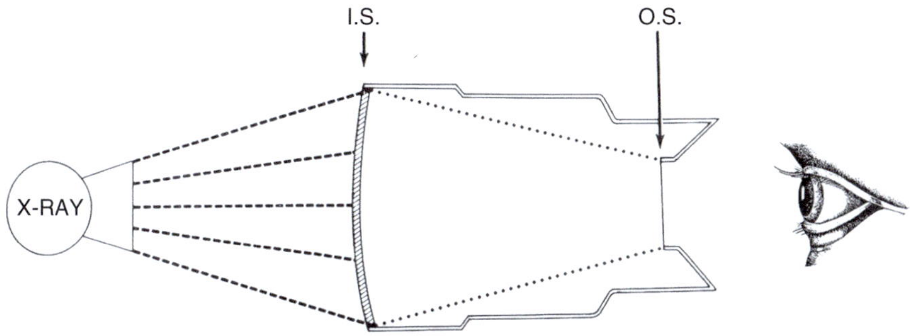

Fig. 1.2 Schematic diagram of an image amplifier. The invisible X-ray beam is converted to light by the fluorescent layer of the input screen (IS). This low-intensity light is transformed electronically to a bright optical image at the output screen (OS). This can be seen through a viewer with the naked eye or recorded with a television camera. Advantages: reduction in radiation, immediate visibility without dark adaptation, and increased visual accuracy compared with the old type of fluoroscopic screening in a subdued light after 30 min of dark adaptation. Reprinted with permission from Berci G, Hamlin JA. Ch 3. Retrieval of retained stones. In: Berci G, Hamlin JA. (eds) *Operative Biliary Radiology*. Baltimore, MD: Williams & Wilkins. 1981

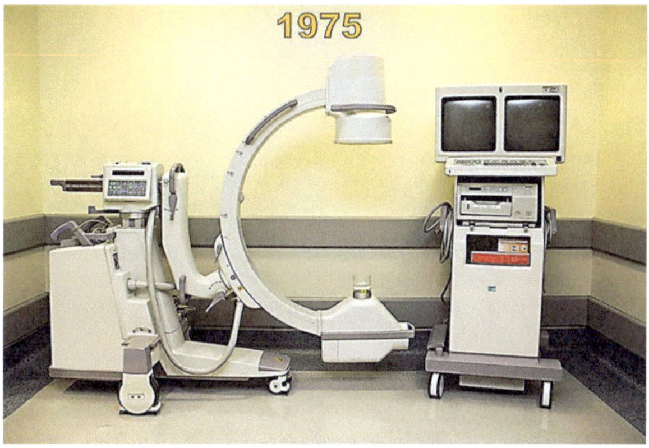

Fig. 1.3 We introduced the mobile image amplifier in 1975, which is available in every hospital performing orthopedic surgery. Reprinted with permission from Cuschieri A, Berci G. Laparoscopic Biliary Surgery. London, UK: Blackwell. 1990

Pierre Mallet-Guy introduced the first mobile image amplifier with video display in 1958 and opened an era of more frequent use of IOC. The immediate image availability, reduction of radiation, and possibility of obtaining films from the important anatomy made it an important adjunct in biliary surgery [36].

Grace and Peckar reported the value of operative cholangiography using an image intensifier and television monitor in 1968 [34].

At my own institution, we first started in 1975 with a mobile image amplifier (Fig. 1.3). This unit is available in every hospital where orthopedic surgery is performed.

The use of lead aprons by the anesthesiologist and circulating nurse is necessary (Fig. 1.4). The surgeon and the scrubbed assistants should stand behind a translucent

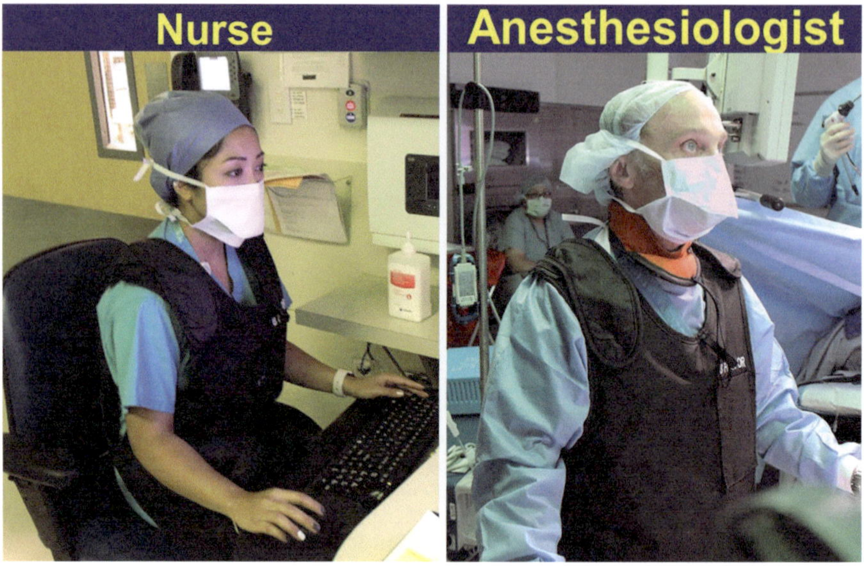

Fig. 1.4 We highly recommend that the circulating nurse and the anesthesiologist should have a lead protective apron when performing IOC. Reprinted with permission from Berci G, Hamlin JA. *Operative Biliary Radiology*. Baltimore, MD: Williams & Wilkins. 1981

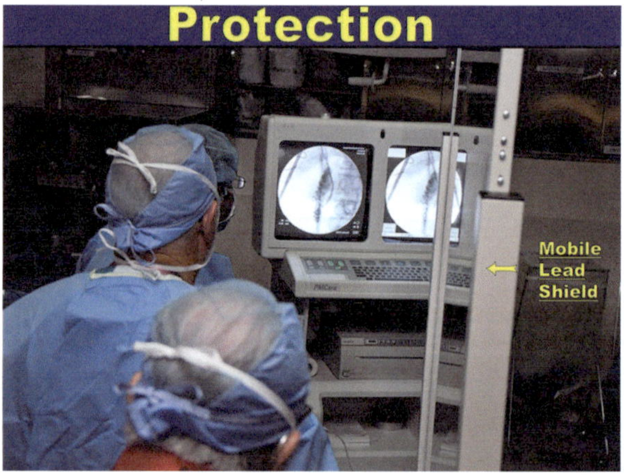

Fig. 1.5 The surgeon, assistant, and scrubbed nurse should be behind a mobile translucent shield. Reprinted with permission from Berci G, Hamlin JA. *Operative Biliary Radiology*. Baltimore, MD: Williams & Wilkins. 1981

mobile lead shield (Fig. 1.5). Practically speaking there will be zero hazard with an approximate distance of 6 ft (Fig. 1.6).

Our radiation officer, Donna Earley, assessed patient exposure, distance of X-ray source to patients, and surgeon and personnel exposure and requested appropriate protection [37]. The National Council of Radiation Protection and Measurements (NCRPM) published a recommendation to be strictly followed [38].

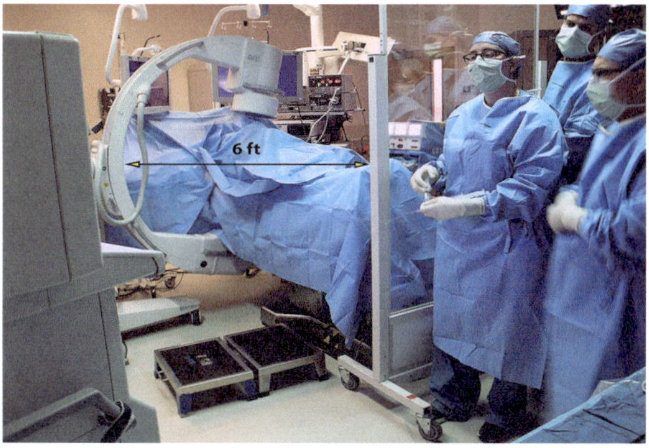

Fig. 1.6 There will almost be zero hazard of radiation exposure with image amplifier and the use of a lead apron with a distance of at least 6 ft. Reprinted with permission from Berci G, Hamlin JA. *Operative Biliary Radiology*. Baltimore, MD: Williams & Wilkins. 1981

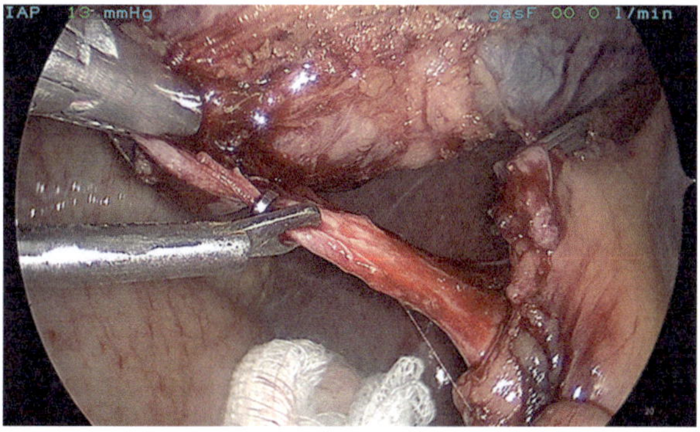

Fig. 1.7 Well-dissected cystic duct has to be clipped under the fundus and carefully incised for the next step

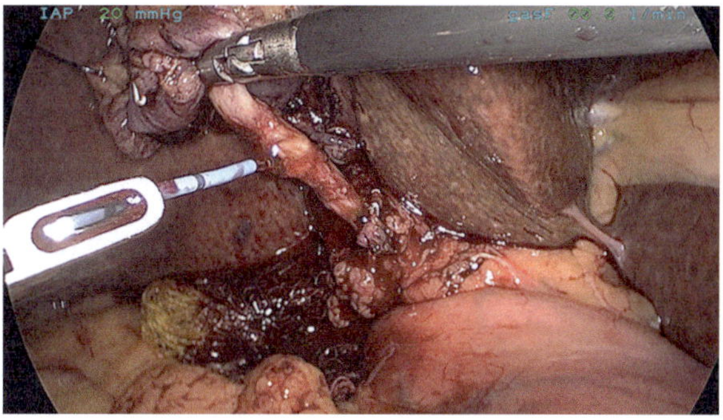

Fig. 1.8 We employed a ureter catheter and introduced with a cholangio grasper through the small hole in the cystic duct and kept the catheter in position by closing the grasper over it

It is also of importance that additional tools for intraoperative cholangiography should be in the room and double-checked by the scrub nurse and surgeon.

After careful exploration and dissection, the Calot's Triangle should be inspected. The cystic duct is identified and clipped below the fundus and incised (Figs. 1.7 and 1.8).

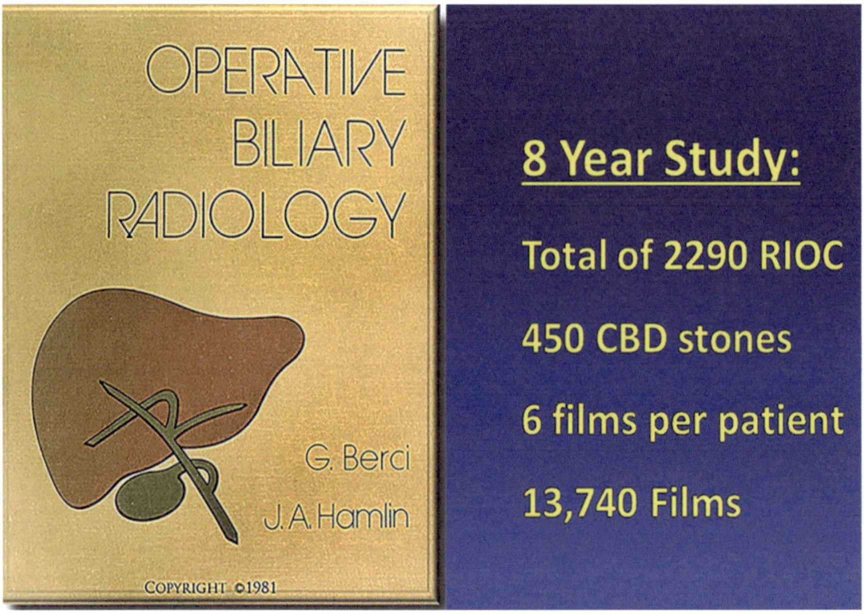

Fig. 1.9 In our first study, we collected 2290 cholangiograms and 450 common bile duct stones and were able to collect and review 13,750 films. A large amount of data was collected and reviewed in our published monograph

A monograph, *Operative Biliary Radiology*, was published with our radiologist, Dr. J. Andrew Hamlin, in 1981. In the first 8 years of study, we were able to collect 2290 cases with 450 CBD stones. Six films per patient were taken. We were able to analyze 13,740 films with Dr. Hamlin (Fig. 1.9) [39].

The Cystic Duct Configuration

We found that in 83% of patients, the cystic duct drained posterior, parallel, spiral, or in the right hepatic duct, and only in 17% drained laterally in the "classical" pattern (Fig. 1.10).

If we pull a short cystic duct more laterally, which is not unusual (Fig. 1.11), it can be easily clipped, e.g., if the short duct drained into a hepatic duct in a very closed position (Fig. 1.12).

Another example is the parallel run of the cystic duct (Fig. 1.13) close to the hepatic duct, which can be easily clipped by mistake.

The tortuous cystic duct can be straightened out by the catheter even if the duct has a spiral configuration. For more details of the anatomy, refer to our monograph *Operative Biliary Radiology* [39].

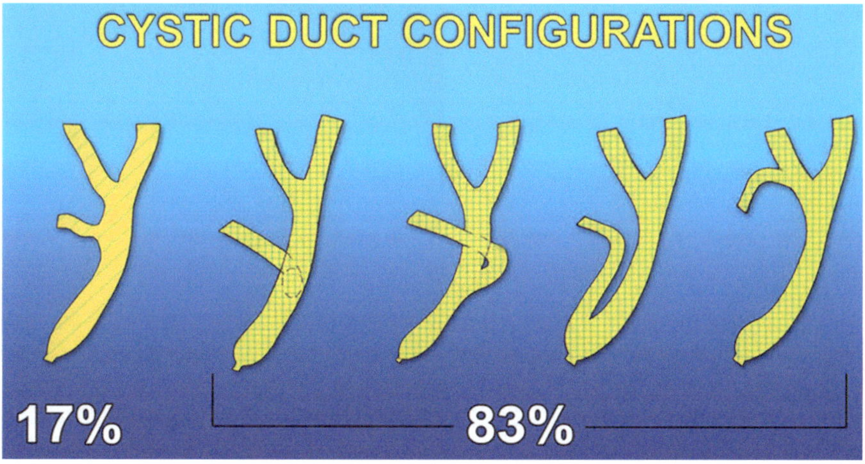

Fig. 1.10 We found that the cystic duct configuration in 83% drained posterior spiral, parallel, or even in the right hepatic and only in 17% drained laterally. Reprinted with permission from Berci G, Hamlin JA. Retrieval of retained stones. In: Berci G, Hamlin JA. (eds) *Operative Biliary Radiology*. Baltimore, MD: Williams & Wilkins. 1981

Fig. 1.11 If the short cystic duct is pulled laterally, you can clip the CBD easily if you do not recognize it in time. Reprinted with permission from Cuschieri A, Berci G. Laparoscopic Biliary Surgery, 2nd ed. London, UK: Blackwell. 1992

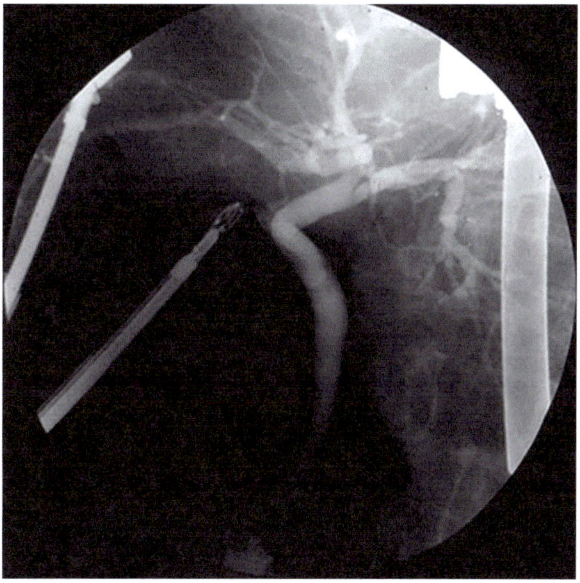

The most important advantage of IOC performed is that these configurations of the biliary system can be discovered during the primary surgery.

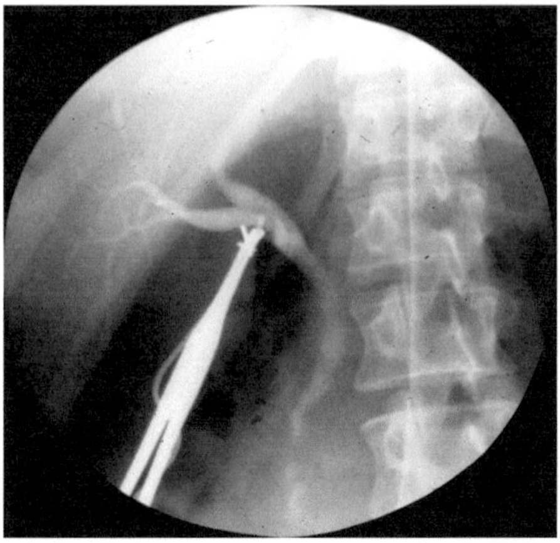

Fig. 1.12 A very short cystic duct draining into the right hepatic duct. If this critical area is not recognized in time, it can be clipped. Reprinted with permission from Cuschieri A, Berci G. Laparoscopic Biliary Surgery, 2nd ed. London, UK: Blackwell. 1992

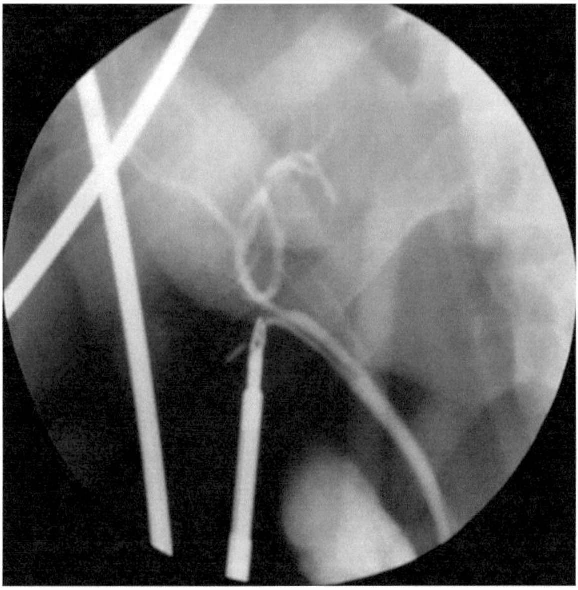

Fig. 1.13 A parallel cystic duct running very near to the CBD can result in clipping of the CBD if the surgeon does not recognize the anatomy. Reprinted with permission from Hamlin J. Ch 3. Anomalies of biliary ductal system. In: Berci G, Cuschieri A (eds). Bile Ducts and Bile Duct Stones. Philadelphia, PA: Saunders. 1996

Normal Anatomy

A non-dilated distal duct is well displayed, including the sphincter area. Some contrast material is also found in the duodenum (Fig. 1.14). In the same patients, after the position of the image amplifier is moved slightly toward the head of the patient, the proximal duct and the anatomy of the hepatic ductal system are also well displayed (Fig. 1.15).

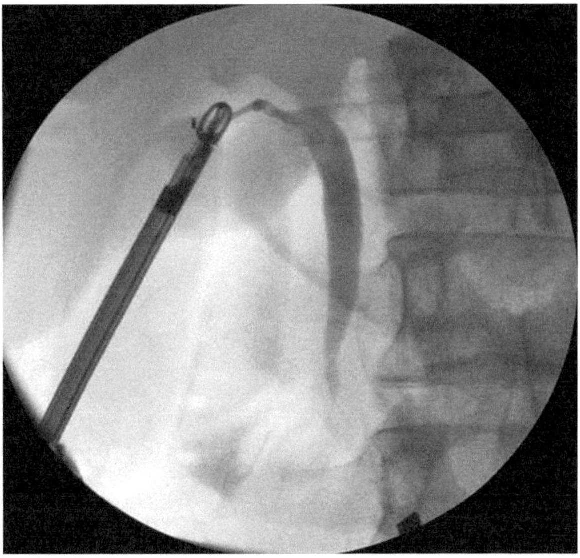

Fig. 1.14 Normal anatomy: make sure that the common bile duct is not covered by the spine, the distal anatomy is well seen with the well-functioning sphincter, and contrast material is observed in the duodenum. Reprinted with permission from Berci G, Hamlin JA. Ch 7. Fluoro-cholangiography. In: Berci G, Hamlin JA. (eds) *Operative Biliary Radiology*. Baltimore, MD: Williams & Wilkins. 1981

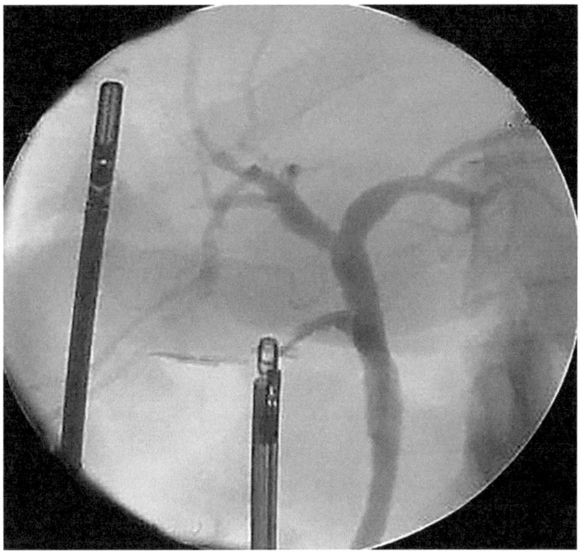

Fig. 1.15 Normal anatomy: to opacify the proximal ductal system, you need perhaps more pressure or two syringes of diluted contrast material to display the entire anatomy of the hepatic ductal system. Reprinted with permission from Berci G, Hamlin JA. Ch 7. Fluoro-cholangiography. In: Berci G, Hamlin JA. (eds) *Operative Biliary Radiology*. Baltimore, MD: Williams & Wilkins. 1981

Extravasation or Leakage of Contrast

Bile duct injuries with the introduction of laparoscopic cholecystectomies unfortunately increased significantly [40]. If IOC is routinely performed, discovering a bile duct injury (BDI) immediately can be lifesaving. The patient can be immediately

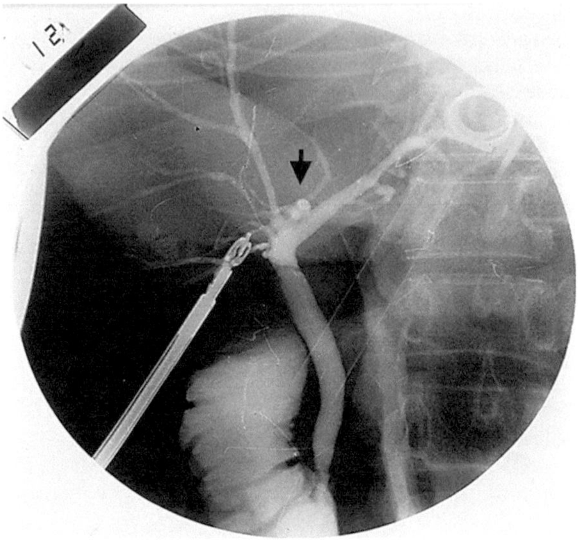

Fig. 1.16 A small amount of extravasation was discovered (arrow); patient was explored and the minor damage was corrected

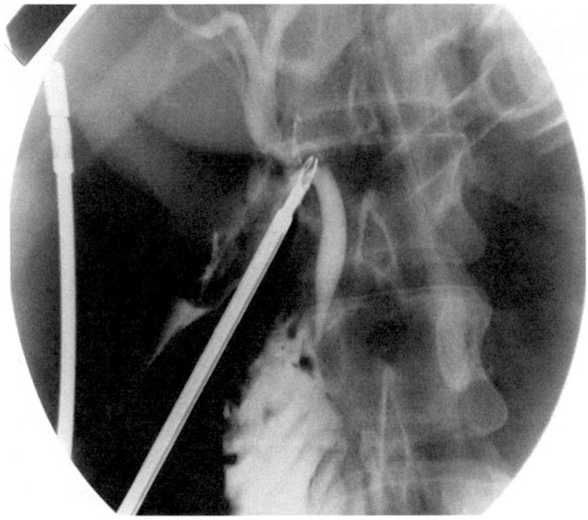

Fig. 1.17 Extravasation of contrast material was detected, patient was immediately explored, and the injury was corrected. Patient avoided a second operation

explored and proper treatment performed (Fig. 1.16). Hence, a second surgery with higher morbidity and mortality is avoided.

Figures 1.17 and 1.18 show contrast extravasation, leading to immediate exploration and repair of the BDI.

In the case shown in Fig. 1.19, contrast material was not seen in the proximal duct because it had been clipped mistakenly. The patient was explored, the clip removed, and the cholangiogram repeated, which showed no damage, and this patient was saved from further complications.

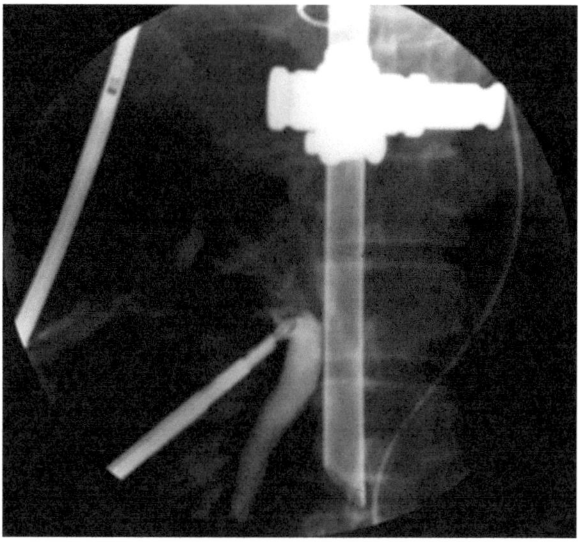

Fig. 1.18 A dilated duct was completely transected, the operator fortunately found a liver surgeon in the house to initiate the appropriate treatment modality, and patient was followed up in 6 months without complications

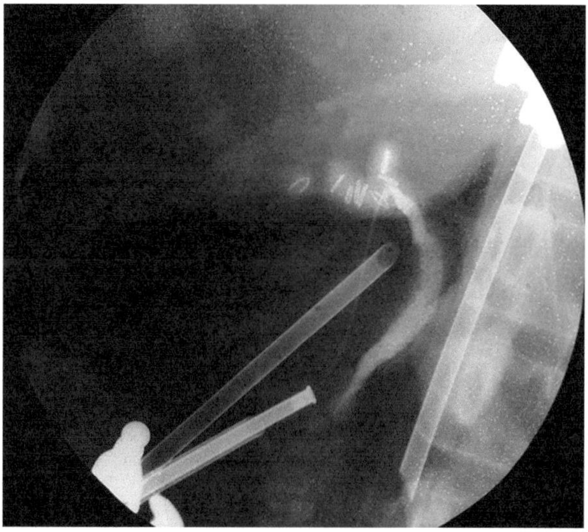

Fig. 1.19 Contrast material was not visible in the proximal hepatic ductal system. Patient was explored and the clip from the duct removed. The cholangiogram showed a normal duct. Patient was followed up for 6 months without complaints

In difficult cases where the dissection of the anatomy is difficult or impossible to continue safely, a *cholecysto-cholangiogram* may be of great help (Fig. 1.20). Two clips should be placed loosely in the area where you are thinking the cystic duct area should be located. A pneumoneedle is inserted into the gallbladder, bile aspirated, and contrast material injected. You can immediately obtain important information about the difficult anatomy and where the cystic duct area will be located. A decision can then be made as to the appropriate next step in the operation.

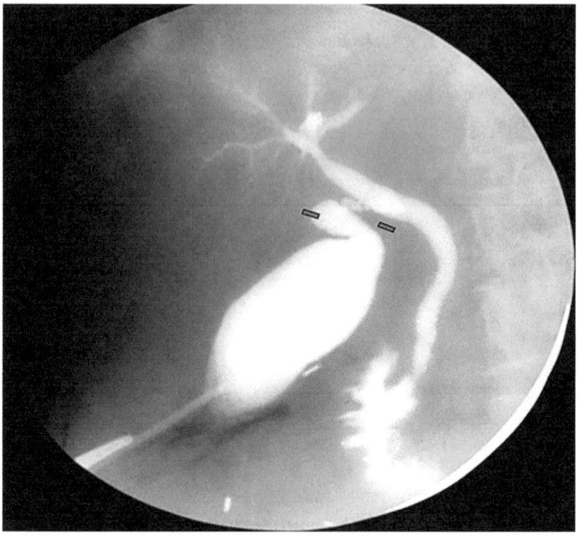

Fig. 1.20 Cholecysto-cholangiogram. This technique may be helpful in difficult cases where the ductal anatomy cannot be recognized because of significant oozing, bleeding, edema, or other problems. It is worthwhile to consider placing two loose clips where you believe the cystic duct will be located and take a pneumo-needle and insert it into the gallbladder. Evacuate some bile and inject contrast material. Information about the anatomy of the critical area will be displayed. Reprinted with permission from Cuschieri A, Berci G. Laparoscopic Biliary Surgery. London, UK: Blackwell. 1990

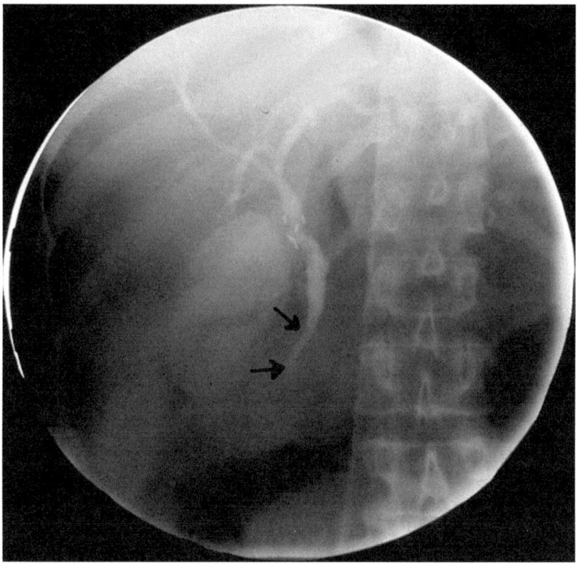

Fig. 1.21 Small gallstones can be easily washed through the sphincter. Administration of one ampule of IV glucagon may help by dilating the ampulla of Vater. Reprinted with permission from Berci G, Cuschieri A (eds) Bile Ducts and Bile Duct Stones. Philadelphia, PA: Saunders. 1996

Common Bile Duct Stones

Small calculi (Fig. 1.21) can be washed through the sphincter. The anesthesiologist should always have in the room glucagon for IV administration, which can relax the sphincter significantly and allow even slightly larger calculi to be easily washed into the duodenum. Larger calculi (Fig. 1.22) in a dilated duct can be removed with the

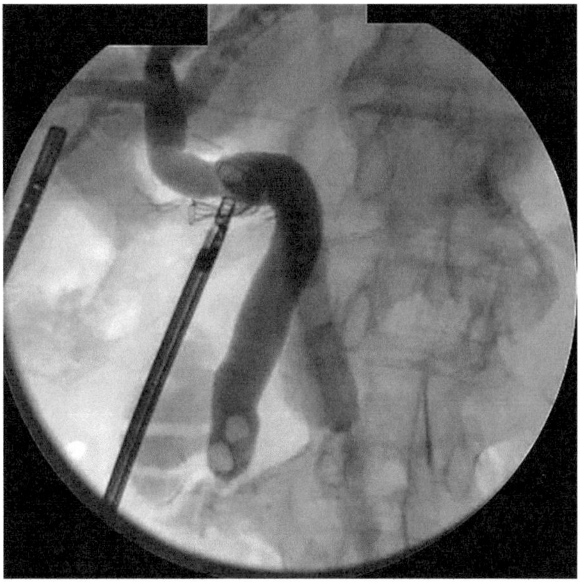

Fig. 1.22 In this dilated CBD duct, two larger calculi were found. Glucagon did not help. The calculi were removed with the choledochoscope. Reprinted with permission from Berci G, Hamlin JA. Ch 7. Fluoro-cholangiography. In: Berci G, Hamlin JA. (eds) *Operative Biliary Radiology*. Baltimore, MD: Williams & Wilkins. 1981

choledochoscope (also see chapter "Biliary Choledochoscopy" in *Operative Biliary Radiology* [39]).

ERCP can be indicated in the preoperative phase with indications in high-risk patients with severe underlying disease, icterus, and/or cholangitis.

Mirizzi syndrome is uncommon; it is a conglomerate of bile and stones that compress the cystic and hepatic ducts. In Fig. 1.23 a small stone is visible in the sphincter area. In these cases, an open procedure should be considered.

Intraoperative Choledochoscopy: Past and Present

When I started biliary surgery, it was clear that our approach to common bile duct exploration was in need of significant improvements. The dilated (empty) duct, misleading laboratory results, and nonexistent radiological support were factors that concluded in disappointing surgical results (see topic "Retained Stones" in reference [31]). First we experimented to convert a blind examination to a visual one using the already existing cystoscope (Nitze, 1873) [41]. It did not prove helpful to insert a straight rigid tube into a curved CBD with a poorly illuminated distal globe. There is nothing more frustrating during the postoperative period than when the patient has to be readmitted with the symptoms of a retained stone. *J. Bakes*, in 1923, developed a small funnel with a mirror on one side and with a larger opening [42]. Light was reflected by a head lamp. It seemed to be too clumsy to be widely accepted (Fig. 1.24).

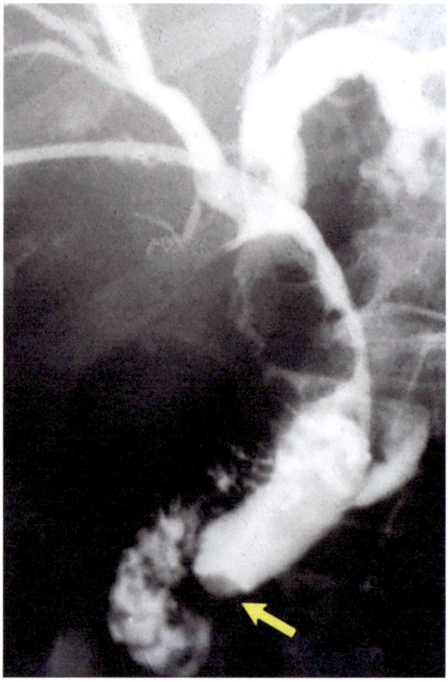

Fig. 1.23 Mirizzi syndrome is uncommon; it is a conglomerate of bile and stones which are compressing the cystic and hepatic ducts. A small stone is visible in the sphincter area. In these cases, an open procedure should be considered. Reprinted with permission from Cuschieri A, Berci G. Laparoscopic Biliary Surgery. London, UK: Blackwell. 1990

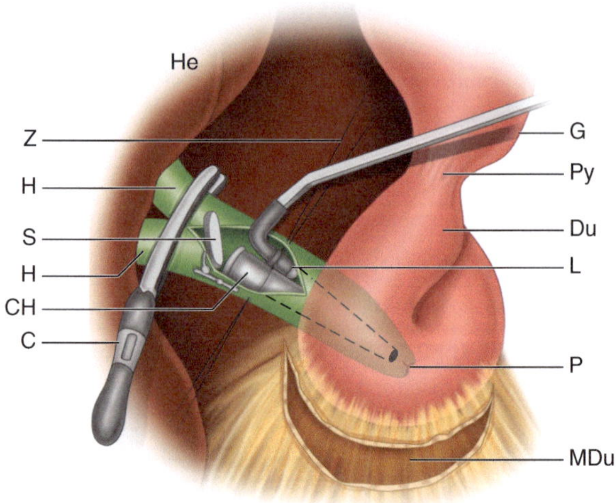

Fig. 1.24 Bakes in 1923 developed a small funnel with a mirror on one side with a larger opening for viewing the interior of the CBD. It was too clumsy to be widely accepted. Reprinted with permission from Bakes J. Die Choledochopapilloskopie, nebst Bemerkungen über Hepaticus drainage und Dilatation der Papille. Archiv fur Klinische Chirurgie. 1923;126:473-483

Monroe McIver, in 1941, employed a rigid right-angled endoscope with an eyepiece and small distal light globe (probably from the cystoscope era) [43]. I could not find published clinical data.

The real pioneer was *Hans Wildegans* from Germany [44]. He employed a cystoscope system with a shorter 60 mm horizontal limb and a 260 mm vertical one in a

60° angled configuration with a built-in eyepiece for viewing. The horizontal tip had a small light bulb. The object had to be observed through the eyepiece, which was in a (dangerous) non-sterile distance from the examiner's eyes. In his monograph in 1960, he reported 150 successful cases out of which 143 had stones removed [44]. Other anomalies were also diagnosed: papillary stenosis, carcinomas, strictures, etc. *Clarence Schein* also reported successful cases in 1963 [45].

The problem with the Wildegans system was the interference with sterility, low light levels, cumbersome viewing, and a monocular dark image.

It was not until a better optical system was described by *Harold Hopkins* that choledochoscopy could be brought into the mainstream [46]. The positive features were obvious, a right-angled version with a 50 mm horizontal and a 160 mm vertical limb with a wide viewing angle, which was easy to introduce. The advantages were the larger image angle and the extremely bright image (both playing a factor for improved perception). A fiber light cable was employed instead of a distal small globe, which sometimes burned out during the examination. It showed great advantages in a multi-institutional study (Fig. 1.25) [47–50].

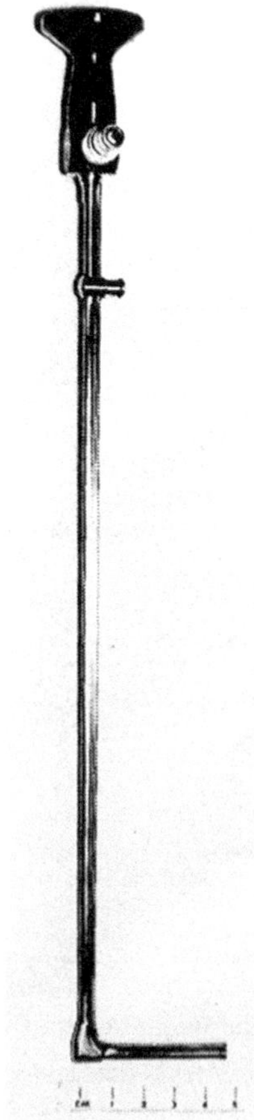

Fig. 1.25 Choledochoscope with a Hopkins rod-lens system was a great advantage, partially because of the right-angle version of the 5 mm horizontal limb with a 160 mm vertical one. The wide wing angle configuration was dominant using a much higher intensive (fiber) light. At a later stage, a removable, sterilizable, wider eyepiece cover was placed on the eyepiece to avoid interfering with sterility if it is touched in the close distance of the view. In a series of 120 cases, the choledochoscope was used. Reprinted with permission from Shore JM, Morgenstern L, Berci G. An improved rigid choledochoscope. Am J Surg. 1971;122: 567-568

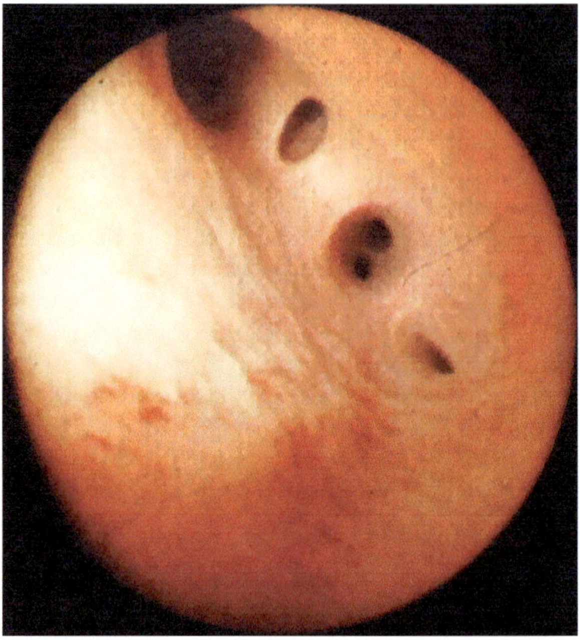

Fig. 1.26 Various opening of the hepatic ductal system is extremely well seen. Reprinted with permission from Cuschieri A, Berci G, Hamlin JA, Paz-Partlow M. *Common Bile Duct Exploration: Intraoperative Investigations in Biliary Tract Surgery*. Boston, MA: Martinus Nijhoff Publishers (Springer). 1984

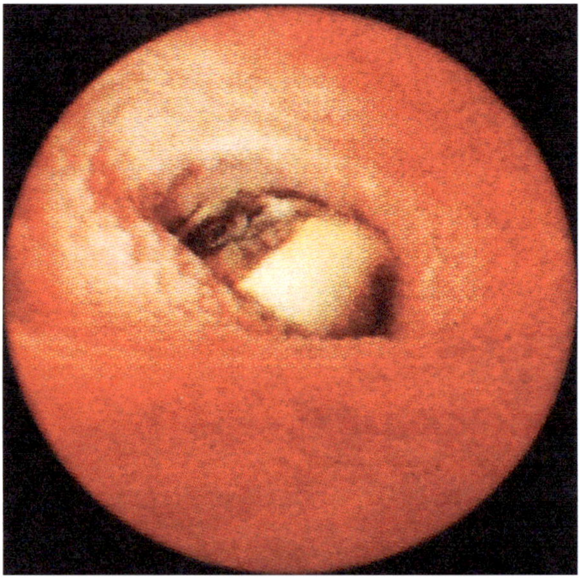

Fig. 1.27 Stone impacted in the sphincter area. Reprinted with permission from Cuschieri A, Berci G, Hamlin JA, Paz-Partlow M. *Common Bile Duct Exploration: Intraoperative Investigations in Biliary Tract Surgery*. Boston, MA: Martinus Nijhoff Publishers (Springer). 1984

With *Alfred Cuschieri*, we produced a monograph on CBD explorations where the advantages of improved choledochoscopy and recordings were well demonstrated (Figs. 1.26, 1.27, 1.28, and 1.29) [51].

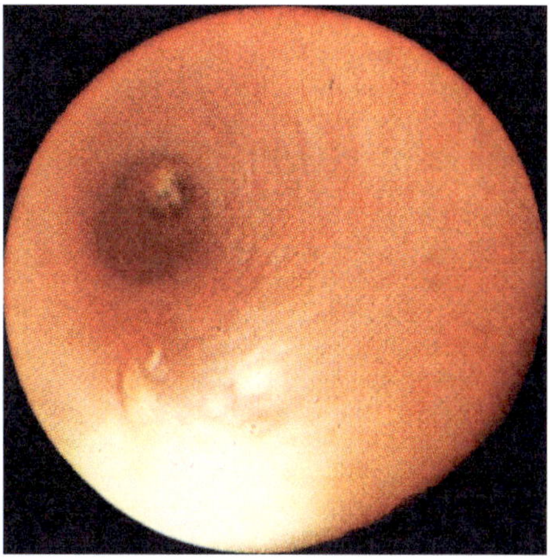

Fig. 1.28 Clear sphincter area. During irrigation the function can be clearly observed. Reprinted with permission from Cuschieri A, Berci G, Hamlin JA, Paz-Partlow M. *Common Bile Duct Exploration: Intraoperative Investigations in Biliary Tract Surgery*. Boston, MA: Martinus Nijhoff Publishers (Springer). 1984

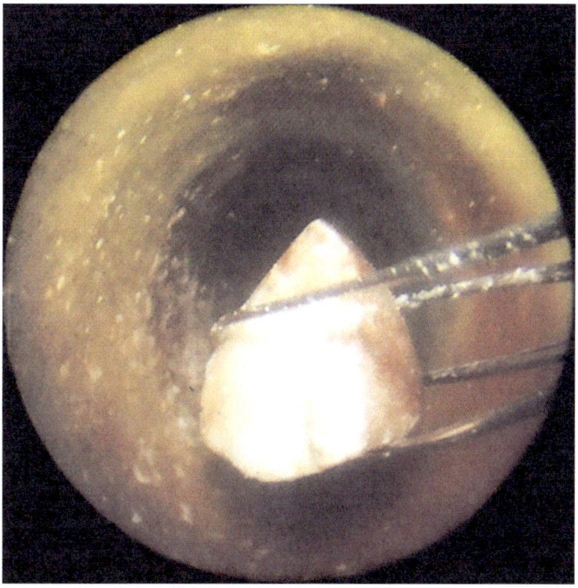

Fig. 1.29 Entrapped stone in the basket. Reprinted with permission from Cuschieri A, Berci G, Hamlin JA, Paz-Partlow M. *Common Bile Duct Exploration: Intraoperative Investigations in Biliary Tract Surgery*. Boston, MA: Martinus Nijhoff Publishers (Springer). 1984

The real breakthrough was the introduction of the choledochoscope with a miniature sterilizable TV camera attached to the eyepiece (Fig. 1.30) [52]. There was no constant fear of interfering with the sterility by touching the eyepiece. A significantly enlarged image on a large TV screen was observed, allowing the possibility to have four hands properly coordinated by the surgeon and assistant. This made the maneuvering and the manipulation of a stone basket and/or balloon catheter much easier and faster and produced better results. It became the tool of choice for coordinating assistants, improving collaboration of nursing staff and visitors, and, last

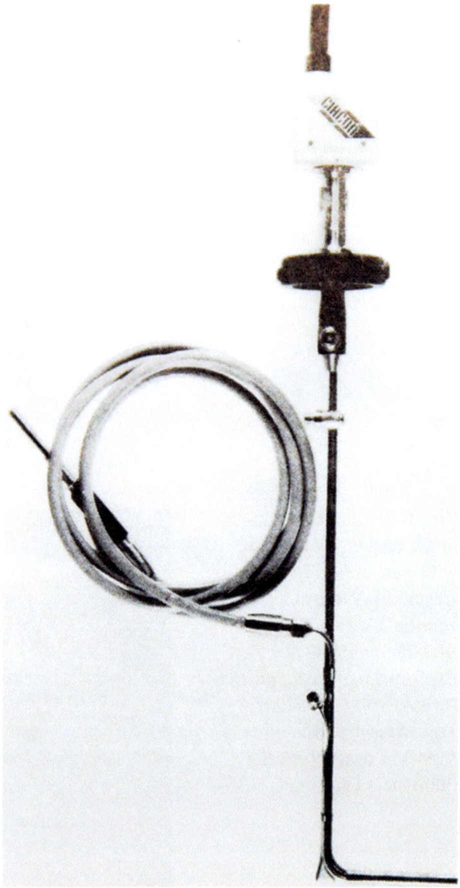

Fig. 1.30 The rigid choledochoscope was attached to a sterilizable miniature TV camera. Problems with interference of sterility were excluded. On a TV screen, the enlarged image could be seen by surgeons and the assistant including the scrubbed nurse. Therefore, coordination of movement was faster and secured. The OR time was reduced. It became the technique of choice for teaching and recording the findings. Reprinted with permission from Berci G, Shulman AG, Morgenstern L, Paz-Partlow M, Cuschieri A, Wood RA. Television choledochoscopy. Surg Gyn Obst. 1985;160:176-177

but not least, the crucial component to create a print or video showing the empty sphincter area or clear hepatic ducts. Another important factor was also the short learning period and the improved results.

The introduction of flexible choledochoscopes was also of help; however, the image quality, brightness of the image, and video capability of the early models were not able to compete with the Hopkins system [53].

The Future

It would be unfair to compose a "prehistorical" chapter on the flexible choledochoscope without mentioning that there are recent improvements in the flexible system, for example, the size of a 2.8 mm scope with a channel but a distal CMOS chip with a high-resolution capacity without a fiber light cable attached and heavy TV camera

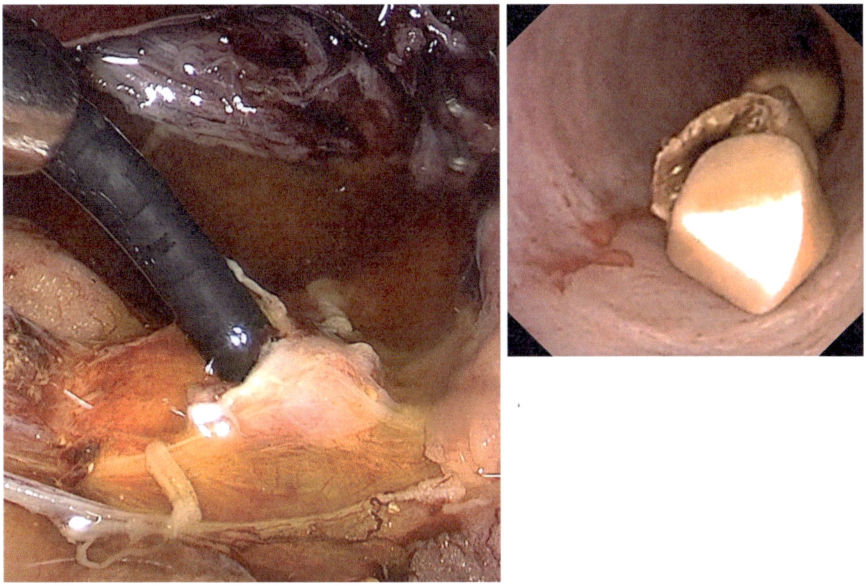

Fig. 1.31 The recent advantages of a miniature (2.8 mm) flexible choledochoscope are obvious. It has a higher resolution, C-MOS chip, has a tip providing a higher resolution and a larger image (K. Storz Company). The tip has a shorter working radius allowing the introduction into the proximal hepatic ductal system which we never had been able to do with previous choledochoscopes. The image on the TV screen is split, and on one side, the surgeon can see the movements of the inserted scope and on the other one the intraluminal anatomy and the manipulation of the basket. The procedure is easier and faster for the surgeons and can save OR time

for easier and faster manipulation, which competes with the previous rigid and flexible fiber models (Fig. 1.31) [54].

The redesign of the tip (smaller radius) makes it also possible to introduce it into the proximal hepatic ductal system, which in the case of a laparoscopic choledochoscopy is another advantage [55].

The video choledochoscope has also economic advantages in saving healthcare costs.

The evolution and development of better miniature, vastly improved, remote-controlled tools for better vision made a significant improvement of the so common complication of biliary ductal surgery, thus allowing the avoidance of a secondary more complicated surgery with higher morbidity, mortality, and significantly higher healthcare costs [55].

The question to be asked is if the data and results are so convincing, why are only a minority of surgeons following these treatment modalities?

The answer is complex, but the major factors are known. One is the very low reimbursement, the lack of time to learn the new techniques, and, of course, in certain cases the low volume.

Let us hope that the newer surgical generation will consider better patient care concepts and will take the time to attend training courses to be introduced to a better treatment modality. The same concept and philosophy apply to the other intraoperative techniques of cholangiography, which are only applied in a small percentage of elective laparoscopic cholecystectomies.

We never can perform surgery without complications, but there are techniques available and published data [16] where the known problems can be reduced to a more acceptable incidence. Important advantages are obvious, the reduction of retained stones and the ability to teach.

Acknowledgment I would like to express my thanks to Marc Arizmendez, Senior Media Specialist and Assistant, and Barbara Rosette and Susan Frederick for helping me to put this chapter together.

References

1. Praderi R, Hess W. Brief history of biliary and pancreatic diseases. In: Hess W, Berci G, editors. Text book of biliary pancreatic diseases, vol. 4. Piccin: Padova; 1997.
2. Bobbs JS. Case of lithotomy of the gallbladder. Indianapolis: Trans Indiana State Med Soc. 1868;18:68.
3. Sims JM. Cholecystostomy in dropsy of the gallbladder. Br Med J. 1879;8:811.
4. Courvoisier LG. Kasuistisch statistiche beitraege. Leipzig: Vogel; 1890.
5. Langenbuch C. Ein fall von extirpation der gallenblase wegen chronischer cholelithiasis. Berl Klin Wschr. 1882;19:725.
6. Ohage J. The surgical treatment of diseases of the gallbladder. Med Newsl. 1886;1:202–6.
7. Hatch TL. Owatonna, Minn. in Northwestern Lancet, St. Paul. 1886. vol. VI, No. 3.
8. Kehr H. Practice der gallenwege-chirurgie. Munchen: Lehmann; 1913.
9. Morgenstern L. Halsted nemesis. Surg Endosc. 1994;8:1165–7.
10. Halsted W. Contribution to the surgery of the bile passages, especially of the common bile duct. Johns Hopkins Hosp Bull. 1900;11:1.
11. Mayo WJ. Some observations on the surgery of the gallbladder and bile ducts. Ann Surg. 1899;30:452.
12. Graham E, Cole W. Roentgenologic examination of the gallbladder preliminary report of a new method utilizing the intravenous injection of tetrabromphenolphthalein. JAMA. 1924;82:613–4.
13. Graham E, Cole W, Copher G, Moore S. Diseases of the gall bladder and bile ducts. Philadelphia: Lea & Febiger; 1928.
14. Reich A. Accidental injection of bile ducts with petrolatum and bismuth paste. JAMA. 1918;71:1555.
15. Tenney CF, Patterson SH. Injection of the bile ducts with bismuth paste. JAMA. 1922;78:171.
16. Mirizzi PL. La Cholangiografia durante las Operaciones de las vias Biliares. Bol Soc Cir Buenos Aires. 1932;16:1133.
17. Mirizzi PL. Operative cholangiography. Surg Gynecol Obstet. 1937;65:702.
18. Hicken NF, Best RR, Hunt HB. Cholangiography. Ann Surg. 1936;103:210.
19. Glenn F. Exploration of the common bile duct. Ann Surg. 1940;112(1):64–79.
20. Colcock BP, Perey B. Exploration of the common bile duct. Surg Gynecol Obstet. 1964;81:20–4.
21. Mack EA, Saito C, Goldfarb S, Crummy AB, Thistle JL, Carson FL, Babayan VK, Hoffman AF. A new agent for gallstone dissolution. Surg Forum. 1978;24:438.

22. Burhenne JJ. Nonoperative retained biliary tract stone extraction. Am J Roentgenol. 1973;117:388–99.
23. Yamakawa T, Mieno K, Nogucki T, Shikata J. An improved choledochofiberscope and non-surgical removal of retained biliary calculi under direct visual control. Gastrointest Endosc. 1976;22:160–4.
24. Berci G, Hamlin JA. A combined fluoroscopic and endoscopic approach for retrieval of retained stones through the T-Tube tract. Surg Gynecol Obstet. 1981;153:237–40.
25. Blumgart LH, Fong Y. Surgery of the liver and bile duct. 3rd ed. New York: Saunders; 2000.
26. Smith S, Engel C, Averhook B, Longmire WP. Problems of retained and recurrent common bile duct stones. JAMA. 1957;164:231–6.
27. Hicken NF, McAllister JA, Walker G. The problems of retained common duct stones. Am J Surg. 1959;97:173–83.
28. Schein CJ, Stern WZ, Jacobson HG. Residual stones. In: Schein CJ, editor. The common bile duct. Springfield: C. C. Thomas; 1966. p. 266–71.
29. Corlette MB, Achatzky S, Ackroyd F. Operative cholangiography and overlooked stones. Arch Surg. 1978;113:729–33.
30. Gartell PC, McGinn FP. Choledochoscopy: are stones missed? A controlled study. Br J Surg. 1984;71:767–70.
31. Cuschieri A, Berci G. Common bile duct exploration. Boston: Martinus-Nijhoff; 1984. p. 54–61.
32. Berci G, Hamlin JA. Retrieval of retained stones. In: Berci G, Hamlin JA, editors. Operative biliary radiology. Baltimore: Williams & Wilkins; 1981. p. 147–58.
33. Lackner J, Volkel L. Die technik der intraoperative cholangiographie unter verwendung des roentgen-bildverstaerker. Roentgenbl. 1957;10:119.
34. Grace RH, Peckar VG. The value of operative cholangiography using an image intensifier and television monitor. Br J Surg. 1968;55:993.
35. Berci G, Hamlin JA. Operative biliary radiology. Baltimore: Williams & Wilkins; 1981. p. 17
36. Mallet-Guy P. Television radioscopy during operations on the biliary passages. Surg Gynecol Obstet. 1958;106(6):747–8.
37. Donna Earley, Chapter 4: Radiation Hazard in Berci G, Hamlin JA. Operative Biliary Radiology. Baltimore: Williams & Wilkins; 1981. p. 23–38.
38. Lee KH. Radiation safety consideration in fluoroscopy. In: Berci G, Cuschieri A, editors. Bile ducts and ductal stones. Philadelphia: Saunders; 1996.
39. Berci G, Hamlin J. Operative biliary radiology. Baltimore: Williams; 1981. p. 202–13.
40. Berci G, Hunter J, Morgenstern L, Arregui M, Brunt M, Carroll B, et al. Laparoscopic cholecystectomy: first do no harm; second, take care of bile duct stones. Surg Endosc. 2013;27(4):1051–4.
41. Nitze M. Eine neu beobachtung und untersuchungsmethode, D. Harnblase. Wien Med Wochenschr. 1879;24:649.
42. Bakes J. Die choledochopapilloskopie, nebst bemerkungen über hepaticus drainage und dilatation der papille. Arch Klinische Chirurgie. 1923;126:473–83.
43. McIver MA. Instrument for visualizing interior of the common duct at operation. Surgery. 1941;9:112.
44. Wildegans H. Die operative gallengangsendoskopie. Munich: Urban & Schwarzenberg; 1960.
45. Schein CJ, Stern WZ, Hurwitt ES, Jacobson HG. Cholangiography and biliary endoscopy as complementary methods of evaluating the bile ducts. Am J Roentgenol Radium Therapy, Nucl Med. 1963;89:864–75.
46. Berci G, Kont LA. A new optical endoscope with special reference to urology. Br J Urol. 1969;41:564–71.
47. Shore JM, Morgenstern L, Berci G. An improved rigid choledochoscope. Am J Surg. 1971;122:567–8.
48. Nora PF, Berci G, Dorazio PA, Kirshenbaum G, Shore JM, Tompkins RK, Wilson SD. Operative choledochoscopy. Am J Surg. 1977;133:105–10.

49. Feliciano D, Mattox K, Jordan G. The value of choledochoscopy in exploration of the common bile duct. Ann Surg. 1980;191:649–53.
50. Rattner DW, Warshaw AL. Impact of choledochoscopy on the management of choledocholithiasis. Experience with 499 common duct explorations at the Massachusetts General Hospital. Ann Surg. 1981;194(1):76–9.
51. Cuschieri A, Berci G, Hamlin JA, Paz-Partlow M. Common bile duct exploration: intraoperative investigations in biliary tract surgery. Boston: Martinus Nijhoff Publishers; 1984.
52. Berci G, Shulman AG, Morgenstern L, Paz-Partlow M, Cuschieri A, Wood RA. Television choledochoscopy. Surg Gynecol Obstet. 1985;160:176–7.
53. Shore JM, Berci G. An improved flexible cholangioscope. Endoscopy. 1976;8:41–2.
54. Phillips P, Berci G, Barber K, Williams J. The role of choledochoscopy: the eternal problem of how to remove a CBD stone. Surg Innov. 2015;22(5):540–5.
55. Phillips E, Berci G, Barber K. The role of the video-choledochoscopy. J Surg Innovation. 2016;23:546–9.

Part II
Preoperative Evaluation

Chapter 2
Current Understanding of Choledocholithiasis: Clinical Presentation and Preoperative Evaluation

Michael Ujiki and H. Mason Hedberg

Incidence and Pathophysiology

Gallstones are extremely common, affecting up to 20% of the population. In those with biliary lithiasis, 20% will also have stones present in the common bile duct (CBD). CBD stones (CBDS) occur when stones formed in the gallbladder migrate into the ductal system (secondary CBDS) or more rarely when stones form in situ within the duct itself (primary CBDS) [1].

Bile Composition

Bile salts and bile acids are the major constituents of normal bile, accounting for 67% of its content. Hepatocyte hydroxylases act upon cholesterol to form primary bile acids. Gut bacteria further modify bile acids into secondary bile acids in the enterohepatic circulation. Bile salts result from conjugation of taurine or glycine to bile acids in hepatocytes. Both bile acids and bile salts are water soluble and act like a detergent to keep free cholesterol in solution. Phospholipids make up 22% of the bile and also help to solubilize cholesterol. Additional components are present in small quantities including protein (4.5%), free cholesterol (4%), conjugated bilirubin (0.3%), and trace amounts of water, electrolytes, and bicarbonate [2].

M. Ujiki, MD, FACS (✉)
Department of Surgery, NorthShore University HealthSystems Evanston Hospital, Evanston, IL, USA
e-mail: mujiki@northshore.org

H. M. Hedberg, MD
Department of Surgery, University of Chicago Medicine, Chicago, IL, USA
e-mail: Herbert.Hedberg@uchospitals.edu

© Springer International Publishing AG, part of Springer Nature 2018
B. F. Santos, N. Soper (eds.), *Choledocholithiasis*,
https://doi.org/10.1007/978-3-319-74503-9_2

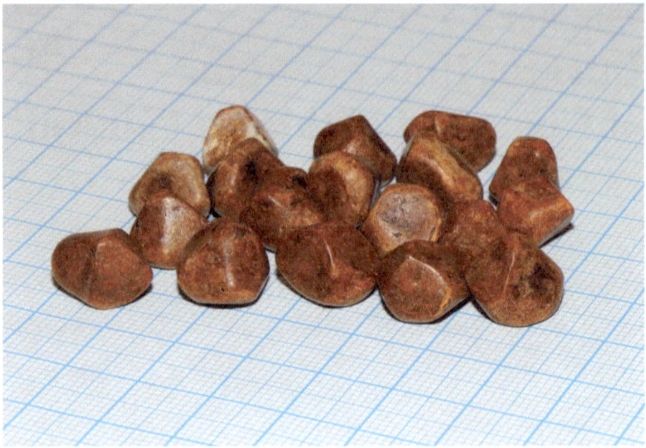

Fig. 2.1 Cholesterol stones. Reprinted under terms of Creative Commons license from George Chernilevsky (own work). https://upload.wikimedia.org/wikipedia/commons/1/17/Human_gallstones_2015_G1.jpg. CC BY-SA 4.0 http://creativecommons.org/licenses/by-sa/4.0

Cholesterol Stones

Cholesterol stones (Fig. 2.1) account for 90% of all gallstones [3]. They form when the bile becomes supersaturated with free cholesterol due either to excess cholesterol in bile (as seen in obesity) or inadequate bile acids/salts. Bile acid/salt deficiency may be caused by:

1. Decreased production (e.g., cirrhosis)
2. Destruction caused by bacterial overgrowth (e.g., autonomic neuropathy)
3. Binding and removal from enterohepatic circulation (e.g., cholestyramine)
4. Lack of reabsorption in the terminal ileum (e.g., Crohn's disease)

Risk Factors for Stone Formation

Major risk factors for cholesterol stones include female sex, age over 40 years of age, obesity, rapid weight loss, and Native American heritage [2]. Specific risk factors are elaborated upon as follows.

Estrogen increases the formation of cholesterol stones by multiple mechanisms. It increases hepatocyte uptake of lipoproteins from the circulation, resulting in a higher percentage of dietary cholesterol excreted in the bile. It upregulates HMG-CoA reductase, the rate-limiting step in endogenous cholesterol synthesis. It also decreases the synthesis of bile acids from cholesterol, further contributing to the supersaturation of the bile with free cholesterol [2]. Given the effect of estrogen, it follows that pregnancy is a well-known lithogenic state. Of note, resolution of sludge and even gallstones may occur in up to 60% and 28% of women, respectively, during the first year postpartum, demonstrating the potentially reversible effect of increased estrogen [4, 5].

Rapid weight loss, defined as more than 1.5 kg body weight lost per week, may occur due to fasting, low-calorie diets, or bariatric surgery. Approximately 30% of individuals with these conditions will form gallstones. In bariatric surgery patients, specific risk factors for stone formation include low fiber or low-calorie diets, prolonged overnight fasting, and gallbladder hypomotility. Following bariatric surgery, a diet containing 7–10 g of daily fat intake improves gallbladder emptying and may combat the formation of symptomatic stones. Taking at least 500 mg ursodeoxycholic acid daily has also been shown to be a cost-effective therapy to prevent gallstone formation after bariatric surgery [5].

Genetics also influences stone formation. Specific populations have been shown to have a high prevalence of gallstones (e.g., up to 65% of Native Americans and up to 35% of Chileans with indigenous backgrounds) [3]. The Swedish Twin Registry, an analysis of 43,141 twin pairs, has revealed that genetics contributes about 25% of the risk of forming gallstones. Recent genome-wide association studies have identified multiple gene abnormalities that may also contribute to stone formation. Variations in the intestinal cholesterol transporter *ABCG8* account for the majority of the estimated 25% genetic risk and may in the future provide an opportunity for personalized medical treatments to decrease this risk [6].

Pigment Stones

Pigment stones (Fig. 2.2) come in two varieties: black and brown. They are composed primarily of calcium bilirubinate, which precipitates from the bile when bilirubin is present in abnormally high concentrations. Black pigment stones are a sign of a chronic extravascular hemolytic process such as hereditary spherocytosis or sickle cell anemia. Brown pigment stones generally form within the bile ducts and biliary tree in the setting of biliary infection and are more common in Asian populations [2].

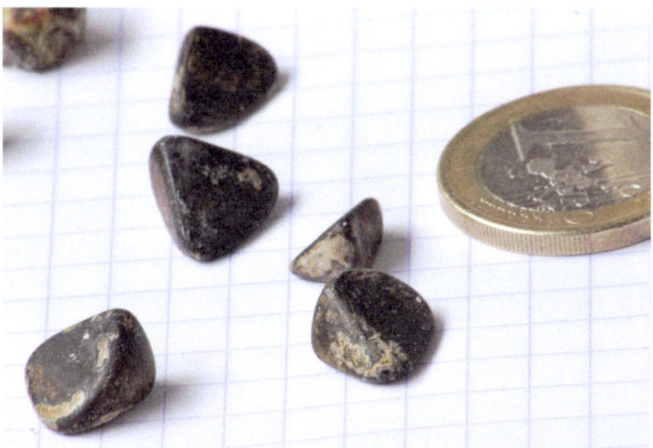

Fig. 2.2 Pigment stones. Reprinted under terms of Creative Commons license from Luk (own work) [FAL]. https://upload.wikimedia.org/wikipedia/commons/0/06/Calculsbiliaires04.JPG. https://creativecommons.org/licenses/by-sa/4.0/

Clinical Syndromes

Choledocholithiasis can produce a wide range of symptoms and pathology, from benign and asymptomatic to life-threatening septic shock. Signs and symptoms are determined by the anatomic level of biliary obstruction and the presence of infection [1]. See Table 2.1 for a summary of clinical syndrome features.

Asymptomatic

CBDS are present in about 4% of the general population, and up to half of these are asymptomatic. The overwhelming majority of these stones are formed in the gallbladder, and stones small enough to pass through the ampulla follow the normal path of the bile into the duodenum [1]. The natural course of asymptomatic CBDS is difficult to study, since stones noted on intraoperative cholangiography traditionally undergo removal. However, recent studies indicate that up to a third of asymptomatic CBDS will pass without intervention after cholecystectomy [7].

Table 2.1 Summary of common bile duct stone (CBDS) syndromes

	Asymptomatic	Biliary colic	Cholangitis	Gallstone pancreatitis
Cause	Passage of small stones through biliary tree without obstruction	Transient obstruction of the biliary tree	Obstruction and infection of the biliary tree, translocation of bacteria and toxins	Obstruction at the ampulla, increased pancreatic duct pressure
Epidemiology	CBDS in 4% of population, half asymptomatic	Most often due to cholelithiasis	~1% with symptomatic gallstones over 5–10-year period	Most common cause of acute pancreatitis
Subjective findings	None	Right upper quadrant pain radiating to back/shoulder, 20–30 min duration	Right upper quadrant pain, radiating to the back/shoulder, chills/rigors	Epigastric pain radiating to back, nausea
Objective findings	Incidental stones on imaging	Transaminases 500–1000 IU in 18%	Fever Leukocytosis Abnormal LFTs	Elevated lipase and/or amylase Abnormal LFTs
Mortality	0%	0%	2.7–10%	Mild: 1–3% Organ failure >48 h: 36% Multiorgan failure within 72 h of onset: >50%

IU international units, *LFTs* liver function tests

Biliary Colic

Biliary colic is defined as episodic, severe epigastric, or right upper quadrant pain of at least 20–30 min in duration. The pain typically radiates to the back or right shoulder and is alleviated with pain medication. Whereas biliary colic is generally attributed to gallstones within the gallbladder, CBD obstruction from stones can present with identical symptoms. Pain from CBDS results from dilation of the biliary tree, and symptoms are generally accompanied by altered hepatic function tests and, on imaging, dilated bile ducts. Passage of the obstructing stone into the duodenum or movement of the stone retrograde into the dilated duct can relieve pressure in the biliary tree and the associated symptoms (Fig. 2.3) [5]. Thus, assuming that a stone has passed because a patient's pain has resolved is not a safe assumption.

Biliary colic itself presents no risk of mortality, and morbidity is limited to pain often requiring narcotic pain medications. However, in one study about half of patients who presented with complicated gallstone disease (pancreatitis, CBDS, or cholecystitis) had prior episodes of biliary colic, so the symptom should be considered a potential harbinger of more serious conditions [8].

Jaundice

The most common cause of obstructive jaundice is choledocholithiasis. Jaundice results from conjugated bilirubin deposits in the skin, mucosa, and sclera; generally, serum bilirubin must be higher than 3 mg/dL for discoloration to be visible [9]. Obstructive CBDS may present with painless jaundice, but more commonly presents with biliary colic symptoms (Fig. 2.4). Morbidity from obstructive stones causing jaundice is limited to itching from bilirubin deposits and generally mild

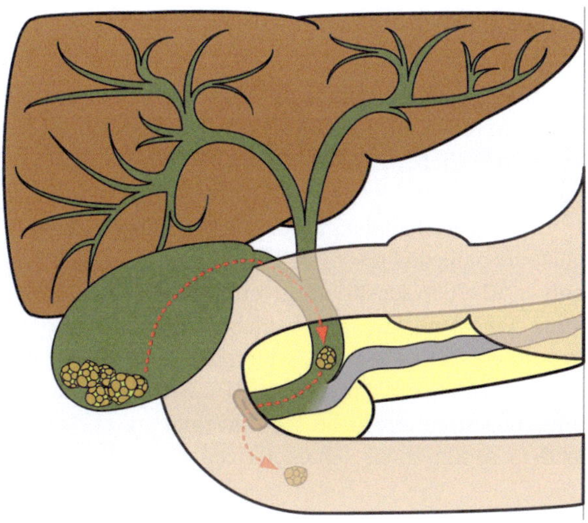

Fig. 2.3 Transient CBDS may be asymptomatic or cause biliary colic

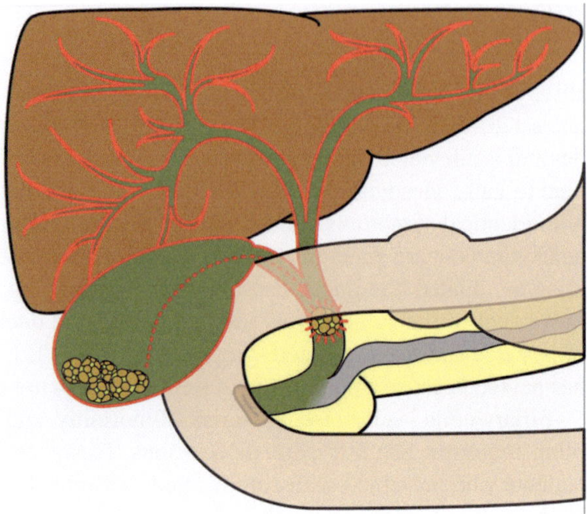

Fig. 2.4 Impacted CBDS can cause pain, gallstone hepatitis, jaundice, and cholangitis

hepatocyte injury due to increased pressure in the biliary system. However, cholestasis increases the risk of infection, and an obstructive stone at the ampulla may cause pancreatitis. These conditions are discussed in detail below.

Cholangitis

The biliary tree is normally protected from infection due to antegrade flow of bile, biliary epithelial tight junctions, and mucosal immunoglobulin A (IgA) [10]. Bactobilia occurs when bacteria from the duodenum traverse the ampulla in a retrograde fashion and is a common finding in asymptomatic individuals with CBDS [11]. Cholangitis occurs when cholestasis is complicated by bacterial infection, with obstructive CBDS being by far the most common cause of cholangitis. Normal pressure within the CBD is 7–14 cm H_2O. When pressure increases to >20 cm H_2O, bacterial cells and toxins can translocate across the biliary epithelium into the systemic circulation causing septic shock. Risk factors for cholangitis include diabetes mellitus, age >70 years, and recent infection outside of the biliary tree [10].

Up to 75% of cholangitis cases present with Charcot's triad: jaundice, right upper quadrant pain, and fever [9]. The presence of Charcot's triad has high specificity, but only a 50–70% sensitivity given that not all patients with cholangitis develop all three symptoms. Laboratory analysis reflects biliary obstruction with elevated liver function tests (LFTs) and systemic inflammation with elevated white blood cell count and C-reactive protein (CRP). Bile duct dilation may occur, and possibly the offending stone might be seen on imaging [12]. Progression of the infection can lead to septic shock, characterized by hypotension and mental status changes.

The addition of these findings to Charcot's triad is known as Reynolds' Pentad and is seen in about 5–7% of cases [10, 11].

According to the Tokyo Guidelines, the diagnosis of cholangitis may be classified as suspected or definite based on criteria and can be classified as severe, moderate, or mild [12]. Diagnostic criteria include:

A. *Systemic inflammation*: fever and/or shaking chills, laboratory evidence of an inflammatory response (leukocytosis or leukopenia, elevated CRP)
B. *Cholestasis*: jaundice (total bilirubin >2 mg/dL), abnormal liver function tests
C. *Imaging*: biliary dilation, evidence of the etiology on imaging (e.g., stone, stricture, or stent)

A diagnosis of cholangitis is suspected if there is the presence of one item from criteria "A," plus one item from criteria "B" or "C." A diagnosis of cholangitis is definite if there is the presence of one item from all three criteria (A, B, and C).

Signs of organ dysfunction in at least one of the following organ systems define severe cholangitis:

- Mental status change
- Hypotension
- PaO_2/FiO_2 >300
- Acute kidney injury
- Elevated prothrombin time (PT) or international normalized ratio (INR)
- Platelet count <100,000

Moderate cholangitis lacks organ dysfunction but includes any two of the following:

- Age >75 years
- White blood cell (WBC) count >12,000 or <4000
- Fever >39 °C or 102.2 °F
- Serum total bilirubin >5 mg/dL
- Serum albumin <70% low normal limit

Mild cholangitis does not meet the above criteria at the time of diagnosis.

Acute obstructive cholangitis due to gallstones is relatively rare on a population level, so its absolute incidence is difficult to determine. One study observed that 0.3–1.6% of individuals with asymptomatic or mildly symptomatic gallstones will develop acute cholangitis over a 5–10-year period. Per the Tokyo Guidelines, about 12.3% of gallstone-related acute cholangitis cases present with some end-organ dysfunction and qualify as severe [13].

Mortality due to cholangitis varies with the severity of disease. Individuals with cholangitis, signs of organ failure, and lack of response to medical management will not survive without prompt biliary decompression, whereas mild to moderate cholangitis may respond well to initial systemic antibiotic therapy. Reported mortality has decreased over time, with >50% mortality reported prior to 1980 and more recent studies citing 2.7–10% mortality rates [14].

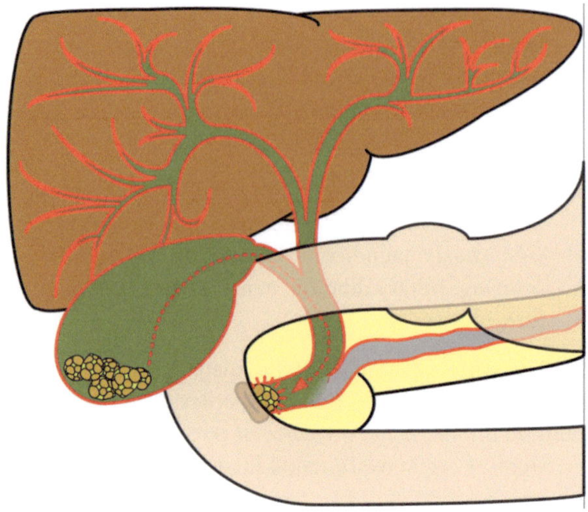

Fig. 2.5 CBDS impacted at the ampulla can cause pain, gallstone hepatitis, and gallstone pancreatitis

Gallstone Pancreatitis

Gallstones are the most common cause of acute pancreatitis in the Western world. The CBD and pancreatic duct converge at the ampulla of Vater, where gallstones following the natural flow of bile may become impacted (Fig. 2.5). The resulting pancreatic duct obstruction leads to intrapancreatic activation of lytic digestive enzymes, inflammation of the pancreas and surrounding tissues, and the classic epigastric pain characteristic of pancreatitis. In most cases the offending stone is impacted only transiently before passing into the duodenum and is not evident on imaging during workup. Fecal gallstones can be found in 90% of individuals diagnosed with gallstone pancreatitis (GSP) and only 10% of the general population. Persistent obstruction from a stone, or ampullary edema after passage of a stone, increases the severity of GSP. Risk factors include female sex, age >60 years, multiple gallstones <5 mm in diameter, a dilated cystic duct, excellent postprandial gallbladder emptying, and possibly anatomic abnormalities of the pancreatic duct such as a non-patent accessory duct [11, 15].

The morbidity and mortality from GSP are dependent upon its severity. There are multiple scoring systems available to stratify the severity of GSP, including the Ranson criteria, Glasgow criteria, and the Acute Physiology and Chronic Health Evaluation II (APACHE-II) scoring system. However, the relatively low incidence of severe GSP lowers the positive predictive value of these clinical tools to less than 50% [11]. Classification by the Ranson criteria is as follows [12]:

- Age >55 years
- Serum glucose >200 mg/dL
- Lactate dehydrogenase (LDH) >350 mg/dL
- Aspartate aminotransferase (AST) >250 units/L
- White blood cell count >16,000

Moderate to severe GSP:

- Four or more Ranson criteria
- Evidence of organ failure

Mild GSP:

- Clinical stability
- Euvolemia
- Blood urea nitrogen (BUN) <15
- Heart rate (HR) <110 bpm
- <4 Ranson criteria

Severe GSP is also predicted by an APACHE-II score greater than 7.

The Atlanta classification is a clinically based tool that associates severe disease with findings of organ failure, gastrointestinal bleeding, pancreatic necrosis/pseudocyst, or systemic complications such as disseminated intravascular coagulation. These clinical factors can carry significant impact on mortality. Mild acute pancreatitis has a mortality rate from 1 to 3%. Of mild cases, 15–25% will develop pancreatic necrosis, and the presence of infected necrotic tissue increases the mortality rate to 30%. Duration of organ failure is also a significant predictor of mortality. Organ failure lasting less than 48 h is associated with a 36% mortality rate, and progressive multisystem organ failure presenting within the first 72 h of initial symptoms carries a mortality rate greater than 50% [11].

Laboratory Studies

Symptomatic Common Bile Duct Stones

The increased pressure of an obstructed biliary tree can cause necrosis of hepatocyte and release of liver transaminases into the circulation, as indicated by increased LFTs on blood chemistry. The destruction of hepatocytes and ensuing inflammation due to obstructive CBDS is called gallstone hepatitis (GSH). In one study of individuals with symptomatic CBDS, GSH was seen with transaminase elevation to 500–1000 IU in 18% of patients, with elevation over 1000 IU seen in 10% of patients. The liver enzymes gamma-glutamyl transpeptidase and alkaline phosphatase can also be elevated, but rise later than transaminases. The absence of LFT elevation within 24 h of biliary colic-like symptoms indicates CBDS are likely not present [5]. A different prospective series of individuals with CBDS identified on endoscopic retrograde cholangiopancreatography (ERCP) found 4.3% of individuals to have GSH (defined as transaminitis >400 IU) in the absence of cholangitis. Of individuals with CBDS, 13.2% had normal LFTs. The authors were able to associate younger age, shorter-lasting and more intense abdominal pain, cholelithiasis, and narrower CBDs with GSH [16].

Cholangitis

Nonspecific laboratory findings of cholangitis include leukocytosis and elevated C-reactive protein and erythrocyte sedimentation rate. LFTs are always abnormal, but elevations vary widely. Cultures of bile in cholangitis are positive in 80–100% of cases. Reports of positive blood cultures range from 21 to 71%. The most commonly isolated organisms are enteric gram-negatives: *Enterococcus*, *Klebsiella*, and *E. coli*. Polymicrobial infections are more common in the setting of prior biliary surgery, in elderly patients, or with severe disease, and cultures can yield anaerobic species such as *Clostridium*. Biliary surgery and biliary stents are associated with infections by hospital-acquired or drug-resistant organisms and fungi [11].

Gallstone Pancreatitis

Serum amylase and/or lipase are elevated three times over the upper limit of normal in GSP. Serum lipase levels peak about 24 h after initial insult, and elevation persists for several days. Amylase begins to rise within 2–12 h after insult and returns to normal within 3–5 days. Degree of elevation does not correlate with disease severity, and trending daily values is not useful for predicting disease progression [11].

Elevated LFTs in patients presenting with acute pancreatitis should raise the suspicion of GSP. Alanine aminotransferase (ALT) elevated over three times the upper limit of normal has a 95% positive predictive value for GSP. However, sensitivity is only 48%, and 10% of individuals with GSP have normal LFTs [11].

Noninvasive Imaging Studies

Identification of CBDS when working up biliary pathology is critical to determine the appropriate course of treatment. Multiple effective imaging modalities exist, each with advantages and disadvantages. Imaging modalities and specific applications are reviewed as follows (see Table 2.2 for a summary of each modality).

Ultrasound

Given availability, portability, and low cost, transabdominal ultrasound (US) is typically the first imaging study employed when working up biliary-type abdominal pain. US has a poor sensitivity of 23–65% for directly visualizing CBDS, but is effective at detecting CBD dilation. However, borderline CBD dilation can have limited clinical significance given the lack of a clear definition of bile duct dilation. Studies exist using anywhere from 5 to 10 mm as an upper limit of normal, and

Table 2.2 Summary of imaging studies for common bile duct stones (CBDS)

	Ultrasound	CT cholangiography	MRCP	Scintigraphy
Efficacy for CBDS	23–65% sensitivity	Sensitivity 85–97%, specificity 88–96%	Sensitivity 93%, specificity 96%	Slightly better than ultrasound
Advantages	Inexpensive, portable, widely available	Less expensive and faster than MRCP	Does not require contrast agents	May pick up CBD obstruction with minimal dilation
Disadvantages	Poor CBDS visualization	15% allergy to contrast	Routine use not cost-effective	Long-duration study
Other	CBD dilation to 7 mm is 92% specific for CBDS	Noncontrast CT efficacy similar to US for CBDS	Can miss stones <5 mm	CBDS indicated by no contrast in the duodenum at 2 h

CT computed tomography, *MRCP* magnetic resonance cholangiopancreatography, *CBD* common bile duct, *US* ultrasound

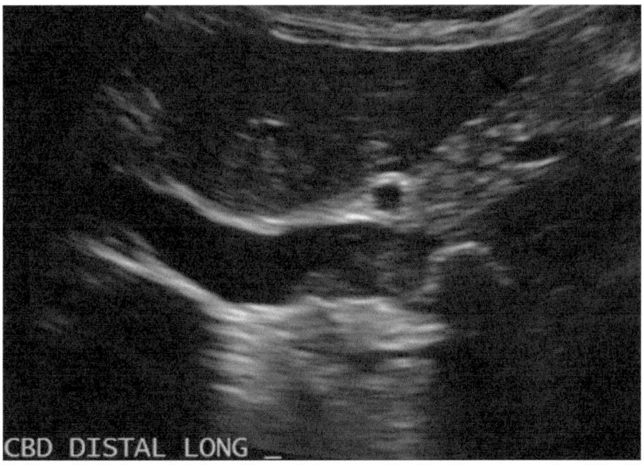

Fig. 2.6 Transverse ultrasound view of the CBD, with echogenic material distally (screen right). During follow-up ERCP, multiple 10–15 mm stones and sludge were removed

dilation of the CBD to 7 mm is 92% specific for CBDS. Initial ultrasonography carries an additional benefit of identifying cholelithiasis and other intra-abdominal pathology [5, 17]. Figure 2.6 shows a relatively rare instance of directly visualizing CBDS with US. Figures 2.7 and 2.8 show dilated intrahepatic and extrahepatic bile ducts, respectively.

Computed Tomography

Similar to US, standard computed tomography (CT) utilizing intravenous and oral contrast has good sensitivity for detecting biliary dilation (Fig. 2.9), but poorly detects CBDS (Fig. 2.10). CT can be advantageous, however, to differentiate other

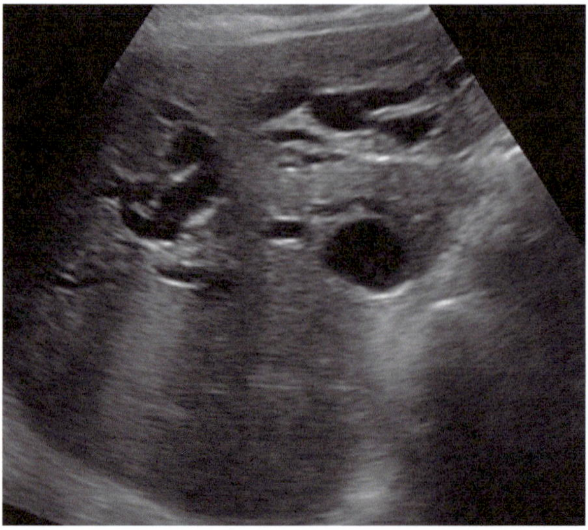

Fig. 2.7 Dilated intrahepatic bile ducts as seen on US

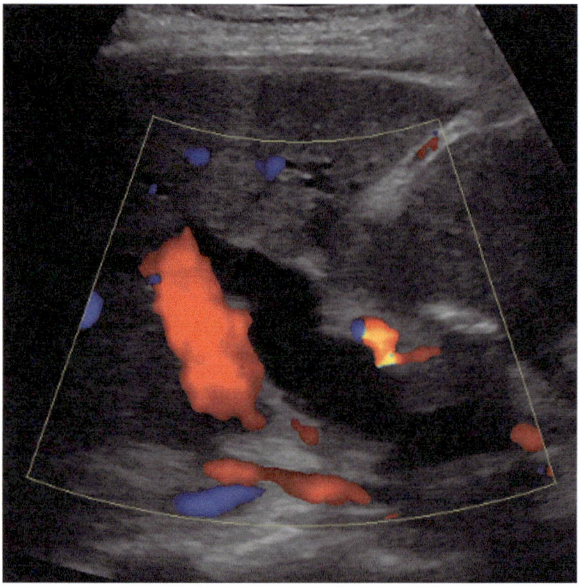

Fig. 2.8 Duplex US differentiating the portal vein (red) from a dilated, 13 mm CBD (black)

causes of CBD obstruction such as malignancy and to evaluate for complications such as pancreatitis or liver abscess. CT cholangiography utilizes oral or intravenous contrast agents specifically excreted into the bile (e.g., intravenous meglumine iotroxate) with three-dimensional (3D) reconstruction of the biliary tree and carries sensitivity of 85–97% and specificity of 88–96% for detecting CBDS. However, poor visualization of intrahepatic ducts, hindered ductal opacification in the setting of jaundice, and an allergy rate of 15% to contrast agents have limited its

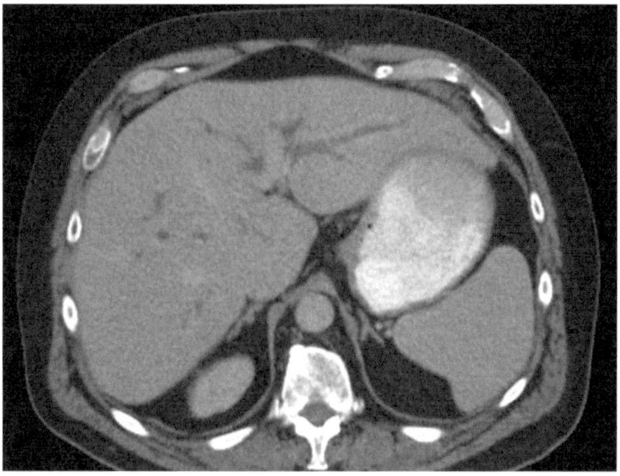

Fig. 2.9 CT with IV contrast demonstrating intrahepatic bile duct dilation. Dilated bile ducts are seen as dark gray tubular structures (in contrast with portal branches, which are contrast-enhanced)

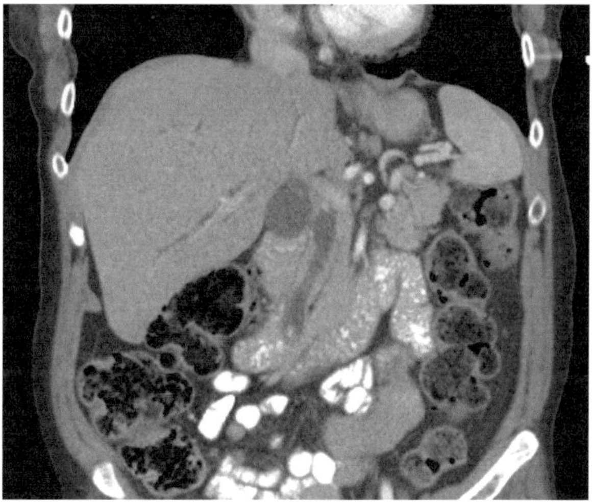

Fig. 2.10 Coronal CT showing a CBD dilated to 13 mm (center, dark gray), with a calcified distal CBDS

widespread use [11]. Currently, only intravenous cholangiography contrast agents are available in the United States. Unfortunately, oral cholecystographic contrast agents, previously widely used in the era of oral cholecystography and with a more acceptable safety profile compared to intravenous cholangiography contrast agents, are no longer available in the United States.

Magnetic Resonance Cholangiopancreatography

Magnetic resonance cholangiopancreatography (MRCP) is a highly effective imaging modality for CBDS (Figs. 2.11 and 2.12). It is noninvasive, does not require contrast, and can be performed without anesthesia. The major drawback is cost, and

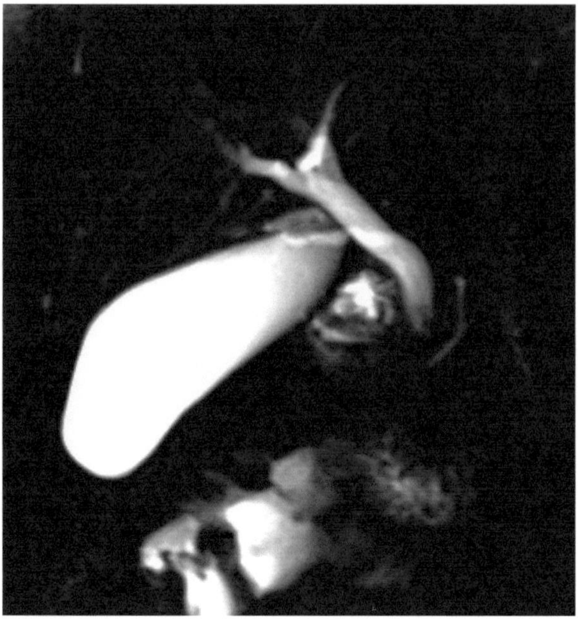

Fig. 2.11 MRCP demonstrating CBD dilation with a distal CBDS

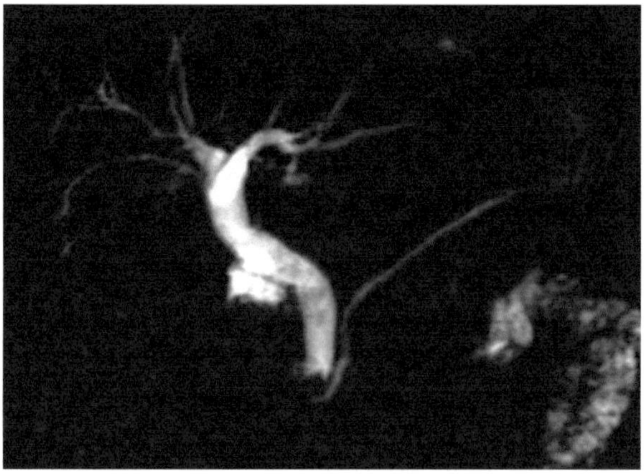

Fig. 2.12 MRCP showing multiple CBDS, with a dilated CBD (10 mm)

routine MRCP for biliary disease without laboratory evidence of CBDS is not cost-effective [18]. Small stone diameter (<5 mm) and peripancreatic edema have been shown to reduce the accuracy of CBDS identification [11, 16–19]. Sensitivity and specificity of MRCP for CBDS are 93% and 96%, respectively [5].

Biliary Scintigraphy

Biliary scintigraphy is not routinely used to evaluate for the presence of CBDS, but signs of choledocholithiasis can be inferred from the information revealed about bile flow through the biliary tract (Fig. 2.13). Findings indicating CBDS include lack of contrast in the duodenum after 2 h and persistent prominence of extrahepatic and intrahepatic ducts 90 min after contrast administration. Accuracy of scintigraphy for detecting CBDS is slightly better than that of US. The ability of scintigraphy to analyze bile flow over time allows it to detect partial CBD obstruction that may not cause significant dilation [17].

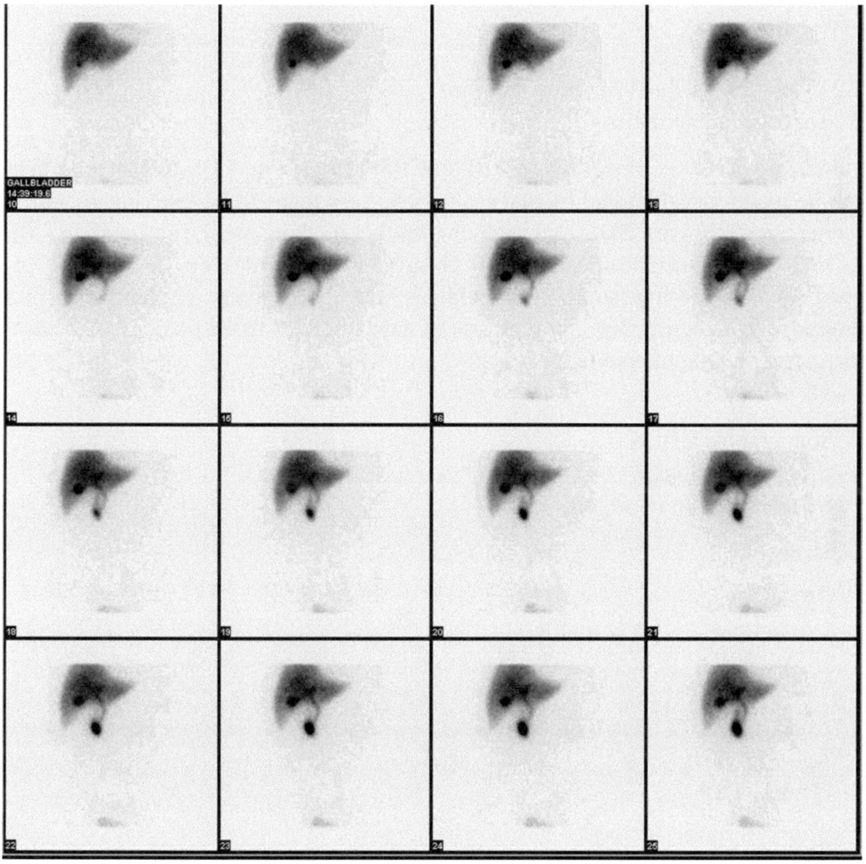

Fig. 2.13 Normal biliary scintigraphy, demonstrating the accumulation of bile in the gallbladder and normal flow through the CBD to the duodenum. Reprinted under terms of Creative Commons license from Myo Han. HIDA scan. https://upload.wikimedia.org/wikipedia/commons/9/94/HIDA.jpg. CC BY 3.0 (http://creativecommons.org/licenses/by/3.0)

Preoperative Prediction Models and their Accuracy

Ability to predict the risk of CBDS during workup for biliary disease can help inform appropriate preoperative imaging studies and interventional management. Several scores have been proposed that draw from clinical, radiological, and laboratory data.

The Lacaine-Huguier score was developed in 1988 and has been validated by multiple prospective trials. It relies only upon clinical and sonographic data in those with calculous cholecystitis, which improves ease of use. The score is calculated as follows:

0.04 * (age) +
1 for biliary colic
3.1 for CBD >12 mm
1.2 if smallest gallbladder stone <10 mm
0.7 for acute cholecystitis

A score of 3.5 or greater carries risk of CBDS from 17 to 85%, and an argument can be made for additional biliary evaluation. Less than 2% of individuals with a score under 3.5 have CBDS, and excluding further imaging may be appropriate [20].

In 2010, the American Society for Gastrointestinal Endoscopy (ASGE) developed a risk score that stratifies individuals with symptomatic cholelithiasis into groups of low, intermediate, or high risk of having CBDS based on clinical, laboratory, and sonographic predictors [21]:

Very strong

- Sonographic CBDS
- Clinical cholangitis
- Serum bilirubin >4 mg/dL

Strong

- CBD >6 mm
- Serum bilirubin 1.8–4 mg/dL

Moderate

- Abnormal LFTs other than bilirubin
- Age >55 years
- Clinical GSP

Risk of CBDS:

Any very strong predictor	High
Both strong predictors	High
No predictors	Low
All others	Intermediate

Category of risk determines the recommended therapeutic and/or imaging approach. A criticism of the ASGE score is that its many predictors create a wide range of intermediate risk patients. A study of 109 individuals falling into the intermediate group found that presence of either "strong" predictor carried a 28% risk of CBDS [22].

Conclusion

Common bile duct stones are present in up to 20% of individuals with cholelithiasis. Half are asymptomatic and pass into the intestine with the normal flow of bile. Clinical manifestations of choledocholithiasis range from biliary colic-type symptoms to severe epigastric pain from gallstone pancreatitis or septic shock from cholangitis. Derangements of liver function tests are expected with cholangitis and are good predictors of choledocholithiasis in the setting of biliary or pancreatic pain. Transabdominal ultrasound is always appropriate when working up biliary disease and with clinical and laboratory data helps inform further workup and management.

References

1. Internal Clinical Guidelines Team (UK). Gallstone disease: diagnosis and management of cholelithiasis, cholecystitis and choledocholithiasis. London: Natl Inst Health Care Excellence (UK). 2014;20(37):13382–401.
2. Goljan EF, editor. Pathology. Philadelphia: Mosby; 2010.
3. Tiderington E, Lee SP, Ko CW. Gallstones: new insights into an old story. F1000Res. 2016;5:1817.
4. Maringhini A, Ciambra M, Baccelliere P, Raimondo M, Orland A, Tine F, Grasso R, Randazzo MA, Barresi L, Gullo D, Musico M, Pagliaro L. Biliary sludge and gallstones in pregnancy: incidence, risk factors, and natural history. Ann Intern Med. 1993;119(2):116–20.
5. Lammert F, Gurusamy K, Ko CW, Miquel JF, Méndez-Sánchez N, Portincasa P, van Erpecum KJ, van Laarhoven CJ, Wang DQ. Gallstones. Nat Rev Dis Primers. 2016;2:16024.
6. Katsika D, Grjibovski A, Einarsson C, Lammert F, Lichtenstein P, Marschall HU. Genetic and environmental influences on symptomatic gallstone disease: a Swedish study of 43,141 twin pairs. Hepatology. 2005;41(5):1138–43.
7. Collins C, Maguire D, Ireland A, Fitzgerald E, O'Sullivan GC. A prospective study of common bile duct calculi in patients undergoing laparoscopic cholecystectomy: natural history of choledocholithiasis revisited. Ann Surg. 2004;239(1):28–33.
8. Besselink MG, Venneman NG, Go PM, Broeders IA, Siersema PD, Gooszen HG, van Erpecum KJ. Is complicated gallstone disease preceded by biliary colic? J Gastrointest Surg. 2009;13(2):312–7.
9. Kathpalia P, Ahn J. Assessment of jaundice in the hospitalized patient. Clin Liver Dis. 2015;19:155–70.
10. Zimmer V, Lammert F. Acute bacterial cholangitis. Viszeralmedizin. 2015;31(3):166–72.
11. Attasaranya S, Fogel EL, Lehman GA. Choledocholithiasis, ascending cholangitis, and gallstone pancreatitis. Med Clin North Am. 2008;92(4):925–60. x

12. Demehri FR, Alam HB. Evidence-based management of common gallstone-related emergencies. J Intensive Care Med. 2016;31(1):3–13.
13. Kimura Y, Takada T, Strasberg SM, Pitt HA, Gouma DJ, Garden OJ, et al. TG13 current terminology, etiology, and epidemiology of acute cholangitis and cholecystitis. J Hepatobiliary Pancreat Sci. 2013;20(1):8–23.
14. Kimura Y, Takada T, Kawarada Y, Nimura Y, Hirata K, Sekimoto M, et al. Definitions, pathophysiology, and epidemiology of acute cholangitis and cholecystitis: Tokyo guidelines. J Hepato-Biliary-Pancreat Surg. 2007;14(1):15–26.
15. Oría A, Cimmino D, Ocampo C, Silva W, Kohan G, Zandalazini H, et al. Early endoscopic intervention versus early conservative management in patients with acute gallstone pancreatitis and biliopancreatic obstruction. Ann Surg. 2007;245(1):10–7.
16. Huh CW, Jang SI, Lim BJ, Kim HW, Kim JK, Park JS, et al. Clinicopathological features of choledocholithiasis patients with high aminotransferase levels without cholangitis. Medicine. 2016;95(42):e5176.
17. Colletti PM, Ralls PW, Lapin SA, Siegel ME, Halls JM. Hepatobiliary imaging in choledocholithiasis: a comparison with ultrasound. Clin Nucl Med. 1986;11(7):482–6.
18. Epelboym I, Winner M, Allendorf JDJ. MRCP is not a cost-effective strategy in the management of silent common bile duct stones. Gastrointest Surg. 2013;17(5):863–71.
19. Polistina FA, Frego M, Bisello M, Manzi E, Vardanega A, Perin B. Accuracy of magnetic resonance cholangiography compared to operative endoscopy in detecting biliary stones, a single center experience and review of literature. World J Radiol. 2015;7(4):70–8.
20. Khalfallah M, Dougaz W, Bedoui R, Bouasker I, Chaker Y, Nouira R, et al. Validation of the Lacaine-Huguier predictive score for choledocholithiasis: prospective study of 380 patients. J Visc Surg. 2012;149(1):e66–72.
21. Maple JT, Ben-Menachem T, Anderson MA, Appalaneni V, Banerjee S, Cash BD, et al. The role of endoscopy in the evaluation of suspected choledocholithiasis. Gastrointest Endosc. 2010;71(1):1–9.
22. Kang J, Paik KH, Lee JC, Kim HW, Lee J, Hwang JH, et al. The Efficacy of clinical predictors for patients with intermediate risk of choledocholithiasis. Digestion. 2016;94(2):100–5.

Chapter 3
Preoperative Decision-Making Algorithm

Arslan Pannu and Ahmad Mirza

Introduction

The incidence of choledocholithiasis varies from around 5% in elective cholecystectomy cases to up to 20% in emergency cases and is observed to rise with increasing age [1–4]. Given this, the European Association of Endoscopic Surgery (EAES) recommends that all patients with cholelithiasis be investigated for choledocholithiasis [5]. The clinical manifestations of choledocholithiasis may vary from asymptomatic stones (incidental finding on bile duct imaging) to biliary colic and to acute, life-threatening presentations such as acute cholangitis and gallstone pancreatitis. The complications related to common bile duct (CBD) stones represent a major burden to health-care services. At the author's institution, the surgeon plays a primary role in the triage, evaluation, and management of patients with common duct stones. The structure of this practice model is well established and will be described for the reader. In addition, this chapter will describe a safe, cost-effective, and widely applicable approach to the management of CBD stone disease.

The discussion in this chapter will focus primarily on the workup and management of patients with syndromes caused by CBD stones. Malignant causes of acute pancreatitis (AP), cholangitis, and jaundice will not be central to this chapter, although it is important for the surgeon to realize there can be considerable overlap in the presentation of benign and malignant conditions of the biliary tract. A brief section will describe warning signs that should prompt the surgeon to consider a malignant etiology, rather than common duct stones as the underlying cause of the patient's presentation.

A. Pannu, MBBS, MRCS
Department of Colorectal/General Surgery, The Royal Oldham Hospital, Manchester, UK
e-mail: Arslan.pannu@nhs.net

A. Mirza, MD, FRCS (✉)
Department of General Surgery, The Pennine Acute Hospitals NHS Trust, Manchester, UK
e-mail: Ahmad.mirza@nhs.net

© Springer International Publishing AG, part of Springer Nature 2018
B. F. Santos, N. Soper (eds.), *Choledocholithiasis*,
https://doi.org/10.1007/978-3-319-74503-9_3

Practice Model of a Specialized Biliary Firm

At our institution all patients with diagnosed or suspected acute biliary pathology are referred to a single specialist firm of biliary surgeons responsible for managing gallstone disease. All referrals are triaged and are reviewed to determine their clinical urgency. The dedicated on-call surgeon for the biliary firm is responsible for directing the evaluation and management of new patients.

A consensus approach for a single surgical firm to take charge of the evaluation and management of patients with biliary emergencies was established following review of prior outcomes of patients with gallstone disease. The protocol was established as a way to streamline the care of such patients. Prior to this approach, patients with suspected bile duct stones were typically subjected to two procedures (endoscopic management followed by cholecystectomy). Some patients underwent negative endoscopic retrograde cholangiopancreatography (ERCP), exposing them to risks without benefit. In addition, preoperative endoscopic management delayed surgical evaluation, and patients wait longer to undergo definitive surgical management. A new approach for the care of biliary patients was formulated after discussion with internal medicine doctors, gastroenterologists, and surgeons. It was agreed in principle that no endoscopic intervention should be carried out without review or discussion of the patient's case with a surgeon from the specialist biliary firm. The objectives of the new approach were to decrease hospital length of stay and readmissions by choosing the optimal treatment approach for each patient, including performance of definitive surgery at the index admission if appropriate. This approach has helped us identify patients who are immediately suited for primary surgical intervention versus those who are best treated with initial endoscopic management or require further noninvasive bile duct imaging.

At our institution, routine intraoperative cholangiography is performed to identify CBD stones thus facilitating the diagnostic algorithm for most patients. The findings of intraoperative bile duct imaging guides further laparoscopic management of bile duct stones. There is dedicated operating room time for biliary emergencies to facilitate scheduling of patients. The high volume of emergency biliary cases also provides an excellent opportunity for our trainees to develop skills in bile duct imaging and laparoscopic bile duct exploration.

Biliary Colic or Acute Cholecystitis

Patients presenting with biliary-type pain should be evaluated with a history and physical exam. In addition to inquiring about the main complaint, it is important to inquire about any episodes of jaundice, dark urine, and acholic stools, as well as to determine whether the patient has experienced unintentional weight loss, as these symptoms either raise a suspicion for common duct stones or alternatively possible malignancy (especially if weight loss is present). Patients should have laboratory studies sent including a complete blood count (CBC), liver function tests (LFTs), and amylase/lipase tests and have an ultrasound of the gallbladder performed. Once a diagnosis of gallstones is confirmed, the patient can usually be categorized according to one of the gallstone disease syndromes (e.g., biliary colic, cholecystitis, pancreatitis, etc.). Most stable patients with biliary colic or cholecystitis are managed with laparoscopic cholecystectomy (LC) with intraoperative imaging and bile duct exploration if necessary (Fig. 3.1). Options when bile duct exploration is unsuccessful or if the surgeon does not perform this

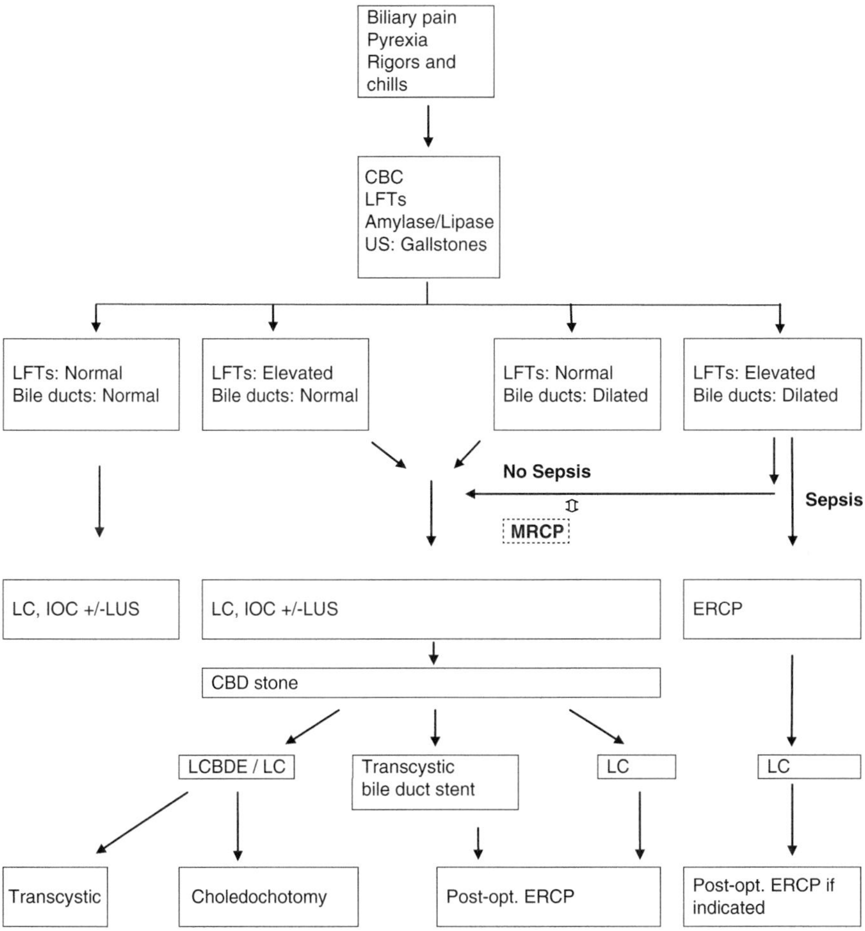

Fig. 3.1 Pathways for diagnosis and management of suspected common bile duct stones. LFTs liver function tests, *CBC* complete blood count, *US* ultrasound scan, *LC* laparoscopic cholecystectomy, *IOC* intraoperative cholangiogram, *MRCP* magnetic resonance cholangiopancreatography, *ERCP* endoscopic retrograde cholangiopancreatography, *LCBDE* laparoscopic common bile duct exploration, *LUS* laparoscopic ultrasound

operation are to proceed with open common duct exploration or postoperative ERCP with or without placement of a biliary stent across the papilla. Placement of a biliary stent facilitates cannulation of the bile duct during postoperative ERCP [5]. In terms of outcomes, the single-stage approach has been well described to have the same efficacy and safety but shorter hospital length of stay and cost compared to two-stage management (ERCP plus cholecystectomy) [6–11]. Unfortunately, the single-stage approach has failed to gain wider acceptability, and despite the documented sensitivity (97%) and specificity (99%) of cholangiography, it too has seen a decline in use in surgical practice [12–18]. These techniques of surgical ductal clearance and cholangiography are user-dependent and improve with experience [19]. It is thus imperative that trainees be exposed to these techniques to develop expertise and that surgeons continue to perform cholangiography to maintain these skills. Even if a surgeon only performs cholangiography (and not common duct exploration), a surgery-first strategy is superior to two-stage management for patients who qualify as intermediate risk according to American Society for Gastrointestinal Endoscopy (ASGE) criteria, with surgery-first patients having a shorter hospital length of stay and fewer additional common duct investigations (endoscopic ultrasound, ERCP, or magnetic resonance cholangiopancreatography [MRCP]) [17].

Gallstone Pancreatitis

Introduction

Gallstones account for 35–75% cases of acute pancreatitis [6–8]. Gallstone-related pancreatitis results from stones passing from the gallbladder via the cystic duct into the common bile duct or rarely, de novo stone formation in the common bile duct. In both cases there is an obstruction at the level of the ampulla of Vater, which causes acute pancreatitis [12].

Patients with a suspected diagnosis of acute pancreatitis should undergo laboratory testing including CBC, complete metabolic panel including LFTs, and amylase/lipase. A right upper quadrant ultrasound should be ordered to determine if gallstones are present, implicating them as the likely etiology if other causes of pancreatitis are absent. The severity of the pancreatitis should be determined using any of a number of well-known scoring systems (described in Chap. 2) and supportive care instituted. Patients with failure of clinical improvement, clinical deterioration, or diagnostic uncertainty should undergo further evaluation with contrast-enhanced computed tomography (CT) to determine if there are further complications such as acute fluid collections, pancreatic necrosis, or peripancreatic complications such as venous thrombosis or pseudoaneurysm formation.

Mild to Moderate Pancreatitis

Most patients will have mild or moderate pancreatitis that improves rapidly with supportive treatment. These patients should be offered cholecystectomy during the same hospital admission after resolution of the episode (Fig. 3.2), since without cholecystectomy recurrent episodes of pancreatitis continue to occur in 25% of patients, and may result in significant morbidity and even mortality in approximately 10% of cases [20–23]. It is important to offer patients a timely cholecystectomy, as, among patients who suffer recurrent attacks, 23.3% have a recurrent attack within 30 days of the previous attack [24]. Same-admission cholecystectomy was compared with interval cholecystectomy (30 days later) in a Dutch, prospective,

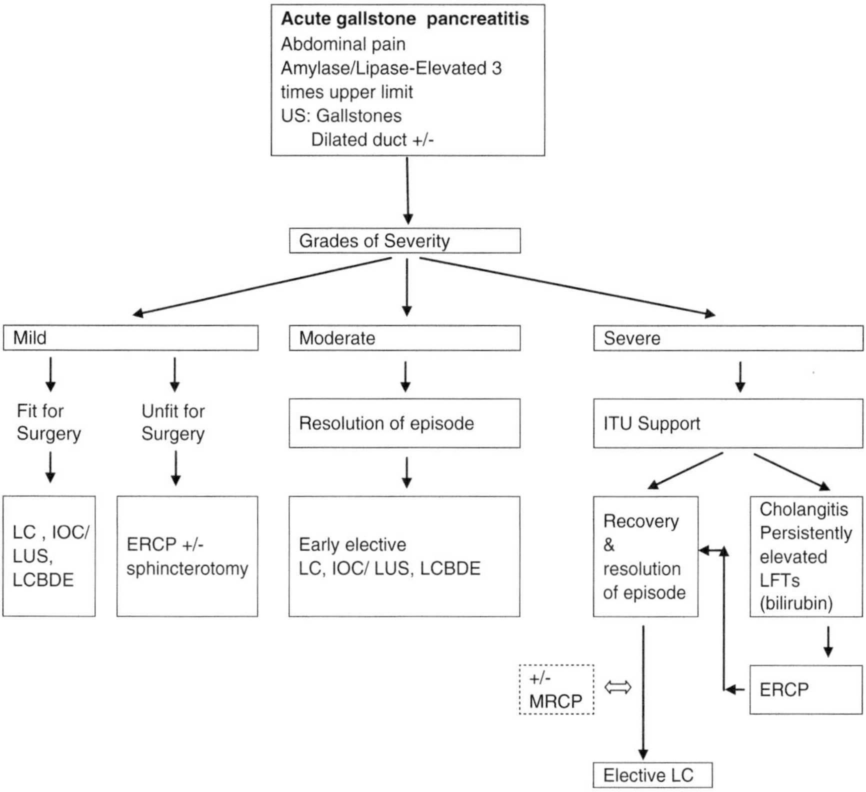

Fig. 3.2 Diagnosis and management of acute gallstone-related pancreatitis. *US* ultrasound scan, *LFTs* liver function tests, *ITU* intensive treatment unit, *ERCP* endoscopic retrograde cholangiopancreatography, *LC* laparoscopic cholecystectomy, *IOC* intraoperative cholangiogram, *LCBDE* laparoscopic common bile duct exploration, *LUS* laparoscopic ultrasound, *MRCP* magnetic resonance cholangiopancreatography

multicenter, randomized controlled trial (PONCHO trial) and was shown to be superior with a decreased risk of gallstone-related complications (5 versus 17%) compared to interval cholecystectomy [25]. Early cholecystectomy has also been shown to be cost-effective and reduces readmissions [12, 26, 27]. In patients who are unfit for surgery, ERCP with sphincterotomy has been shown to have a benefit in reducing the risk of recurrent pancreatitis (8.2%) compared to observation alone (17.1%) at 2 years and should be recommended [28]. Despite these data and guidelines recommending surgery during the same admission for gallstone pancreatitis patients, there continues to be poor adherence among the medical community in ensuring that patients receive recommended care [29–33]. A study of Medicare patients in the United States, for example, shows that only 57% of patients actually get same-admission cholecystectomy, and among patients who never receive cholecystectomy, 55% are never evaluated by a surgeon, and only 28% of those undergo ERCP for risk reduction [34]. At our institution, patients undergo same-admission cholecystectomy with routine intraoperative biliary imaging. If patients refuse surgery during the same admission, they are discharged with a plan for interval cholecystectomy and intraoperative bile duct imaging within 2 weeks to reduce the chance of a recurrent episode.

Severe or Complicated Pancreatitis

Patients with severe pancreatitis require intensive care unit (ICU) support and are not fit for immediate surgery (Fig. 3.2). A delay of at least 6 weeks is recommended in patients with severe acute pancreatitis, pancreatic necrosis, or large peripancreatic collections before consideration for cholecystectomy, as earlier intervention may result in a higher incidence of septic complications and infected peripancreatic fluid collections [29, 35].

Magnetic Resonance Cholangiopancreatography

The role of MRCP in the care of gallstone pancreatitis patients should be limited, as it adds unnecessary costs and delays to care. In centers where surgeons perform intraoperative imaging such as ours, there is no role for routine preoperative MRCP [19, 36, 37]. Its use should be limited to cases in which there is diagnostic uncertainty or to centers in which intraoperative imaging is not done as a way of determining which patients should undergo therapeutic ERCP [38].

Role of Endoscopic Retrograde Cholangiopancreatography

Likewise, the role of ERCP in the care of gallstone pancreatitis patients should be limited and is best understood if one considers the natural history of the disease. In most circumstances the gallstones pass spontaneously through the ampulla of Vater [39], with almost 50% of patients having passed their stones within 24 h of the onset of symptoms [40]. Thus, routine preoperative ERCP in cases of uncomplicated acute pancreatitis cannot be recommended as it adds cost, lengthens hospital stay, and may be harmful [40]. The only situations in which ERCP should be utilized preoperatively are for patients with severe gallstone-induced pancreatitis with obstructed and deranged liver function tests or cholangitis [29, 40, 41]. Intraoperative ERCP has been described as an option when a surgeon feels uncomfortable performing common bile duct exploration but has gained less popularity because of its logistical challenges. Postoperative ERCP is a good salvage option and is best reserved for patients with positive intraoperative imaging in which bile duct exploration cannot be performed or is unsuccessful.

Acute Cholangitis

Common duct stones are a frequent cause of acute cholangitis, responsible for 28–70% of cases [41–43]. The diagnosis of acute cholangitis should be suspected based on presenting complaints such as right upper quadrant pain, fevers, and jaundice (Charcot's triad), even though this triad may be present in only 50–75% of cases [43]. Patients should have laboratory studies sent, including a CBC, and comprehensive metabolic panel including LFTs, C-reactive protein (CRP), and coagulation studies and also biliary imaging. Ultrasonography is a good initial test to evaluate the gallbladder and bile ducts, and even though it is not very sensitive for common duct stones, it can show indirect signs of biliary obstruction such as dilated biliary ducts. The Tokyo guidelines (discussed in Chap. 2) provide specific diagnostic criteria and severity classification for cholangitis based on the results of this initial workup [44, 45]. Additional imaging tests such as MRCP or CT are generally not necessary unless there is a suspicion for malignancy or diagnostic uncertainty.

The pathway described in Fig. 3.3 provides general guidelines for the management of acute cholangitis patients and is primarily based on the severity of the acute cholangitis. Most patients will respond to initial antibiotic therapy and other supportive measures, but the underlying etiology (common duct stones) ultimately needs to be addressed. The two goals in the care of these patients are to clear the bile duct of stones and to remove the source of the stones: the gallbladder.

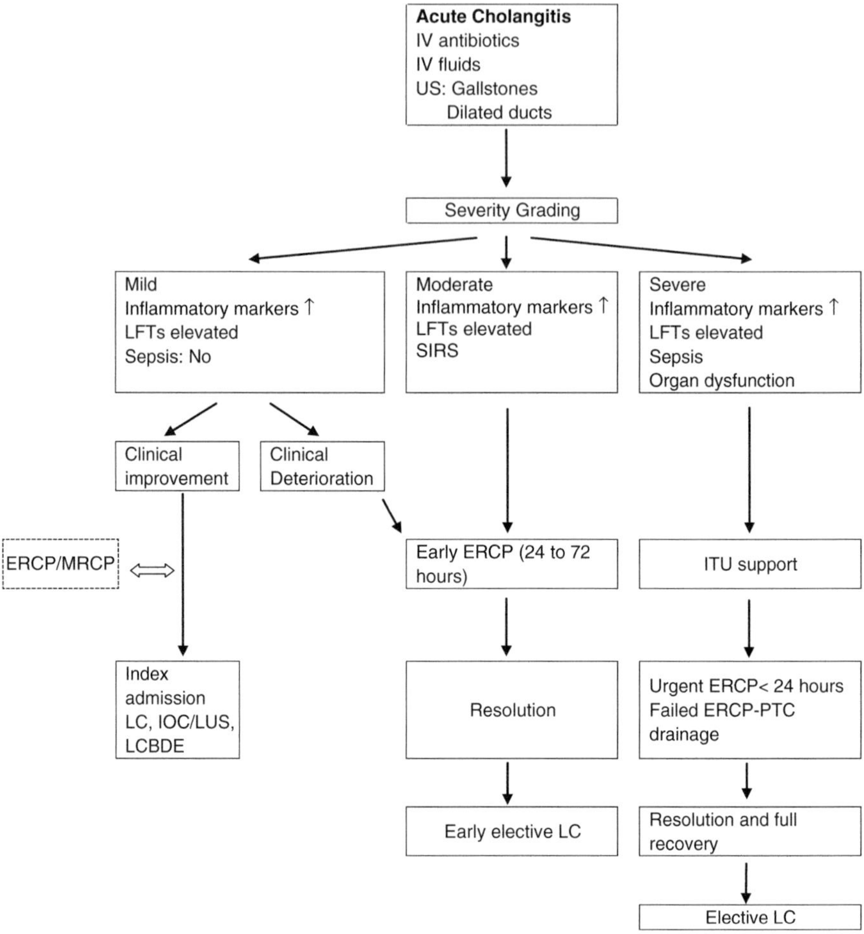

Fig. 3.3 Disease severity guides management of patients with gallstone-related acute cholangitis. *IV* intravenous, *US* ultrasound scan, *LFTs* liver function tests, *SIRS* systemic inflammatory response syndrome, *ERCP* endoscopic retrograde cholangiopancreatography, *ITU* intensive treatment unit, *LC* laparoscopic cholecystectomy, *IOC* intraoperative cholangiogram, *LCBDE* laparoscopic common bile duct exploration, *PTC* percutaneous transhepatic cholangiogram, *LUS* laparoscopic ultrasound, *SIRS* severe inflammatory response syndrome

Mild Cholangitis

Most patients with mild cholangitis will clinically improve with supportive care and should be offered cholecystectomy with intraoperative imaging (and bile duct exploration if necessary) during the same admission. In hospitals without bile duct exploration or intraoperative imaging capabilities, preoperative ERCP (with or without MRCP) to clear the biliary tree followed by cholecystectomy is a reasonable alternative. As is true for gallstone pancreatitis, interval cholecystectomy is important and should be offered if the patient is of suitable operative risk. Patients who do not undergo cholecystectomy long term and who only have endoscopic sphincterotomy are at risk for further episodes of recurrent biliary disease, readmissions, and increased mortality [23, 46].

Moderate to Severe Cholangitis

For patients with moderate to severe acute cholangitis, ERCP is the initial procedure of choice as these patients may have hemodynamic instability and sepsis, which makes them poor candidates for surgery. The need to perform either urgent (<24 h) or early (<72 h) endoscopic decompression should depend on the disease severity, the patient's response, and the availability of local resources [47]. Patients with severe disease requiring organ support and failure of response to intravenous antibiotics will require urgent (<24 h) biliary decompression [48, 49]. In this group of patients, outcome will be considerably worse without prompt biliary drainage [49]. Likewise, patients with moderate cholangitis who fail to improve after 24 h require early (<72 h) endoscopic biliary decompression [47–49].

Alternatives to Endoscopic Decompression

In patients who fail an ERCP or in whom ERCP could not be performed (e.g., inability to cannulate, unstable patient, altered anatomy from gastric bypass, esophageal stricture, gastric outlet obstruction, etc.), percutaneous transhepatic cholangiography (PTC) is a salvage option. Both ERCP and PTC can be employed for stone extraction and stent placement. However, the success of stone extraction via PTC is inferior to ERCP, and repeated attempts may be required to clear the duct [50]. Nevertheless, even if decompression alone is achieved with PTC, this may be enough to stabilize the patient and proceed with a combined rendezvous approach where a wire is passed through the PTC drain into the duodenum to assist with cannulation via ERCP. Endoscopic ultrasound (EUS)-guided transenteric biliary drainage is also an alternative when both ERCP and PTC fail to achieve biliary decompression, but at present only a few centers are performing this technique [51, 52]. Surgical biliary drainage is an option of last resort as it is associated with increased morbidity and mortality and is rarely required nowadays given the availability of ERCP or PTC [53]. Physicians caring for patients with severe cholangitis at hospitals with no facilities to perform ERCP or PTC should consider transfer of these patients to regional specialist units that have these capabilities if the patient is stable [44].

Interval Cholecystectomy

Patients with moderate to severe cholangitis who undergo successful endoscopic clearance should eventually have cholecystectomy to reduce the risk of recurrent problems. The timing of interval cholecystectomy is unclear, but a minimum period of 1 week to a maximum of 6 weeks following endoscopic sphincterotomy is recommended for LC to be performed [23, 54, 55]. This approach has been identified to decrease morbidity and hospital stay [23, 54]. Patients with multi-system organ complications should wait until full recovery is achieved before consideration for elective surgery.

Management of Choledocholithiasis in Patients with Altered Anatomy

The management of choledocholithiasis in patients with altered anatomy, such as following Roux-en-Y gastric bypass (RYGB) or Billroth II reconstruction, is both a diagnostic and therapeutic challenge. Although the estimated rate of choledocholithiasis following RYGB may only be 0.4%, the rate of de- novo gallstone formation is around 40%, and with the increasing utilization of bariatric surgery, many of these patients are now seen by general surgeons for biliary complaints [56]. In patients with altered anatomy, the length of Roux limb or afferent limb limits the access of conventional endoscopes to the biliary tree, making ERCP difficult or impossible without advanced techniques such as balloon enteroscopy or surgically assisted access [57, 58].

Patients presenting with biliary symptoms should have the same initial evaluation as for any biliary patient as previously mentioned (history and physical exam, labs, and ultrasound). MRCP should also be considered in the initial evaluation of these patients, as it can help in cases of diagnostic uncertainty and may help in planning interventions (e.g., ensuring ERCP is available if needed).

Patients with Gallbladder In Situ

Patients with a gallbladder still in situ should initially be managed according to the appropriate algorithms for each clinical syndrome as previously discussed (Fig. 3.4). For hemodynamically unstable patients requiring emergent biliary drainage, consideration should be given to either PTC, surgically assisted ERCP, or surgical drainage via common duct exploration if expertise is available. If the patient is deemed appropriate to proceed with cholecystectomy, the operation should be planned with some additional considerations. The easiest situation is if the surgeon performs routine intraoperative imaging and is capable of performing common duct

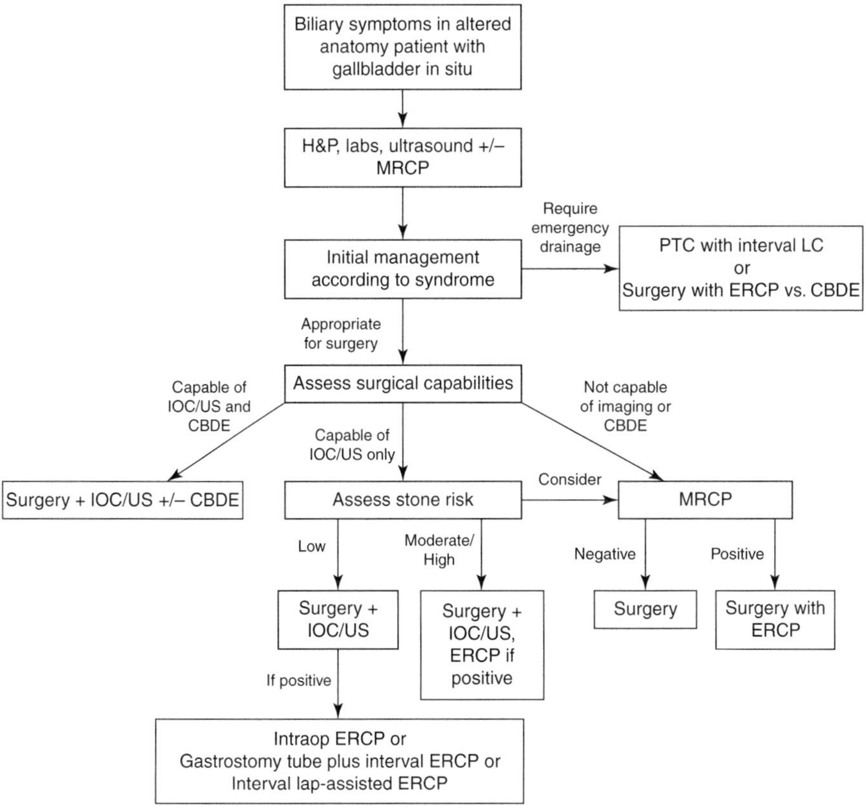

Fig. 3.4 Management of patients with altered anatomy presenting with suspected CBD stone and gallbladder in situ. *H&P* history and physical exam, *US* ultrasound, *CBDE* common bile duct exploration, *PTC* percutaneous transhepatic cholangiogram, *MRCP* magnetic resonance cholangiopancreatography, *LC* laparoscopic cholecystectomy, *ERCP* endoscopic retrograde cholangiopancreatography, *IOC* intraoperative cholangiogram

exploration if necessary; these cases can proceed straight to surgery. If the surgeon does not perform common duct exploration, but is capable of performing intraoperative imaging, a determination should be made as to the preoperative risk of choledocholithiasis (based on clinical, laboratory, and ultrasound findings). If the risk is low, the surgeon should proceed to surgery with intraoperative imaging. In the unlikely scenario that the intraoperative imaging is positive, an intraoperative ERCP may be performed if available. If ERCP is not immediately available, the surgeon may place a gastrostomy tube for interval ERCP access (in the case of prior gastric bypass), or the surgeon may elect to close and plan for an interval laparoscopic-assisted ERCP. If intraoperative imaging is not available, or if there is any suspicion of possible choledocholithiasis, a preoperative MRCP can be performed (if not already done), and plans for surgically assisted ERCP at the time of cholecystectomy can be made if the MRCP is positive.

Patients with Previous Cholecystectomy

Patients with a history of previous cholecystectomy should have the same initial evaluation and management according to the clinical syndrome (Fig. 3.5). Patients requiring emergent drainage can be treated with PTC or surgically assisted ERCP or common duct exploration if not available. Stable patients with positive imaging may proceed to various treatments, including surgically assisted ERCP, percutaneous transhepatic stone extraction, common duct exploration, endoscopic ultrasound-guided extraction, or other hybrid techniques, which have all been described with variable success [59–62]. Currently, there are no guidelines or recommendations as to the optimal approach [56]. The management decisions for these complex patients have to be individualized and may require comprehensive multidisciplinary team discussion with consideration of the specific problem at hand, the clinical condition of the patient, and the expertise and resources available [59]. Consultation with or transfer to a specialist center should be considered for these complex patients.

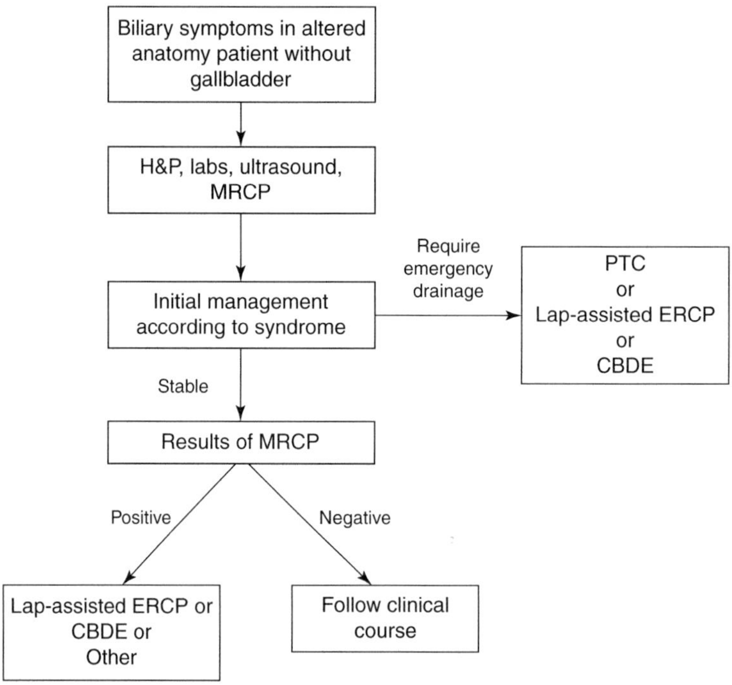

Fig. 3.5 Management of patients with altered anatomy presenting with suspected CBD stone with history of prior cholecystectomy. *H&P* history and physical exam, *CBDE* common bile duct exploration, *PTC* percutaneous transhepatic cholangiogram, *MRCP* magnetic resonance cholangiopancreatography, *ERCP* endoscopic retrograde cholangiopancreatography

Jaundice and Suspected Malignancy

Patients presenting with jaundice (without typical biliary pain symptoms), weight loss, or in whom otherwise a suspicion of malignancy exists should be thoroughly investigated. It is important to differentiate between medical and surgical causes of jaundice to initiate appropriate management. All patients should undergo routine investigations as outlined in Fig. 3.6, including right upper quadrant ultrasound and a CT scan of the abdomen and pelvis [63]. If no cause is identified on initial imaging, in order to further assess biliary anatomy in the setting of jaundice, MRCP should be performed [64]. Endoscopic ultrasonography and/or ERCP is useful when the aforementioned investigations have either been inconclusive or further assessment of jaundice, biliary dilatation of unclear etiology, or examination of the pancreas is required [65, 66]. Given the complex evaluation and decision-making required for patients with malignancy or jaundice, most hospitals in the United Kingdom are in the process of implementing a dedicated jaundice pathway. This involves a joint effort by primary care physicians, radiologists, gastroenterologists, and surgeons to complete investigations, establish a diagnosis, and initiate treatment in an expedited fashion [67–69].

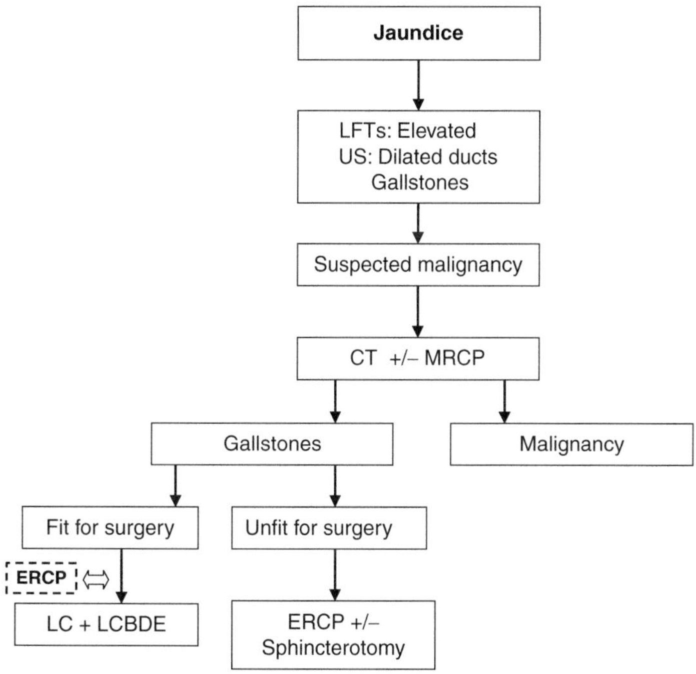

Fig. 3.6 Diagnosis and management of patients presenting with jaundice. *US* ultrasound scan, *LFTs* liver function tests, *CT* computed tomography, *MRCP* magnetic resonance cholangiopancreatography, *ERCP* endoscopic retrograde cholangiopancreatography, *LC* laparoscopic cholecystectomy, *LCBDE* laparoscopic common bile duct exploration

Summary/Key Points

- Management of common bile duct stones is both a diagnostic and therapeutic challenge.
- Patients with uncomplicated gallstone pancreatitis do not routinely require pre-operative ERCP.
- Patients with acute severe pancreatitis should be considered for surgery once they have fully recovered.
- Urgent ERCP should be performed in <24 h in acute severe cholangitis to improve morbidity and decrease mortality.
- Management of choledocholithiasis in patients with altered anatomy is complex and often requires multidisciplinary discussion and coordination of care.
- All patients with jaundice or a suspicion of malignancy should be thoroughly investigated to identify underlying pathology and initiate management appropriately.

References

1. Collins C, Maguire D, Ireland A, Fitzgerald E, O'Sullivan GC. A prospective study of common bile duct calculi in patients undergoing laparoscopic cholecystectomy: natural history of choledocholithiasis revisited. Ann Surg. 2004;239(1):28–33.
2. Hunter JG. Laparoscopic transcystic common bile duct exploration. Am J Surg. 1992;163(1):53–6. discussion 57–58
3. Petelin JB. Laparoscopic common bile duct exploration. Surg Endosc. 2003;17(11):1705–15.
4. Shojaiefard A, Esmaeilzadeh M, Ghafouri A, Mehrabi A. Various techniques for the surgical treatment of common bile duct stones: a meta review. Gastroenterol Res Pract. 2009;2009:840208.
5. Martin CJ, Cox MR, Vaccaro L. Laparoscopic transcystic bile duct stenting in the management of common bile duct stones. ANZ J Surg. 2002;72(4):258–64.
6. Cuschieri A, Lezoche E , Morino M , Croce E, Lacy A, Toouli J, Faggioni A, , Ribeiro VM, Jakimowicz J, Visa J, Hanna GB.. E.A.E.S. multicenter prospective randomized trial comparing two-stage vs single-stage management of patients with gallstone disease and ductal calculi. Surg Endosc 1999;13(10):952-957.
7. Bansal VK, Misra MC, Rajan K, Kilambi R, Kumar S, Krishna A, Kumar A, Pandav CS, Subramaniam R, Arora MK, Garg PK. Single-stage laparoscopic common bile duct exploration and cholecystectomy versus two-stage endoscopic stone extraction followed by laparoscopic cholecystectomy for patients with concomitant gallbladder stones and common bile duct stones: a randomized controlled trial. Surg Endosc. 2014;28(3):875–85.
8. Rogers SJ, Cello JP, Horn JK, Siperstein AE, Schecter WP, Campbell AR, Mackersie RC, Rodas A, Kreuwel HT, Harris HW. Prospective randomized trial of LC + LCBDE vs ERCP/S+LC for common bile duct stone disease. Arch Surg. 2010;145:28–33.
9. Koc B, Karahan S, Adas G, Tutal F, Guven H, Ozsoy A. Comparison of laparoscopic common bile duct exploration and endoscopic retrograde cholangiopancreatography plus laparoscopic cholecystectomy for choledocholithiasis: a prospective randomized study. Am J Surg. 2013;206:457–63.
10. Noble H, Tranter S, Chesworth T, Norton S, Thompson M. A randomized, clinical trial to compare endoscopic sphincterotomy and subsequent laparoscopic cholecystectomy with primary

laparoscopic bile duct exploration during cholecystectomy in higher risk patients with choledocholithiasis. J Laparoendosc Adv Surg Tech A. 2009;19:713–20.

11. Rhodes M, Sussman L, Cohen L, Lewis MP. Randomised trial of laparoscopic exploration of common bile duct versus postoperative endoscopic retrograde cholangiography for common bile duct stones. Lancet. 1998;351:159–61.
12. Isla A, Griniatsos J, Rodway A. Single-stage definitive laparoscopic management in mild acute biliary pancreatitis. J Laparoendosc Adv Surg Tech A. 2003;13(2):77–81.
13. Banks PA, Bollen TL, Dervenis C, Gooszen HG, Johnson CD, Sarr MG, et al. Classification of acute pancreatitis--2012: revision of the Atlanta classification and definitions by international consensus. Gut. 2013;62(1):102–11.
14. Ito K, Ito H, Whang EE. Timing of cholecystectomy for biliary pancreatitis: do the data support current guidelines? J Gastrointest Surg. 2008;12(12):2164–70.
15. Kharbutli B, Velanovich V. Management of preoperatively suspected choledocholithiasis: a decision analysis. J Gastrointest Surg. 2008;12(11):1973–80.
16. Kimura Y, Arata S, Takada T, Hirata K, Yoshida M, Mayumi T, et al. Gallstone-induced acute pancreatitis. J Hepatobiliary Pancreat Sci. 2010;17(1):60–9.
17. Iranmanesh P, Frossard JL, Mugnier-Konrad B, Morel P, Majno P, Nguyen-Tang T, et al. Initial cholecystectomy vs sequential common duct endoscopic assessment and subsequent cholecystectomy for suspected gallstone migration: a randomized clinical trial. JAMA. 2014;312(2):137–44.
18. Altieri MS, Yang J, Obeid N, Zhu C, Talamini M, Pryor A. Increasing bile duct injury and decreasing utilization of intraoperative cholangiogram and common bile duct exploration over 14 years: an analysis of outcomes in New York State. Surg Endosc. 2017;32(2):667–74. https://doi.org/10.1007/s00464-017-5719-2.
19. Nassar AH, Mirza A, Qandeel H, Ahmed Z, Zino S. Fluorocholangiography: Reincarnation in the laparoscopic era-evaluation of intra-operative cholangiography in 3635 laparoscopic cholecystectomies. Surg Endosc. 2016;30(5):1804–11.
20. Cameron DR, Goodman AJ. Delayed cholecystectomy for gallstone pancreatitis: re-admissions and outcomes. Ann R Coll Surg Engl. 2004;86(5):358–62.
21. Sandzen B, Rosenmuller M, Haapamaki MM, Nilsson E, Stenlund HC, Oman M. First attack of acute pancreatitis in sweden 1988 - 2003: incidence, aetiological classification, procedures and mortality - a register study. BMC Gastroenterol. 2009;9:18.
22. Moreau JA, Zinsmeister AR, Melton LJ 3rd, DiMagno EP. Gallstone pancreatitis and the effect of cholecystectomy: a population-based cohort study. Mayo Clin Proc. 1988;63(5):466–73.
23. McAlister VC, Davenport E, Renouf E. Cholecystectomy deferral in patients with endoscopic sphincterotomy. Cochrane Database Syst Rev. 2007;4:CD006233.
24. Hernandez V, Pascual I, Almela P, Anon R, Herreros B, Sanchiz V, Minguez M, Benages A. Recurrence of acute gallstone pancreatitis and relationship with cholecystectomy or endoscopic sphincterotomy. Am J Gastroenterol. 2004;99(12):2417–23.
25. da Costa DW, Bouwense SA, Schepers NJ, Besselink MG, van Santvoort HC, van Brunschot S, Dutch Pancreatitis Study Group, et al. Same-admission versus interval cholecystectomy for mild gallstone pancreatitis (PONCHO): a multicentre randomised controlled trial. Lancet. 2015;386(10000):1261–8.
26. Targarona EM, Balague C, Espert JJ, Perez Ayuso RM, Ros E, Navarro S, et al. Laparoscopic treatment of acute biliary pancreatitis. Int Surg. 1995;80(4):365–8.
27. Stromberg C, Nilsson M. Nationwide study of the treatment of common bile duct stones in sweden between 1965 and 2009. Br J Surg. 2011;98(12):1766–74.
28. Hwang SS, Li BH, Haigh PI. Gallstone pancreatitis without cholecystectomy. JAMA Surg. 2013;148(9):867–72.
29. Working Group IAP/APA Acute Pancreatitis Guidelines. IAP/APA evidence-based guidelines for the management of acute pancreatitis. Pancreatology. 2013;13(4 Suppl 2):e1–15.
30. Anonymous. UK guidelines for the management of acute pancreatitis. Gut. 2005;54 (Suppl 3):iii1–9.

31. Forsmark CE, Baillie J. AGA Institute technical review on acute pancreatitis. Rev Gastroenterol Mex. 2007;72(3):257–85.
32. Uhl W, Warshaw A, Imrie C, Bassi C, McKay CJ, Lankisch PG, et al. IAP guidelines for the surgical management of acute pancreatitis. Pancreatology. 2002;2(6):565–73.
33. Kimura Y, Takada T, Kawarada Y, Hirata K, Mayumi T, Yoshida M, et al. JPN guidelines for the management of acute pancreatitis: treatment of gallstone-induced acute pancreatitis. J Hepato-Biliary-Pancreat Surg. 2006;13(1):56–60.
34. Trust MD, Sheffield KM, Boyd CA, Benarroch-Gampel J, Zhang D, Townsend CM Jr, Riall TS. Gallstone pancreatitis in older patients: are we operating enough? Surgery. 2011;150(3):515–25.
35. Nealon WH, Bawduniak J, Walser EM. Appropriate timing of cholecystectomy in patients who present with moderate to severe gallstone-associated acute pancreatitis with peripancreatic fluid collections. Ann Surg. 2004;239(6):741–9. discussion 749–751
36. Hanif F, Ahmed Z, Samie MA, Nassar AH. Laparoscopic transcystic bile duct exploration: The treatment of first choice for common bile duct stones. Surg Endosc. 2010;24(7):1552–6.
37. Gough V, Stephens N, Ahmed Z, Nassar AH. Intrahepatic choledochoscopy during transcystic common bile duct exploration; technique, feasibility and value. Surg Endosc. 2012;26(11):3190–4.
38. Darge K, Anupindi S. Pancreatitis and the role of US, MRCP and ERCP. Pediatr Radiol. 2009;39(Suppl 2):S153–7.
39. Uhl W, Muller CA, Krahenbuhl L, Schmid SW, Scholzel S, Buchler MW. Acute gallstone pancreatitis: timing of laparoscopic cholecystectomy in mild and severe disease. Surg Endosc. 1999;13(11):1070–6.
40. Folsch UR, Nitsche R, Ludtke R, Hilgers RA, Creutzfeldt W. Early ERCP and papillotomy compared with conservative treatment for acute biliary pancreatitis. The German Study Group on Acute Biliary Pancreatitis. N Engl J Med. 1997;336(4):237–42.
41. van Santvoort HC, Besselink MG, de Vries AC, Boermeester MA, Fischer K, Bollen TL, et al. Early endoscopic retrograde cholangiopancreatography in predicted severe acute biliary pancreatitis: a prospective multicenter study. Ann Surg. 2009;250(1):68–75.
42. Saik RP, Greenburg AG, Farris JM, Peskin GW. Spectrum of cholangitis. Am J Surg. 1975;130(2):143–50.
43. Huibregtse K, Carr-Locke DL, Cremer M, Domschke W, Fockens P, Foerster E, et al. Biliary stent occlusion--a problem solved with self-expanding metal stents? European Wallstent Study Group. Endoscopy. 1992;24(5):391–4.
44. Okamoto K, Takada T, Strasberg SM, Solomkin JS, Pitt HA, Garden OJ, et al. Tg13 management bundles for acute cholangitis and cholecystitis. J Hepatobiliary Pancreat Sci. 2013;20(1):55–9.
45. Takada T, Strasberg SM, Solomkin JS, Pitt HA, Gomi H, Yoshida M, et al. Tg13: updated tokyo guidelines for the management of acute cholangitis and cholecystitis. J Hepatobiliary Pancreat Sci. 2013;20(1):1–7.
46. Boerma D, Rauws EA, Keulemans YC, Janssen IM, Bolwerk CJ, Timmer R, et al. Wait-and-see policy or laparoscopic cholecystectomy after endoscopic sphincterotomy for bile-duct stones: a randomised trial. Lancet. 2002;360(9335):761–5.
47. Maple JT, Ikenberry SO, Anderson MA, Appalaneni V, Decker GA, Committee ASOP, et al. The role of endoscopy in the management of choledocholithiasis. Gastrointest Endosc. 2011;74(4):731–44.
48. Bornman PC, van Beljon JI, Krige JE. Management of cholangitis. J Hepato-Biliary-Pancreat Surg. 2003;10(6):406–14.
49. Boender J, Nix GA, de Ridder MA, Dees J, Schutte HE, van Buuren HR, et al. Endoscopic sphincterotomy and biliary drainage in patients with cholangitis due to common bile duct stones. Am J Gastroenterol. 1995;90(2):233–8.
50. van der Velden JJ, Berger MY, Bonjer HJ, Brakel K, Lameris JS. Percutaneous treatment of bile duct stones in patients treated unsuccessfully with endoscopic retrograde procedures. Gastrointest Endosc. 2000;51(4 Pt 1):418–22.

51. Minaga K, Kitano M, Imai H, Yamao K, Kamata K, Miyata T, et al. Urgent endoscopic ultrasound-guided choledochoduodenostomy for acute obstructive suppurative cholangitis-induced sepsis. World J Gastroenterol. 2016;22(16):4264–9.
52. Artifon EL, Takada J, Okawa L, Moura EG, Sakai P. EUS-guided choledochoduodenostomy for biliary drainage in unresectable pancreatic cancer: a case series. JOP. 2010;11(6):597–600.
53. McNabb-Baltar J, Trinh QD, Barkun AN. Biliary drainage method and temporal trends in patients admitted with cholangitis: a national audit. Can J Gastroenterol. 2013;27(9):513–8.
54. Schiphorst AH, Besselink MG, Boerma D, Timmer R, Wiezer MJ, van Erpecum KJ, et al. Timing of cholecystectomy after endoscopic sphincterotomy for common bile duct stones. Surg Endosc. 2008;22(9):2046–50.
55. Li VK, Yum JL, Yeung YP. Optimal timing of elective laparoscopic cholecystectomy after acute cholangitis and subsequent clearance of choledocholithiasis. Am J Surg. 2010;200(4):483–8.
56. Kini S, Kannan U. Effect of bariatric surgery on future general surgical procedures. J Minim Access Surg. 2011;7(2):126–31.
57. Evans JA, Muthusamy VR, Acosta RD, Bruining DH, Chandrasekhara V, American Society for Gastrointestinal Endoscopy Standards of Practice C, et al. The role of endoscopy in the bariatric surgery patient. Gastrointest Endosc. 2015;81(5):1063–72.
58. Committee ASoP. The role of endoscopy in the bariatric surgery patient. Surg Endosc. 2015;29(5):1007–17.
59. Ahmed AR, Husain S, Saad N, Patel NC, Waldman DL, O'Malley W. Accessing the common bile duct after roux-en-y gastric bypass. Surg Obes Relat Dis. 2007;3(6):640–3.
60. Snauwaert C, Laukens P, Dillemans B, Himpens J, De Looze D, Deprez PH, et al. Laparoscopy-assisted transgastric endoscopic retrograde cholangiopancreatography in bariatric roux-en-y gastric bypass patients. Endosc Int Open. 2015;3(5):E458–63.
61. Saleem A, Levy MJ, Petersen BT, Que FG, Baron TH. Laparoscopic assisted ERCP in roux-en-y gastric bypass (RYGB) surgery patients. J Gastrointest Surg. 2012;16(1):203–8.
62. Bowman E, Greenberg J, Garren M, Guda N, Rajca B, Benson M, et al. Laparoscopic-assisted ercp and eus in patients with prior roux-en-y gastric bypass surgery: a dual-center case series experience. Surg Endosc. 2016;30(10):4647–52.
63. Williams EJ, Green J, Beckingham I, Parks R, Martin D, Lombard M, et al. Guidelines on the management of common bile duct stones (CBDS). Gut. 2008;57(7):1004–21.
64. Lacitignola S, Minardi M. Management of common bile duct stones: a ten-year experience at a tertiary care center. JSLS. 2008;12(1):62–5.
65. Shah JN, Bhat YM, Hamerski CM, Kane SD, Binmoeller KF. Feasibility of nonradiation eus-based ercp in patients with uncomplicated choledocholithiasis (with video). Gastrointest Endosc. 2016;84(5):764–9.
66. Verma D, Kapadia A, Eisen GM, Adler DG. EUS vs MRCP for detection of choledocholithiasis. Gastrointest Endosc. 2006;64(2):248–54.
67. Anonymous. British society of gastroenterology (2009) acute jaundice. 2009. www.bsg.org.uk.
68. Anonymous. Ashford and St. Peter's hospitals NHS Foundation Trust (2011) painless obstructive jaundice. Ambulatory emergency care pathways. Ashford and St. Peter's Hospitals NHS Foundation Trust. 2011. www.asphnhs.uk.
69. Mitchell J, Hussaini H, McGovern D, Farrow R, Maskell G, Dalton H. The "jaundice hotline" for the rapid assessment of patients with jaundice. BMJ. 2002;325(7357):213–5.

Part III
Operative Techniques

Chapter 4
Intraoperative Cholangiography

Matthew B. Bloom and Edward H. Phillips

Introduction

Prior to the advent of biliary imaging in the late 1800s, bile duct exploration was based on direct operative palpation of the bile duct. This approach led to unnecessary duct exploration in roughly half of the cases. Missed and retained common duct stones were the greatest cause of morbidity and mortality in biliary disease. The introduction of operative cholangiography by Mirizzi in 1937 [1] represented a major technological advance. It reduced both the rate of negative bile duct exploration and the incidence of retained bile duct stones after exploration.

With the advent of endoscopic retrograde cholangiopancreatography/endoscopic sphincterotomy (ERCP/ES) in 1974, surgeons began to place less reliance on operative cholangiography, as the static cholangiography available at that time was both time-consuming and not very accurate. By the time of the adoption of laparoscopy in the 1990s, many surgeons were not trained to perform cholangiography, nor did they possess the skills necessary to perform laparoscopic duct explorations. As a direct result, there was a surge in number of ERCPs that were obtained preoperatively, and the majority were negative. The stones that were identified were removed by endoscopic means. So in this post-laparoscopic era, why should we perform a cholangiogram?

The performance of an intraoperative cholangiogram (IOC) permits the real-time identification of common duct stones, which may be immediately addressed during cholecystectomy or immediately after surgery. If a properly performed cholangiogram is negative, unnecessary tests can be avoided postoperatively if patients continue to have symptoms or develop new ones. In addition, the identification of unusual anatomy and/or the prompt recognition of erroneously placed clips, ductal

M. B. Bloom, MD, MS (✉) · E. H. Phillips, MD
Department of Surgery, Cedars-Sinai Medical Center, Los Angeles, CA, USA
e-mail: Matthew.bloom@cshs.org; Edward.Phillips@cshs.org

© Springer International Publishing AG, part of Springer Nature 2018

B. F. Santos, N. Soper (eds.), *Choledocholithiasis*,
https://doi.org/10.1007/978-3-319-74503-9_4

injuries, and/or transections can be identified and corrected at the time of the original operation, which results in better outcomes [2–5].

Performing IOC does not need to be a lengthy, frustrating, or difficult procedure. Portable digital fluoroscopes are readily available in operating rooms (ORs) capable of supporting cholangiography. When performed routinely, IOC is seamlessly incorporated into the flow of the operation. The equipment is on the table ready to go, and both the operating room staff know how to help and the radiology techs are better trained. Additionally, the radiologists will have more experience in reading and interpreting the images. If a strict selective approach is adopted, the surgeon and staff may not have developed the skills to perform a cholangiogram when a difficult case is encountered.

Rationale and Benefits of Routine Use

Whether or not cholangiography should be performed routinely or "when necessary" has been debated for years. Improvements in technology, especially mobile fluoroscopy machines, have made the procedure faster and safer to perform and permit a more accurate assessment of the bile ducts.

The rationale for performing cholangiography is that it affords:

1. A roadmap of the anatomy of the biliary tree prior to transection/division of the cystic duct
2. The intraoperative identification of bile duct injury
3. Demonstration of the presence of biliary stones that can then be flushed into the duodenum or removed at the time of cholecystectomy
4. Greater experience in performing and interpreting cholangiograms and performing laparoscopic common bile duct explorations in teaching programs, which is critical to producing well-trained surgeons

Large population-based studies have demonstrated that routine cholangiography is associated with lower rates of bile duct injuries [6–9], while others have suggested that its routine use is unnecessary and results in extra costs and additional procedures [10, 11]. A meta-analysis of 40 studies revealed that with the routine use of IOC, the incidence of intraoperative common bile duct (CBD) injuries was 0.21% versus 0.43% with its selective use. Furthermore, the rate of immediate diagnosis of these injuries at the time of the primary operation was 87% vs 45% [12]. The large recent Swedish Inpatient Registry study [6] of 152,776 patients demonstrated that those surgeons who performed cholangiography had lower rates of bile duct injury. Whether this represents greater awareness of anatomy or skill in common duct exploration is unknown. More recently, in a study of 856 consecutive patients compared before and after the adoption of routine cholangiography, the rate of major bile duct injury fell from 1.9% to 0% ($p = 0.004$, $n = 435$ routine IOC vs $n = 421$ selective IOC) [13].

Still, there is controversy as to whether a cholangiogram can provide adequate information to prevent injuries, such as visualizing the cystic duct insertion on the right hepatic duct or identifying a cystic duct that spirals across the common bile duct. A clear road map of a specific patient's anatomy can demonstrate one of the several variations in ductal configurations (Fig. 4.1). Only 17% of cystic ducts drain directly into the common bile duct at a 90° angle. The overwhelming majority drain posteriorly, spirally, or parallel to the common duct, or they drain directly into the right hepatic duct [14, 15]. As the single most important factor responsible for the creation of bile duct injuries is the misinterpretation of the patient's anatomy, accurate anatomic knowledge prior to further dissection or clip placement can avoid injury (Fig. 4.2) [16, 17].

In the case of a bile duct injury identified during surgery, the ability to treat the injury during the primary procedure reduces the greater morbidity associated with its late recognition and treatment [18]. A clip placed across the common duct, for example, can be immediately removed. Partial transection may be treated with the placement of a biliary stent across the injured area and primary closure. A more complete transection injury may require immediate or delayed hepaticojejunostomy reconstruction by a surgeon with this specific expertise. If not immediately available at the time of the primary operation, drainage, ligation, or tube drainage and referral to the care of a surgical team with expertise in repair of complex biliary injuries are recommended. The delayed recognition of bile duct injuries is associated with a mortality rate of 11% and risks severe morbidity that for some is lifelong and may

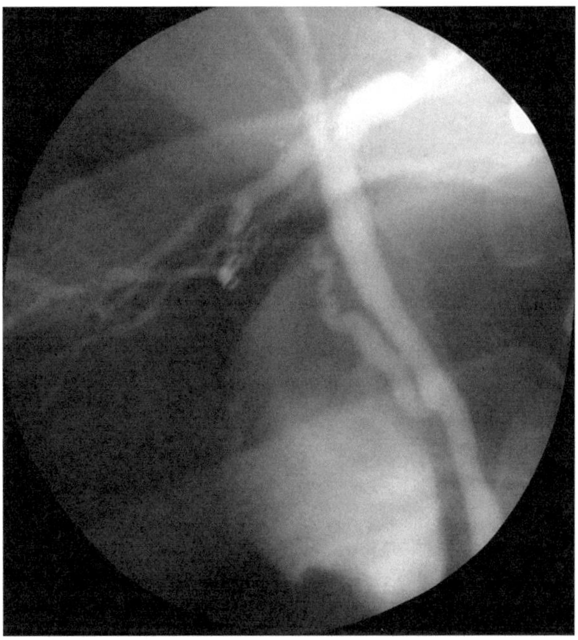

Fig. 4.1 A normal variant of cystic duct configuration that runs parallel to the common bile duct

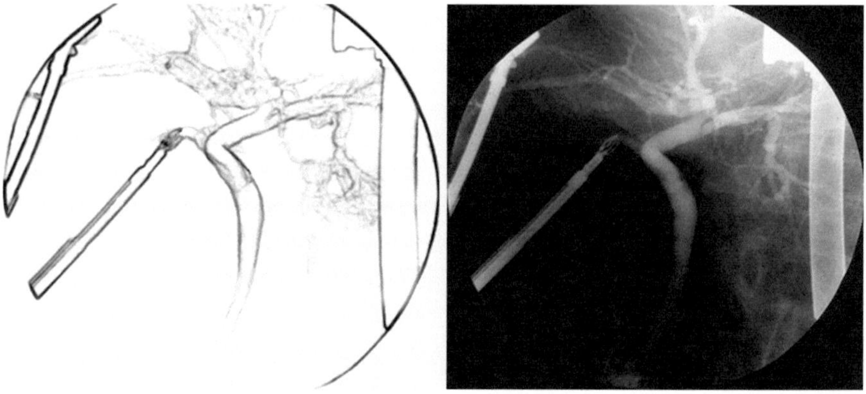

Fig. 4.2 Providing normal lateral retraction when there is a short cystic duct can tent the common bile duct laterally, making it easy to inadvertently clip or transect

require multiple corrective operations and/or procedures such as balloon dilation and stenting [19].

While several authors have noted the increased immediate cost associated with performing "unnecessary" cholangiograms, it has been estimated that performing routine IOC would prevent 2.5 deaths for every 10,000 patients at a cost of $390,000 per life saved. From a purely financial perspective, this more than makes up for the additional cost of the procedure, making it more financially attractive to perform than not [20]. This cost analysis did not include the potential for even greater economic savings to be realized if fewer postoperative magnetic resonance cholangiopancreatographies (MRCPs)/ERCPs are ordered because intraoperative cholangiography has been performed for the workup of the 5–25% of patients who continue to experience pain symptoms postoperatively [21].

The discovery of biliary stones during the cholangiogram allows for their treatment at the time of surgery or more accurately guides postoperative therapy [13]. Approximately 2–12% of patients will have unsuspected choledocholithiasis found on a routine IOC, which would be missed with thoughtful selective cholangiography [10, 22–24]. Small stones may be flushed with warm saline, often with the additional use of glucagon. The majority of the remainder may be removed through laparoscopic ductal exploration: either via transcystic or choledochotomy. Unsuspected duct stones tend to be smaller and fewer than in a symptomatic patient and are the perfect cases to hone one's laparoscopic duct exploration skills. Again, by identifying these stones and treating them at the time of operation, the patient is spared an additional ERCP/ES procedure. ERCP/ES carries a 3–6% risk of pancreatitis and a 1% risk of bleeding, perforation, or stricture and requires additional follow-up and possibly still more procedures for the placement and subsequent removal of biliary stents and/or treatment of duodenoscope-based carbapenem-resistant *Enterobacteriaceae* transmission. Reduced hospital length of stay and cost savings are achieved when stones are treated in a single procedure during cholecystectomy, compared to preoperative or postoperative ERCP/ES [25, 26].

The performance of IOC is facilitated by a support staff who are familiar with the setup of the equipment and the procedural steps and a surgical team with experience and confidence in interpreting the fluoroscopic images. Both are only achieved through the repetition that is achieved with a protocol of routine cholangiography. The experience gained from multiple cases will be called upon during difficult ones. When cholangiography is only occasionally performed, the skills needed by the entire team for the critical and challenging cases may not be developed. With repetition, a cholangiogram can be completed quickly, with no disruption of the flow of the operation. The performance of routine cholangiography also sets the stage for the acquisition of more difficult laparoscopic skills such as ductal exploration or placement of a biliary stent [27, 28]. This is particularly relevant in teaching institutions [29].

Technique

An intraoperative cholangiogram can be performed quickly and reliably when all the members of the OR staff are familiar both with the equipment required and the proper setup of materials. Having a dedicated instrument tray that includes a laminated photograph of the required equipment makes reprocessing, prepackaging, and assembly more reliable (Fig. 4.3a, b). A list of recommended equipment is provided (Table 4.1).

Back Table Prepare a 50/50 mixture of saline and contrast material such as Omnipaque (Novaplus) or the iso-osmolar Visipaque (Novaplus), and fill two 30 ml syringes with mixture. Connect a three-way stopcock to the extension tubing (the ideal length is 96 in.), one of the filled 30 ml syringes and to a third syringe filled with saline, and label them. Connect the other end of the extension tubing to the cholangiocatheter. It is of utmost importance that care is taken not to introduce air bubbles into the system. It is easier to take your time and avoid introduction of air bubbles than getting rid of them. Flush the tubing with the saline syringe while tapping the tubing with a hemostat to remove any trapped air bubbles, and set it aside.

Ductotomy Once the cystic duct has been identified, place a clip across the proximal cystic duct-gallbladder junction. Make a partial anterior ductotomy distal to the clip, taking care not to transect the duct entirely. Ideally, bile will start to flow out of the ductotomy, but if not, small stones and debris should be milked proximally into the incision and removed. To flush debris and stones out of the cystic ductotomy, carefully place a grasper from the patient's left side, down toward the duodenum, gently apply medial pressure, and sweep upward along the porta hepatis and the common bile duct. If this does not ultimately produce bile, the cystic duct can be gently squeezed in a distal to proximal direction using a blunt grasper to milk contents toward the opening. This maneuver should be followed by gently sweeping the common duct/porta hepatis again.

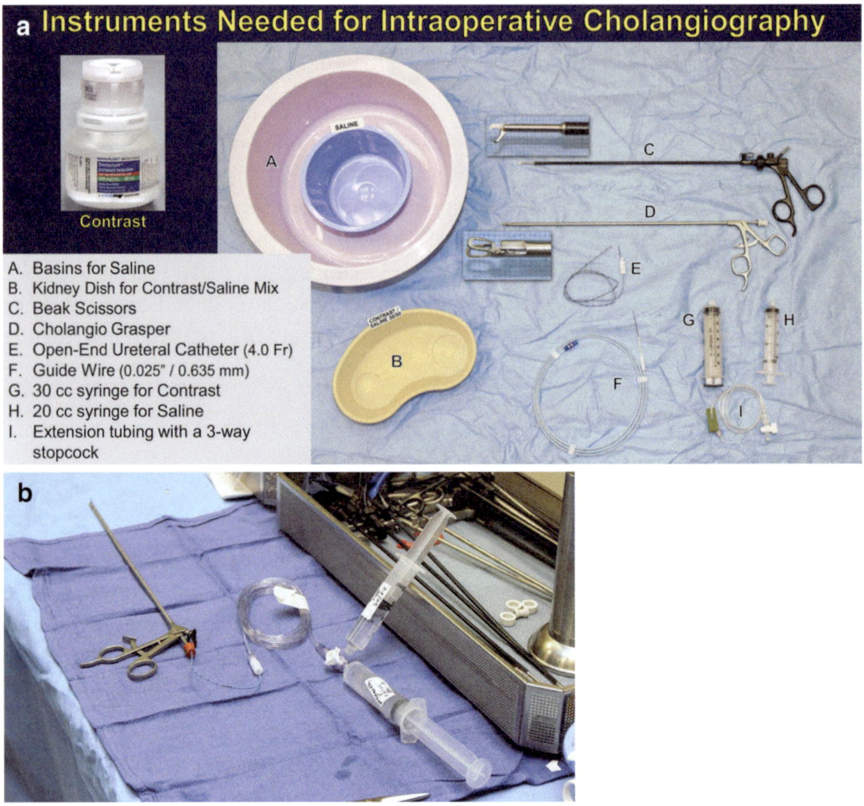

Fig. 4.3 (**a**) The equipment for performing a cholangiogram, and (**b**) its setup on the back table

Table 4.1 Recommended equipment for intraoperative cholangiogram

Recommended materials
Contrast media, such as Omnipaque (Novaplus) or iso-osmolar Visipaque (Novaplus)
Glucagon 1 mg IV; wait for 3 min, OK to repeat
Saline mixed 50/50 with contrast material
1 × 20 ml syringe, 2 × 30 ml syringes
Extension tubing, 96 in. length
Three-way stopcock
Catheter (e.g., 4Fr ureteral catheter, balloon-tip catheter, or Taut cholangiocatheter)
Clamp device (e.g., cholangioclamp, Kumar device)
Endo scissors

Selection of Cholangiogram Catheter A variety of cholangiocatheters may be used, but the 4Fr end-hole ureteral catheter works well and is very inexpensive. If a ureteral catheter is employed, the cystic duct will need to be secured around it, either by clamping with a cholangiography fixation forceps/clamp or with a simple clip applied across the cystic duct. Other variations include the slightly barbed Taut catheter or balloon catheters, which secure themselves by insufflation against the cystic duct wall, or the Kumar clamp for injecting into the gallbladder itself.

Retraction upon the gallbladder/cystic duct varies depending on the site of introduction of the cholangiogram catheter. Placing it through the right upper quadrant port usually provides the best angle for insertion. Alternatively, the catheter may be introduced via the subxiphoid port. Another effective way to introduce a cholangiogram catheter without using an additional working port is to insert a #14 gauge angiocatheter through the abdominal wall in the right upper quadrant. For right upper quadrant insertion, the gallbladder/cystic duct junction should be retracted laterally to present the duct under gentle tension. The incision in the cystic duct should take into account where the duct will ultimately be ligated and the location of the valves. Sharp hooked scissors or micro-scissors are preferred. The optimal angle of entry of the catheter into the duct will be approximately 130°. The act of inserting the catheter into the duct with a grasper is made easier by the availability of additional working ports or the use of an angiocatheter that allows for a two-handed technique.

The injection of saline should be possible without leaking or extreme resistance. If it is not, the catheter should be reinserted. If a cholangiography fixation forceps has been used, its handle should be propped up against a pile of folded sterile towels and the handle clamped in a secure position to avoid any further traction on the duct. The tubing should be clamped securely to the surgical drapes to avoid inadvertent traction. A sterile half drape should be placed over the operative field, or a clear plastic sterile mobile C-arm cover should be used. The sterile drape is less expensive: The area over the patient's xiphoid process can be marked with a twist in the cover drape to aid the placement of the C-arm and reduce the number of images needed to locate the duct. If the cholangiogram catheter is approximately one-third the distance from the top of the image and half of the vertebral bodies are visible on the right side of the image in a vertical fashion, the C-arm is in good position to view the early filling phase of the distal duct where most of the stones are found.

Injection While placing the cholangiocatheter in the cystic duct, saline should be slowly dripped through the catheter so that air or CO_2 is not instilled in the duct. Once the catheter is secured in the cystic duct, the saline syringe should be carefully replaced with a second 30 ml contrast-filled syringe so as to not introduce any bubbles into the three-way stopcock and cholangiogram tubing. After securing the cholangiogram clamp or catheter and the sterile drape or cover placed, the C-arm should be brought into the operative field from the patient's right side, if possible. The table should be brought back to a neutral position and then rolled 10–15° away from the top of the C-arm if it is on the patient's right side. This rotates the patient's vertebrae

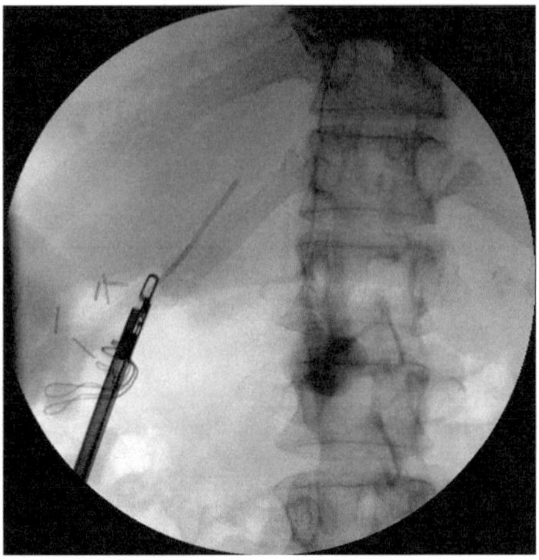

Fig. 4.4 The first static image with very little contrast injected

out of the plane of the image, so that the biliary tree is not superimposed over the bony structures, making interpretation of the images easier. Once OR personnel are appropriately shielded and at a safe distance from the C-arm, a localizing image over the area of the twist in the drape is obtained. Additional images may be required to direct and orient the C-arm image so that a view of the cystic duct, common bile duct, and duodenum is in the field.

At first, only a few milliliters of contrast material should be injected under live fluoroscopy, and video or a static image should be captured (Fig. 4.4). Injecting too much contrast too early may obscure any filling defects from small stones. Under live fluoroscopy, additional contrast is injected, which should fill the common duct distally, and flow freely into the duodenum. Once again, delivering too much contrast too soon can obscure the filling defects from stones. The C-arm can magnify areas of interest to allow for easier interpretation. After dye is observed in the duodenum, the C-arm should be repositioned for viewing the intrahepatic region. Both the left and right hepatic ducts must be visualized (Fig. 4.5). This is aided by placing the patient in a Trendelenburg position to promote retrograde filling. A final still image, without magnification, is taken of the entire biliary tree and duodenum to conclude the cholangiogram (Fig. 4.6). A checklist of critical findings such as contrast in the duodenum and intrahepatic bile ducts can be helpful.

Completion If a common duct stone has been identified, an exploration of the common duct can be performed at this time (Fig. 4.7). Small stones and debris identified at the ampulla can often be flushed into the duodenum by injecting contrast or saline under pressure. This procedure is aided by asking the anesthesiologist to inject glucagon 1 mg intravenously, which promotes the relaxation of the smooth muscle of the sphincter of Oddi. Wait 3 min for this effect to take place. This glucagon injection may be repeated once. Other techniques such as antegrade balloon dilation of the ampullae followed by flushing, common duct exploration by transcystic wire basket retrieval under fluoroscopic guidance, biliary endoscopy via the

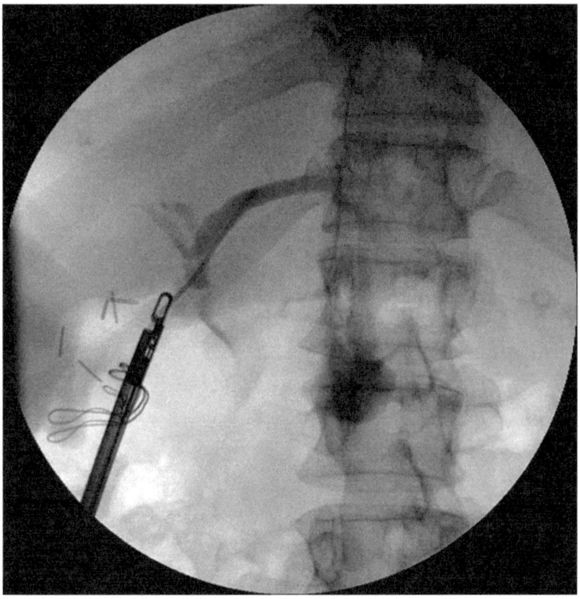

Fig. 4.5 Early filling of the hepatic ducts with contrast

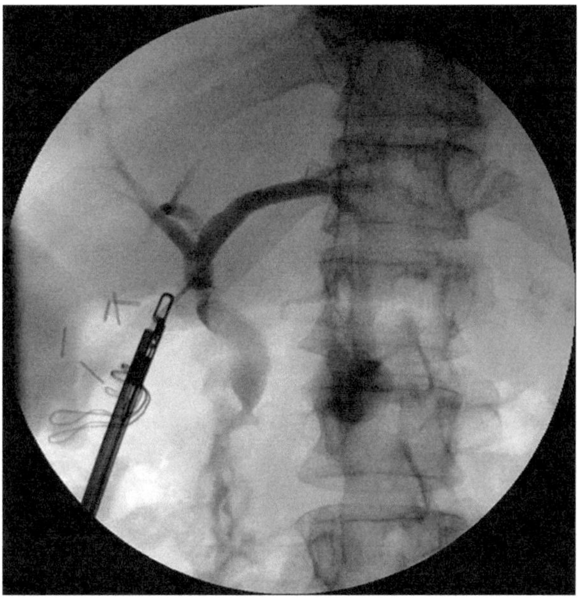

Fig. 4.6 The completion cholangiogram shows that both sets of intrahepatic ducts are visualized, and contrast is seen to flow into the duodenum

cystic duct, or choledochotomy can be performed (see subsequent chapters). If the cholangiogram was unremarkable, the catheter is removed under direct laparoscopic visualization, and the cystic duct can be clipped or ligated distal to the cystotomy. If the cholangiogram was abnormal due to a bile leak or an obstructing clip, this is the time to recognize a possible iatrogenic error and address it (Fig. 4.8).

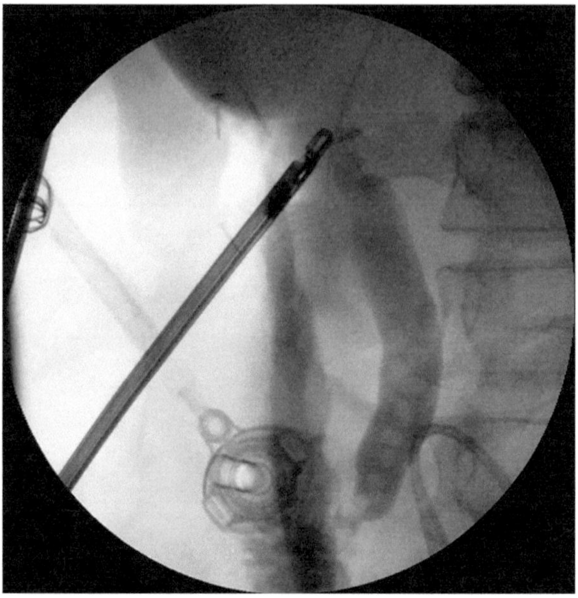

Fig. 4.7 Multiple stones are observed in the distal common bile duct

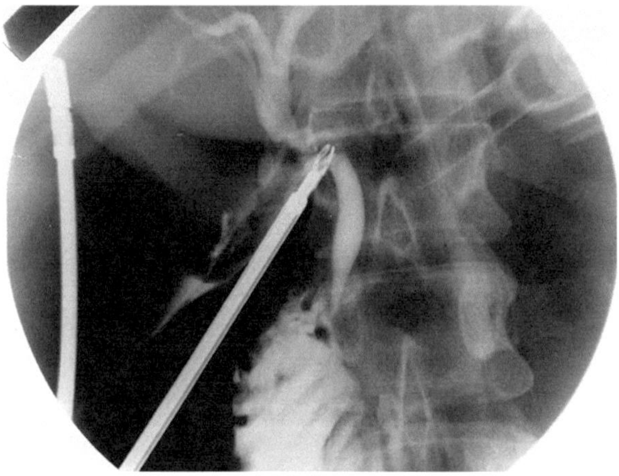

Fig. 4.8 Extravasation of contrast is seen and must be immediately managed

Intraoperative Cholangiogram Interpretation: Pearls and Pitfalls

While the proper performance of a cholangiogram is necessary, its correct interpretation is essential. Even when a cholangiogram has been obtained, its misinterpretation may result in causing or missing a major ductal injury.

Difficulties in placing the catheter into the cystic duct:

1. *Valves*: One must ensure to instrument the true lumen of the duct, and not a false passage or valve fold. The internal valves of Heister of the cystic duct may

prevent the passage of a cholangiocatheter. These valves may be opened by carefully inserting micro-scissors into the ductotomy in a closed fashion and pushing them gently through the obstructing valve. When a valve is encountered, it may be sharply incised with micro-scissors, or one may choose to relocate the ductotomy to the distal side of the valve. Be aware that if the micro-scissors are opened too wide to dilate or disrupt the valve, they can lacerate the wall of the cystic duct.

2. *Size of the duct*: If the duct is small, usually a more distal dissection will find a larger diameter cystic duct. If that is not the case, performing a cholecystogram is usually a safer option.
3. *Stones and debris within the cystic duct*: These can usually be teased out through the ductotomy with a gentle sweeping motion of the closed blunt grasper along the porta hepatis and common and cystic duct. The cystic duct (and stones within) may be gently crushed by the jaws of an atraumatic blunt grasper and its stones milked out as well. It is not ideal to push the stone into the common duct with the cholangiogram catheter (or have it fall into the common duct post cholecystectomy), so returning clear bile with the reflux maneuver is important. Even if the cystic duct cannot be safely identified, a cholecysto-cholangiogram can still be performed via the gallbladder (Fig. 4.9). This technique is commonly used in the infant or pediatric population where small size makes cannulation of the cystic duct more difficult [30]. Localizing clips can be placed in the area overlying where the cystic duct/common duct is thought to be. Then, the gallbladder is pierced with a needle. Bile is aspirated and in its place contrast is injected as in a routine cholangiogram.
4. *Inability to identify the cystic duct, porta hepatis, or critical view of safety*: Another alternative is to divide the gallbladder transversely midway up on the

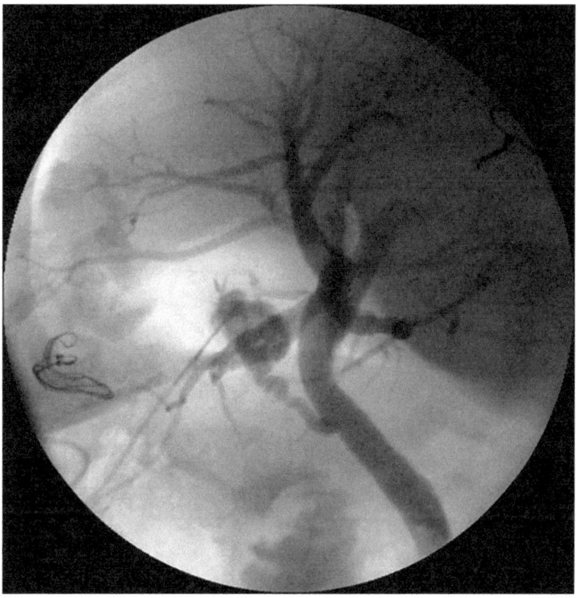

Fig. 4.9 A cholecysto-cholangiogram is performed by injecting contrast into the gallbladder when identification of the cystic duct is difficult

body of the gallbladder, being careful to control the spillage of gallbladder contents by placing a sponge in Morrison's pouch and a specimen bag adjacent to the liver. Once the gallbladder is divided and contents removed, inspection from within the lumen of the opened gallbladder can identify the cystic duct origin, and a cholangiocatheter can be inserted from within the gallbladder. Lastly, a 25-gauge needle can be inserted into what is thought to be the common duct. If the bile is aspirated, cholangiogram can be performed. If blood is aspirated, the needle should be withdrawn and pressure applied until bleeding stops.

Cholangiogram interpretation:

1. *Inability to visualize the proximal bile ducts on cholangiography*: The most common error of this type is the interpretation of the lower biliary tree as normal without the opacification of the hepatic ducts. This may occur if the common bile duct has been instrumented or a clip has been placed so that contrast cannot flow into the hepatic ducts. When only the lower portion of the ducts are visualized, the catheter may be repositioned, erroneously placed clips may be removed, or the patient placed in a Trendelenburg declination and/or intravenous morphine can be administered to increase sphincter of Oddi tone, in an effort to demonstrate cranial flow. Additionally, a blunt grasper can be used with gentle lateral to medial pressure on the distal common bile duct/porta hepatis while contrast is injected. The grasper is then removed and an X-ray taken. Also, intravenous (IV) Demerol can be administered to raise the sphincter pressure if the duct is emptying too quickly to fill the upper ducts. If the hepatic ducts still cannot be visualized, corrective surgical action should be considered immediately.
2. *Inability to visualize the duodenum on cholangiography*: The first step should be asking the anesthesiologist to inject 1 mg of glucagon IV, which promotes the relaxation of the smooth muscle of the sphincter of Oddi. Wait for 3 min for this effect and attempt the cholangiogram again. Another 1 mg of IV glucagon may be repeated once. Sometimes, contrast does not enter the duodenum because the contrast cannot be injected with appropriate force. Assure that the tubing, catheter, or cystic duct is not kinked. If OK, exchange the contrast-filled 30 ml syringe with a 20 or 10 ml syringe, which allows greater force to be applied. If there is still no contrast exiting the bile duct, transcystic choledochoscopy can be employed. Judgment is needed if the common duct is small. Allowing a small stone to pass spontaneously may be the safer choice, but the patient needs close follow-up.
3. *Air bubbles* vs *stones*: Bubbles that are introduced into the biliary tree may mimic the appearance of stones. These bubbles can usually be differentiated by the parallel motion observed when rapidly injecting and withdrawing the syringe. Additionally, placing the patient in a reverse Trendelenburg position should cause the bubbles to float proximally toward the liver, whereas calculi would not. Also, air bubbles tend to move in the duct more rapidly during flushing than stones, and air bubbles deform as they enter the smaller intrahepatic ducts. Avoidance is the easier approach. The attention of the operating staff must be directed to ensuring that any air bubbles that are seen in the syringes and the tubing are flushed out with saline prior to the equipment being handed to the surgeon, but the surgeon should personally inspect the tubing and syringes prior to use.

Intraoperative Near-Infrared Fluorescent Cholangiography

Fluorescence cholangiography is a recently developed technique for imaging the extrahepatic biliary tree without the need for ductotomy. It employs an indocyanine green (ICG) fluorophore, which absorbs near-infrared irradiation between 790 and 805 nm and re-emits it at an excitation wavelength of 835 nm. ICG is typically administered as a single intravenous dose approximately 1 h prior to the start of surgery. It then binds to plasma proteins and remains within the intravascular space until it is metabolized by the liver and excreted into the biliary system 15–20 min after administration [31].

Near-infrared fluorescent cholangiography (NIRFC) has been suggested as an alternative technique to IOC for the safe and easy intraoperative recognition of biliary anatomy and avoidance of ductal injury. It provides a real-time assessment of extrahepatic biliary anatomy and can be done rapidly without the use of ionizing radiation [32]. One cost analysis has suggested that its use results in significant cost savings per case, it is quicker to perform, and the surgical team enjoys an increased ease of use, when compared to standard cholangiography [33].

However, there are several important limitations to NIRFC that may impact its overall usefulness. Despite excellent results in non-inflamed cases, the performance of NIRFC decreases in the presence of inflammation, due in part to the limited depth of tissue penetration of near-IR light of 5–10 mm [32, 34]. In symptomatic cholelithiasis without acute inflammation, rates of visualization have been reported to be 93% for the cystic duct, 88% for the common hepatic duct, and 91% for the common bile duct prior to dissection of Calot's triangle [35], but in a second study, this dropped to 91.6%, 75%, and 79.1% in the presence of acute cholecystitis [36].

A second drawback of this new technology is that it will not provide visualization of most common bile duct stones because the fluorescent light cannot be detected from within the intrapancreatic portion of the CBD [36]. It is also difficult to distinguish small stones. For these reasons, the role of NIRFC in the management of patients with choledocholithiasis remains to be demonstrated.

Conclusion

The intraoperative cholangiogram provides important information concerning the precise anatomy of the biliary tree. This knowledge minimizes the risk of bile duct injury. The cholangiogram also helps the surgeon recognize any bile duct injuries at the time of operation, and this prompt recognition decreases morbidity and mortality. Also, by identifying common duct stones and treating them at the time of surgery, rather than as a separate procedure, the patient is spared additional days in the hospital, additional procedures, and the potential for additional complications.

The routine performance of IOC by a team familiar with the procedure is a quick and painless process. The knowledge and skills developed by regular performance of the procedure will help the surgeon make the best choices during difficult cases and are the first step in developing more advanced laparoscopic biliary surgical skills. At the least, perform routine cholangiography until both your and your team's skills have been perfected. Properly performing and interpreting cholangiograms can be an important step in the performance of a safe laparoscopic cholecystectomy, and these are important skills to be imparted to surgical trainees.

References

1. Mirizzi PL. Operative cholangiography. Surg Gynecol Obstet. 1937;16:702.
2. Kullman E, Borch K, Lindstrom E, Svanvik J, Anderberg B. Value of routine intraoperative cholangiography in detecting aberrant bile ducts and bile duct injuries during laparoscopic cholecystectomy. Br J Surg. 1996;83(2):171–5.
3. Fletcher DR, Hobbs MST, Tan P, Valinsky LJ, Hockey RL, Pikora TJ, et al. Complications of cholecystectomy: risks of the laparoscopic approach and protective effects of operative cholangiography: a population-based study. Ann Surg. 1999;229(4):449–57.
4. Carroll BJ, Friedman RL, Liberman MA, Phillips EH. Routine cholangiography reduces sequelae of common bile duct injuries. Surg Endosc. 1996;10(12):1194–7.
5. Phillips EH, Berci G, Carroll B, Daykhovsky L, Sackier J, Pazpartlow M. The importance of intraoperative cholangiography during laparoscopic cholecystectomy. Am Surg. 1990;56(12):792–5.
6. Waage A, Nilsson M. Iatrogenic bile duct injury: a population-based study of 152 776 cholecystectomies in the swedish inpatient registry. Arch Surg. 2006;141(12):1207–13.
7. Alvarez FA, de Santibanes M, Palavecino M, Claria RS, Mazza O, Arbues G, et al. Impact of routine intraoperative cholangiography during laparoscopic cholecystectomy on bile duct injury. Br J Surg. 2014;101(6):677–84.
8. Buddingh KT, Nieuwenhuijs VB, van Buuren L, Hulscher JBF, de Jong JS, van Dam GM. Intraoperative assessment of biliary anatomy for prevention of bile duct injury: a review of current and future patient safety interventions. Surg Endosc. 2011;25(8):2449–61.
9. Nickkholgh A, Soltaniyekta S, Kalbasi H. Routine versus selective intraoperative cholangiography during laparoscopic cholecystectomy: a survey of 2,130 patients undergoing laparoscopic cholecystectomy. Surg Endosc. 2006;20(6):868–74.
10. Overby DW, Apelgren KN, Richardson W, Fanelli R. Sages guidelines for the clinical application of laparoscopic biliary tract surgery. Surg Endosc. 2010;24(10):2368–86.
11. Wu SC, Chen FC, Lo CJ. Selective intraoperative cholangiography and single-stage management of common bile duct stone in laparoscopic cholecystectomy. World J Surg. 2005;29(11):1402–8.
12. Ludwig K, Bernhardt J, Steffen H, Lorenz D. Contribution of intraoperative cholangiography to incidence and outcome of common bile duct injuries during laparoscopic cholecystectomy. Surg Endosc. 2002;16(7):1098–104.
13. Buddingh KT, Weersma RK, Savenije RA, van Dam GM, Nieuwenhuijs VB. Lower rate of major bile duct injury and increased intraoperative management of common bile duct stones after implementation of routine intraoperative cholangiography. J Am Coll Surg. 2011;213(2):267–74.
14. Berci G, Hamlin JA. Operative biliary radiology. Baltimore: Williams & Wilkins; 1981.
15. Berci G. Biliary ductal anatomy and anomalies. The role of intraoperative cholangiography during laparoscopic cholecystectomy. Surg Clin North Am. 1992;72(5):1069–75.
16. Debru E, Dawson A, Leibman S, Richardson M, Glen L, Hollinshead J, et al. Does routine intraoperative cholangiography prevent bile duct transection? Surg Endosc. 2005;19(4):589–93.
17. Kholdebarin R, Boetto J, Harnish JL, Urbach DR. Risk factors for bile duct injury during laparoscopic cholecystectomy: a case-control study. Surg Innov. 2008;15(2):114–9.

18. Savader SJ, Lillemoe KD, Prescott CA, Winick AB, Venbrux AC, Lund GB, et al. Laparoscopic cholecystectomy-related bile duct injuries: a health and financial disaster. Ann Surg. 1997;225(3):268–73.
19. Kern KA. Medicolegal analysis of bile duct injury during open cholecystectomy and abdominal surgery. Am J Surg. 1994;168(3):217–22.
20. Flum DR, Flowers C, Veenstra DL. A cost-effectiveness analysis of intraoperative cholangiography in the prevention of bile duct injury during laparoscopic cholecystectomy. J Am Coll Surg. 2003;196(3):385–93.
21. Lublin M, Crawford DL, Hiatt JR, Phillips EH. Symptoms before and after laparoscopic cholecystectomy for gallstones. Am Surg. 2004;70(10):863–6.
22. Lacitignola S, Minardi M. Management of common bile duct stones: a ten-year experience at a tertiary care center. JSLS. 2008;12(1):62–5.
23. Bertolin-Bernades R, Sabater-Orti L, Calvete-Chornet J, Camps-Vilata B, Cassinello-Fernandez N, Oviedo-Bravo M, et al. Mild acute biliary pancreatitis vs cholelithiasis: are there differences in the rate of choledocholithiasis? J Gastrointest Surg. 2007;11(7):875–9.
24. Phillips EH. Routine versus selective intraoperative cholangiography. Am J Surg. 1993;165(4):505–7.
25. Urbach DR, Khajanchee YS, Jobe BA, Standage BA, Hansen PD, Swanstrom LL. Cost-effective management of common bile duct stones: a decision analysis of the use of endoscopic retrograde cholangiopancreatography (ERCP), intraoperative cholangiography, and laparoscopic bile duct exploration. Surg Endosc. 2001;15(1):4–13.
26. Kenny R, Richardson J, McGlone ER, Reddy M, Khan OA. Laparoscopic common bile duct exploration versus pre or post-operative ERCP for common bile duct stones in patients undergoing cholecystectomy: is there any difference? Int J Surg. 2014;12(9):989–93.
27. Soper NJ, Brunt LM. The case for routine operative cholangiography during laparoscopic cholecystectomy. Surg Clin North Am. 1994;74(4):953–9.
28. Paganini AM, Guerrieri M, Sarnari J, De Sanctis A, D'Ambrosio G, Lezoche G, et al. Thirteen years' experience with laparoscopic transcystic common bile duct exploration for stones. Effectiveness and long-term results. Surg Endosc. 2007;21(1):34–40.
29. Massarweh NN, Devlin A, Elrod JA, Symons RG, Flum DR. Surgeon knowledge, behavior, and opinions regarding intraoperative cholangiography. J Am Coll Surg. 2008;207(6):821–30.
30. Seleem MI, Al-Hashemy AM, Meshref SS. Mini-laparoscopic cholecystectomy in children under 10 years of age with sickle cell disease. ANZ J Surg. 2005;75(7):562–5.
31. Cherrick GR, Stein SW, Leevy CM, Davidson CS. Indocyanine green: observations on its physical properties, plasma decay, and hepatic extraction. J Clin Invest. 1960;39:592–600.
32. Boni L, David G, Mangano A, Dionigi G, Rausei S, Spampatti S, et al. Clinical applications of indocyanine green (ICG) enhanced fluorescence in laparoscopic surgery. Surg Endosc. 2015;29(7):2046–55.
33. Dip FD, Asbun D, Rosales-Velderrain A, Lo Menzo E, Simpfendorfer CH, Szomstein S, et al. Cost analysis and effectiveness comparing the routine use of intraoperative fluorescent cholangiography with fluoroscopic cholangiogram in patients undergoing laparoscopic cholecystectomy. Surg Endosc. 2014;28(6):1838–43.
34. Ishizawa T, Kaneko J, Inoue Y, Takemura N, Seyama Y, Aoki T, et al. Application of fluorescent cholangiography to single-incision laparoscopic cholecystectomy. Surg Endosc. 2011;25(8):2631–6.
35. Spinoglio G, Priora F, Bianchi PP, Lucido FS, Licciardello A, Maglione V, et al. Real-time near-infrared (NIR) fluorescent cholangiography in single-site robotic cholecystectomy (SSRC): a single-institutional prospective study. Surg Endosc. 2013;27(6):2156–62.
36. Kim NS, Jin HY, Kim EY, Hong TH. Cystic duct variation detected by near-infrared fluorescent cholangiography during laparoscopic cholecystectomy. Ann Surg Treat Res. 2017;92(1):47–50.

Chapter 5
Intraoperative Ultrasound During Laparoscopic Cholecystectomy: An Alternative to Cholangiography

Juaquito M. Jorge and Nathaniel J. Soper

Introduction

Ultrasound has long been used as an anatomic and diagnostic guide during surgery of the liver and biliary tree. The introduction of B-mode ultrasound technology in the 1970s allowed for real-time viewing of two-dimensional (2D) sonographic images, which facilitated its use in a variety of contexts including open cholecystectomy to evaluate the common bile duct (CBD) for stones and define ductal and vascular anatomy [1–3]. However, due to the relative ease of access to tactile manipulation and exploration of the CBD, neither ultrasound nor intraoperative cholangiography (IOC) was routinely employed during cholecystectomy in the open surgical era. The rapid adoption of laparoscopic cholecystectomy in the early 1990s was initially associated with a sharp increase in the rate of CBD injury [4]. A call to remedy this increase in severe complications, in addition to the need for a reliable method for assessing for choledocholithiasis laparoscopically, brought about a renewed interest in both intraoperative laparoscopic ultrasound (LUS) and IOC. While debate still exists regarding the utility of these modalities in decreasing rates of CBD injury, there is no doubt that they are valuable tools that have advanced surgeons' understanding and appreciation of the anatomic relationships of the biliary tree when viewed and approached laparoscopically.

Electronic supplementary material The online version of this chapter (doi: 10.1007/978-3-319-74503-9_5) contains supplementary material, which is available to authorized users.

J. M. Jorge, MD (✉)
Department of Surgery, University of South Florida, Tampa General Hospital, Tampa, FL, USA

N. J. Soper, MD
Department of Surgery, Northwestern University, Chicago, IL, USA
e-mail: nsoper@nmh.org

© Springer International Publishing AG, part of Springer Nature 2018

B. F. Santos, N. Soper (eds.), *Choledocholithiasis*,
https://doi.org/10.1007/978-3-319-74503-9_5

Currently, LUS and IOC each exist as excellent options for both detecting CBD stones and delineating anatomy during laparoscopic cholecystectomy. LUS offers several distinct advantages including a lack of radiation and contrast dye, the ability to perform repeat examinations without the need to cannulate the cystic duct, and comparatively superior time and cost-effectiveness. Additionally, because laparoscopy is a surface imaging modality, LUS allows an assessment of structures beyond the visible surface. This chapter describes the techniques for performing LUS during laparoscopic cholecystectomy and interpreting the resulting sonographic images. The text also provides a review of the available clinical data regarding the effectiveness of LUS, both alone and in comparison with IOC.

Indications

The use of ultrasound during laparoscopic cholecystectomy serves two main functions: the identification of CBD stones and the examination and confirmation of biliary and vascular anatomy. LUS can be used selectively or in a routine fashion in regard to both functions. When applied in a selective manner (similar to selective IOC), LUS is employed when there is a preoperative or intraoperative suspicion of choledocholithiasis. This evaluation can be based on a number of preoperative factors, including jaundice, elevated bilirubin or transaminase levels, a dilated CBD or common duct stones seen on transabdominal ultrasound, or an elevated lipase level or history of gallstone pancreatitis. Intraoperatively, observation of a dilated CBD or cystic duct, and/or the presence of stones within the cystic duct, can also alert to the presence of choledocholithiasis. When applied selectively for anatomic identification, LUS is used when a question exists regarding the anatomic orientation of the hepatocystic triangle, to confirm the location of the CBD and common hepatic duct in relation to the plane of dissection or to confirm an aberrant ductal or vascular configuration that is identified during initial dissection.

We advocate a routine approach to the use of LUS during laparoscopic cholecystectomy, in which a LUS examination is performed during every case regardless of preoperative suspicion of choledocholithiasis or the ease of intraoperative anatomic identification. There are several advantages to a routine usage approach. It allows the surgeon to more quickly amass an extensive LUS experience and gain familiarity with the sonographic appearance of normal ductal anatomy. This allows for greater confidence in interpreting LUS images during difficult and potentially stressful cases, such as those with inflammatory conditions or aberrant anatomy. If surgical trainees are assisting in the cases, routine use gives them increased exposure to the techniques of LUS and allows for enhanced cognitive correlation of the anatomy seen laparoscopically with a second visualization modality. Additionally, a protocol of routine LUS use allows the other operating room staff to become familiar with the procedure and its associated technology and guarantees that the necessary equipment will be available during the case.

Equipment

Modern laparoscopic ultrasound probes are designed to enable efficient and reliable intraoperative use. We use a probe with a 10 mm diameter that can be inserted through standard 10 or 11 mm laparoscopic trocars (type 8666 transducer, BK Medical, Herlev, Denmark), although several other similar probes are commercially available [5]. Probes use primarily B-mode (i.e., two-dimensional) ultrasound, with frequencies between 5 and 10 MHz [6]. The most commonly used frequencies during laparoscopic evaluation of the biliary system are 7 and 7.5 MHz. A linear or curvilinear ultrasound array between 3 and 7 cm in length is optimal.

Probes with both vertically and horizontally deflectable tips are helpful in obtaining variable viewing angles and most incorporate Doppler sonography to simultaneously overlay flow measurements onto the primary sonographic image. This feature is useful in differentiating between bile ducts and adjacent vasculature, especially when imaging the biliary tree proximal to the bifurcation of the common hepatic duct and proper hepatic artery. Modern probes can be sterilized after each usage, obviating the need for sterile probe covers, which can tear causing contamination of the operative field and are often difficult to introduce through laparoscopic trocars.

Essential to efficient use of LUS is an endoscopic operating suite equipped to transmit two images to the viewing monitors simultaneously, in a "picture in picture" display (Fig. 5.1). This allows the surgeon to correlate the ultrasound images with their anatomic position laparoscopically, as well as to efficiently maneuver the LUS probe in the operative field. Additionally, the ability to record both the laparoscopic and sonographic images is helpful for medical documentation and retrospective teaching purposes.

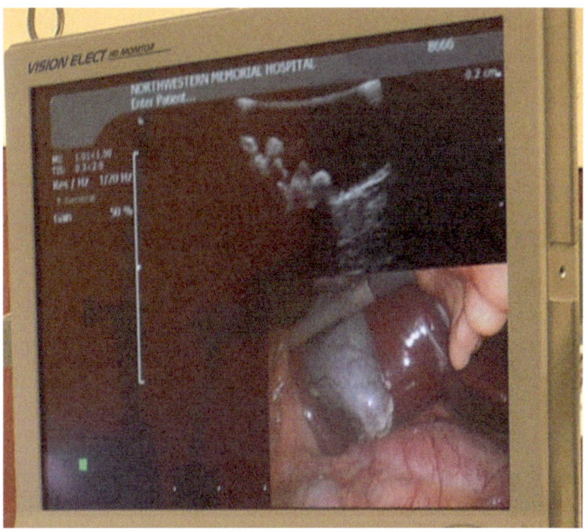

Fig. 5.1 The operating room monitor is configured to show the sonographic and laparoscopic images simultaneously in a "picture in picture" view (Reprinted with permission from Teitelbaum EN, Soper NJ. Ch 13. Intraoperative Ultrasound During Laparoscopic Cholecystectomy. In: Hagopian EJ, Machi J (eds). Abdominal Ultrasound for Surgeons. New York, NY: Springer Science + Business Media. 2014)

Laparoscopic Ultrasound Technique

Initial Dissection

Although some authors have described the use of LUS during laparoscopic cholecystectomy immediately upon establishing the pneumoperitoneum, during routine cases we prefer to perform an initial dissection of the hepatocystic triangle prior to sonographic examination. Using a standard four-port technique, a combination of blunt and electrocautery dissection is used to remove all of the fibrous and fatty tissue from the hepatocystic triangle in order to establish a "critical view of safety" [7]. Reserving use of LUS until after this dissection has been performed offers several advantages. The most important is that a meticulous and thorough dissection is the most essential means to prevent CBD injury [4]. By completing this dissection prior to the LUS examination, the surgeon does not run the risk of being misled by a seemingly normal anatomic configuration on ultrasound. Additionally, opening the hepatocystic triangle via dissection allows for an easier and more complete LUS examination. The gallbladder is freed from the inferior aspects of its peritoneal attachments to the liver bed, enabling retraction of the infundibulum further laterally from the cystic duct-CBD junction. This allows for easier LUS identification and delineation of the ductal structures and enables the surgeon to manipulate the infundibulum with more mobility during LUS to create a variety of viewing angles.

If there is uncertainty regarding the anatomy during the course of the dissection to create a "critical view," LUS can be employed earlier to examine the ducts in relation to the area in question. In the case of a difficult or confusing dissection, LUS and IOC can be employed conjointly to establish a more robust anatomic examination. However, LUS and IOC should be only considered tools that provide additional information, rather than definitive evaluations. If any uncertainty exists regarding the anatomic relationships of the critical ductal and/or vascular structures after the use of these modalities, the surgeon should not hesitate to convert to an open procedure in order to ensure optimal safety.

Intraoperative Scanning

Once a dissection to the "critical view" has been completed, the ultrasound probe is connected to the scanner, and the monitors are switched to a "picture in picture" view. Using the standard "American" four-port configuration, the ultrasound probe can be introduced through either the epigastric or umbilical trocar. While we prefer the epigastric technique (Video 5.1), each method has its own advantages and disadvantages. Often when a certain structure or segment of the CBD cannot be visualized via one trocar, the probe position must be switched, and some authors have advocated routine imaging from both orientations in every case. While we have found this to be infrequently necessary, surgeons must have a good familiarity with both techniques.

Epigastric Scanning Technique

When scanning through the epigastric trocar, the surgeon stands on the patient's left side and manipulates the probe with his or her right hand, while the left hand retracts the gallbladder infundibulum using a grasper placed through the more medial of the two right subcostal trocars. The assistant retracts the gallbladder fundus superiorly over the liver through the lateral subcostal trocar and operates the camera. The probe is inserted in the direction of the gallbladder, with the scanning array facing posteriorly. It is helpful to hold the probe with your index finger positioned on the side opposite to the scanning array in order to maintain spatial orientation during subsequent probe maneuvering.

The probe is first positioned directly over the gallbladder wall. The sonographic depth of field and gain can then be adjusted to optimize the image. Fluid inside the gallbladder should appear anechoic (i.e., black), and any stones should be hyperechoic (i.e., white) and create "shadowing" in the sonographic field beyond their location (Fig. 5.2). When scanning through the gallbladder, other pathologies such as polyps can be identified. In contrast to stones, polyps will appear less hyper-

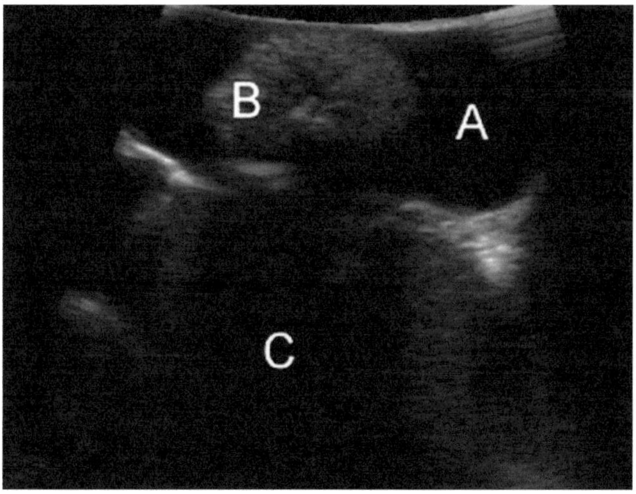

Fig. 5.2 The gallbladder is imaged, showing hypoechoic gallbladder fluid (A), a large hyperechoic stone (B), and sonographic shadowing (C) created by the stone (Reprinted with permission from Teitelbaum EN, Soper NJ. Ch 13. Intraoperative Ultrasound During Laparoscopic Cholecystectomy. In: Hagopian EJ, Machi J (eds). Abdominal Ultrasound for Surgeons. New York, NY: Springer Science + Business Media. 2014)

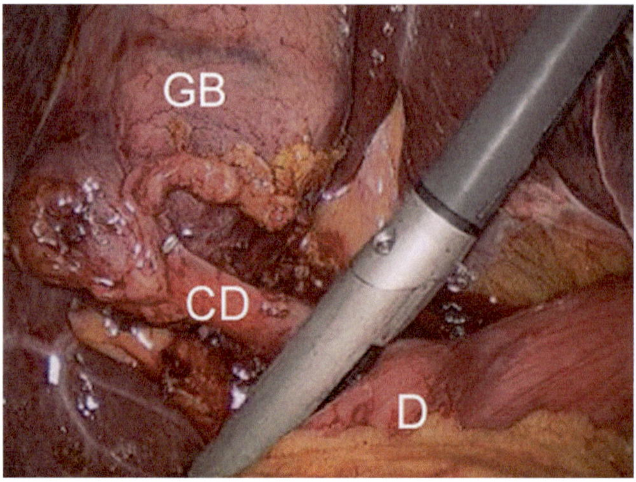

Fig. 5.3 The starting position for imaging the biliary tree when scanning through the epigastric trocar. The probe is placed over the midportion of hepatoduodenal ligament, superior to the duodenum (D) and inferior to the cystic duct (CD) and gallbladder (GB) (Reprinted with permission from Teitelbaum EN, Soper NJ. Ch 13. Intraoperative Ultrasound During Laparoscopic Cholecystectomy. In: Hagopian EJ, Machi J (eds). Abdominal Ultrasound for Surgeons. New York, NY: Springer Science + Business Media. 2014)

echoic, will not create shadowing, may exhibit blood flow on Doppler, and will not fall to a dependent location within the gallbladder.

Once the sonographic view has been fine-tuned and the gallbladder inspected, the probe is placed over the midportion of the hepatoduodenal ligament with the scanning array facing posteriorly (Fig. 5.3). The probe is then manipulated in order to visualize the portal triad structures: the CBD, proper hepatic artery, and portal vein. The probe is positioned perpendicular to the hepatoduodenal ligament, and as a result, all three structures are seen in a transverse orientation and appear as circles on the sonographic image. The CBD and hepatic artery are usually smaller in diameter and aligned in the same anterior-posterior plane, ventral to the larger portal vein. This normal configuration creates a so-called "Mickey Mouse head" sonographic appearance (Fig. 5.4).

The probe is then moved caudad down the hepatoduodenal ligament and toward the duodenum in order to scan the length of the CBD. During this step the surgeon should slide the probe slowly while only moving in a single plane without rotation. This will allow for visualizing the entire length of the suprapancreatic CBD and minimize the risk of skipping over a segment of duct that contains a stone. The probe should rest gently on the hepatoduodenal ligament during this step. If too much pressure is applied, the CBD will be compressed and obscured from view. Conversely, if the probe is lifted off the surface of the ligament, the acoustic window and sonographic image will be lost. This can be an issue in very thin patients in whom the hepatoduodenal ligament is devoid of fat. To remedy this problem, saline can be infused to flood the right upper quadrant and act as an acoustic coupler in

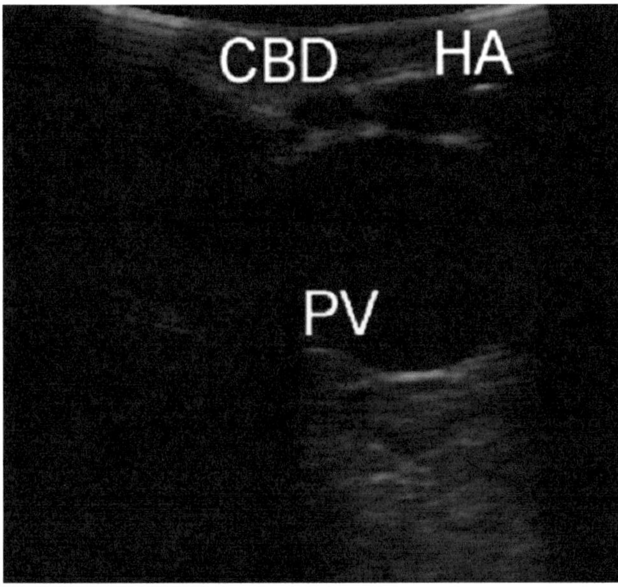

Fig. 5.4 The portal triad is visualized, creating a "Mickey Mouse head" appearance of the common bile duct (CBD) and proper hepatic artery (HA) anteriorly and portal vein (PV) posteriorly, all seen in transverse section (Reprinted with permission from Teitelbaum EN, Soper NJ. Ch 13. Intraoperative Ultrasound During Laparoscopic Cholecystectomy. In: Hagopian EJ, Machi J (eds). Abdominal Ultrasound for Surgeons. New York, NY: Springer Science + Business Media. 2014)

order to create a better acoustic window [8]. However, in actual practice we have found this to be rarely necessary, as well as adding additional time.

As the CBD is sequentially imaged, the surgeon should be primarily looking for intraductal stones and sludge. Stones appear intensely hyperechoic and create acoustic shadowing on the side opposite to the scanning array (i.e., toward the bottom side of the sonographic image) (Fig. 5.5). Once detected, the diameter of a stone can be measured using the sonographic caliper function. This can be helpful in determining the most effective means of stone removal via laparoscopic or open CBD exploration or endoscopic retrograde cholangiopancreatography (ERCP). Sludge is defined as echogenic intraductal debris consisting of particles less than 2 mm in diameter, which does not usually result in shadowing [9]. During our initial experience with LUS, we would attempt to treat all findings of CBD sludge with flushing via a catheter introduced into the cystic duct [10]. However, we have found this sludge to most often be of no clinical consequence and now reserve intervention for cases in which it is causing biliary obstruction or pancreatitis [11].

After imaging of its suprapancreatic portion, the CBD is followed distally as it enters the pancreatic parenchyma. As the CBD enters the pancreas, its path deviates to the patient's right side, toward the ampulla of Vater. In order to follow the duct along this course, the LUS probe is held in a stationary position abutting the superior edge of the duodenum and slowly rotated in a clockwise direction. With this

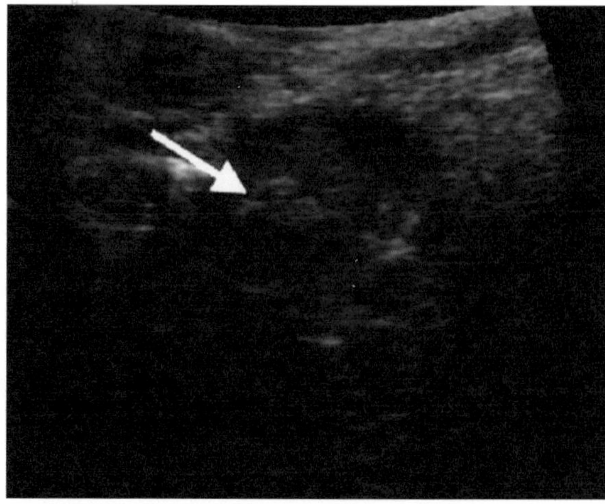

Fig. 5.5 A hyperechoic stone (arrow) visualized within the common bile duct (Reprinted with permission from Teitelbaum EN, Soper NJ. Ch 13. Intraoperative Ultrasound During Laparoscopic Cholecystectomy. In: Hagopian EJ, Machi J (eds). Abdominal Ultrasound for Surgeons. New York, NY: Springer Science + Business Media. 2014)

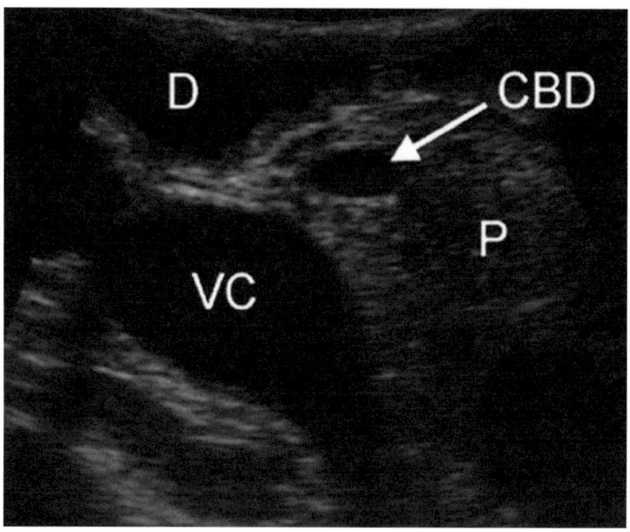

Fig. 5.6 The common bile duct (CBD) is seen traversing the relatively hyperechoic pancreatic parenchyma (P). The duodenum (D) anteriorly and inferior vena cava (VC) posteriorly are also visualized (Reprinted with permission from Teitelbaum EN, Soper NJ. Ch 13. Intraoperative Ultrasound During Laparoscopic Cholecystectomy. In: Hagopian EJ, Machi J (eds). Abdominal Ultrasound for Surgeons. New York, NY: Springer Science + Business Media. 2014)

motion, the CBD should be kept in a transverse orientation on the sonographic image (Fig. 5.6). The duct should be followed until its entrance into the duodenum. The muscular sphincter of the ampulla can often be seen as a hypoechoic ring surrounding the distal most segment of the duct (Fig. 5.7). Additionally, the pancreatic duct can often be seen traversing the pancreas inferior to the CBD. In certain patients a long common segment of CBD-pancreatic duct exists and can be documented

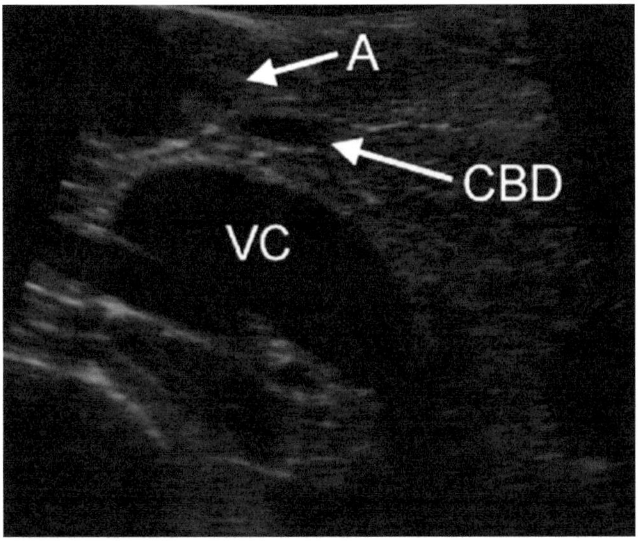

Fig. 5.7 The distal common bile duct (CBD) is seen just as it enters the duodenum through the ampulla of Vater (A). The inferior vena cava (VC) is seen posterior to the pancreas (Reprinted with permission from Teitelbaum EN, Soper NJ. Ch 13. Intraoperative Ultrasound During Laparoscopic Cholecystectomy. In: Hagopian EJ, Machi J (eds). Abdominal Ultrasound for Surgeons. New York, NY: Springer Science + Business Media. 2014)

sonographically, which may predispose to the development of gallstone pancreatitis.

Pancreatic tissue is relatively hyperechoic compared with the fatty tissue of the hepatoduodenal ligament. This can make detection of CBD stones more difficult in the ductal segment within the pancreas. In many series, rates of complete visualization and stone detection in the distal, intrapancreatic CBD are lower than the suprapancreatic portion, and some authors have described imaging of the distal CBD as the "Achilles heel" of LUS during laparoscopic cholecystectomy [12–14]. If visualization of the distal CBD is inadequate, several maneuvers can be performed to improve the image quality. Usually, simply placing the LUS probe directly on the duodenum with the transducer directed posteriorly and scanning while exerting gentle downward pressure (to displace air) will result in excellent imaging of the intrapancreatic CBD. If this maneuver does not provide adequate visualization, saline can be instilled into the stomach and duodenum via a nasogastric tube, creating a better acoustic window. The probe can also be repositioned through the umbilical trocar if epigastric visualization is insufficient. In patients with a narrow CBD, saline can be injected into the duct via a catheter introduced through a cystic ductotomy. This acts to dilate the CBD and may enable better visualization of distal CBD stones but requires the same ductotomy and cannulation as an IOC.

After the entire length of the CBD has been satisfactorily evaluated for the presence of stones, attention is turned to examining the anatomy of the hepatocystic

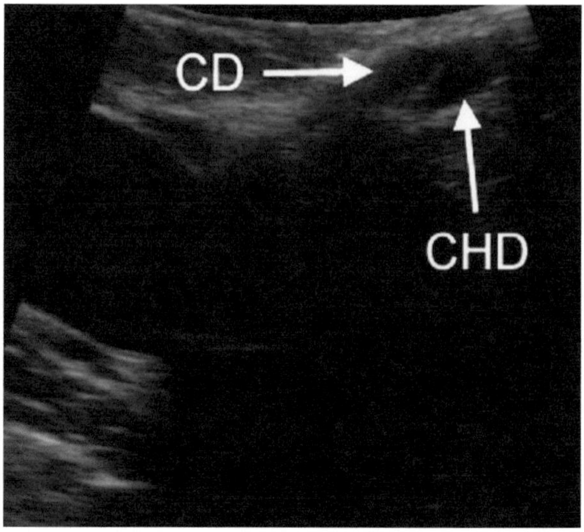

Fig. 5.8 The cystic duct (CD) and common hepatic duct (CHD) are imaged just as they join to form the common bile duct (Reprinted with permission from Teitelbaum EN, Soper NJ. Ch 13. Intraoperative Ultrasound During Laparoscopic Cholecystectomy. In: Hagopian EJ, Machi J (eds). Abdominal Ultrasound for Surgeons. New York, NY: Springer Science + Business Media. 2014)

triangle. The probe is returned to its original position above the hepatoduodenal ligament and then moved cephalad until the junction between the CBD and cystic duct is visualized (Fig. 5.8). The location of this junction is noted on the laparoscopic image to ensure that the anatomic assumptions made after the initial dissection to a "critical view of safety" were in fact correct. LUS can also be used to measure the length of the cystic duct, to ensure adequate space for clip application. To do this, the gallbladder infundibulum is retracted laterally, to orient the cystic duct perpendicular to the CBD. A longitudinal image of the cystic duct can occasionally be obtained and its length measured directly using the sonographic caliper function. If the anatomy does not allow for a longitudinal view, the cystic duct length can be estimated by flooding the right upper quadrant with saline and scanning down the gallbladder in transverse section until the transition from infundibulum to narrow cystic duct is observed. The distance from this point (i.e., the origin of the cystic duct) to the transverse image of the CBD to the right of the sonographic image is then measured. Using this technique, a study determined the measured cystic duct length to be within 5 mm of the length determined by either IOC or complete dissection of the cystic duct to the CBD junction in 87% of cases [15].

After examining the cystic duct and cystic-CBD junction, the probe is slid further cephalad to visualize the common hepatic duct and right and left hepatic ducts. Often during this step the liver edge obstructs the probe when scanning through the epigastric trocar. If this occurs, the probe tip can be flexed to the right to create a longitudinal view of the hepatic ducts.

Umbilical Scanning Technique

In contrast to the transverse views seen when scanning through the epigastric trocar, the umbilical technique creates longitudinal images of the CBD. This allows for entire segments of the duct to be viewed simultaneously, and for this reason it is the preferred technique of many authors [12, 13]. However, scanning from an umbilical position requires removal and reinsertion of the laparoscope through the epigastric trocar. With the laparoscope viewing cephalad to caudad and the monitors positioned toward the head of the table, the movements of the probe are seen in a "mirror image" and are counterintuitive. This makes probe maneuvering awkward, especially for those new to the technique, and can therefore lengthen the time required to perform the examination. For this reason we prefer epigastric scanning, although surgeons should become proficient in both techniques as often a certain segment of the CBD cannot be viewed via the initial approach.

Umbilical scanning begins with the gallbladder released from both fundal and infundibular retraction. The probe is positioned over the liver, and the gallbladder is visualized using segment V as an acoustic window. As in the epigastric technique, this view is used to adjust the sonographic image, and the gallbladder is examined for stones and polyps. The probe is then moved medially over liver segment IV, and the confluence of the hepatic ducts and hepatic arteries is visualized. Use of Doppler mode to identify arterial flow can be helpful in orienting the anatomy proximal to the branching of these structures.

Once the common hepatic duct has been identified, it is examined for stones and sludge. With the probe entering through the umbilical trocar, the hepatic duct and CBD will be seen in longitudinal section (Fig. 5.9). The more proximal portion of the duct will appear toward the left side of the sonographic image using typical settings. In order to examine the entire width of the ducts, the probe is slowly rotated back and forth. Once a segment of the duct has been scanned in its entirety, the probe is slid caudad in order to scan distally. As the CBD enters the pancreatic head, its sonographic image will switch from longitudinal to oblique, as the duct curves to the patient's right side and into the duodenum.

Once the CBD has been scanned completely for stones, the anatomy of the cystic duct-CBD junction is examined. To obtain this view, the gallbladder should be regrasped and the infundibulum retracted laterally. From the umbilical trocar, the cystic duct can be seen in transverse section and followed along its length. It can be more difficult to identify the cystic-CBD junction using the umbilical scanning technique because often the two structures cannot be visualized concurrently. This can be remedied by deflecting the probe tip to the left in order to obtain an image of both the cystic duct and CBD in transverse section, in a sense replicating the view obtained via epigastric scanning.

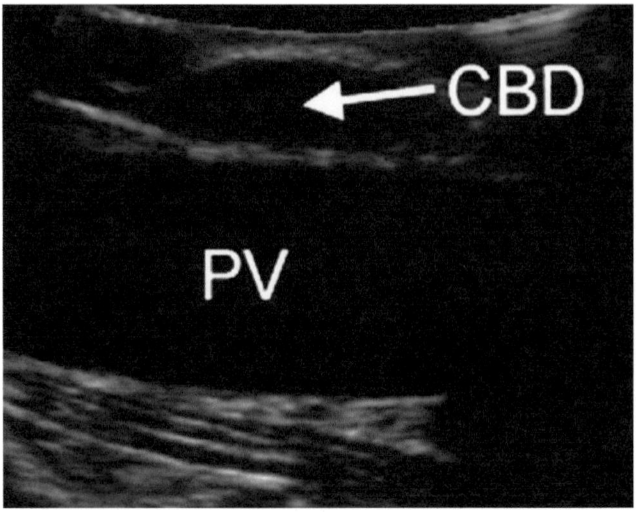

Fig. 5.9 The common bile duct (CBD) and portal vein (PV) seen in longitudinal section when scanning through the umbilical trocar (Reprinted with permission from Teitelbaum EN, Soper NJ. Ch 13. Intraoperative Ultrasound During Laparoscopic Cholecystectomy. In: Hagopian EJ, Machi J (eds). Abdominal Ultrasound for Surgeons. New York, NY: Springer Science + Business Media. 2014)

Clinical Outcomes and Comparison with Intraoperative Cholangiography

As LUS and IOC are generally used for the same two purposes, detecting CBD stones and identifying biliary anatomy, it is natural that the two modalities should be compared in regard to their efficacy in these tasks. However, while it is necessary to know the relative strengths and weaknesses of each technique, surgeons should not become solely reliant on one or the other. In some instances, it is necessary to use both imaging methods during a single operation in order to confirm the presence of choledocholithiasis or interpret confusing or aberrant anatomy. For this reason, routine practice with both methods is recommended, especially during a surgeon's early experience and when teaching surgical trainees.

LUS has several discrete advantages as compared with IOC. LUS does not use radiation and thus can be performed safely during pregnancy without exposing operating room personnel to potentially harmful radiation; furthermore, there is no need for assistance from a dedicated radiology technician. No contrast dye is used, which contraindicates IOC for patients with iodine allergy. IOC also requires cannulation of the cystic duct and therefore poses a risk of CBD injury if the biliary anatomy has been misinterpreted on initial dissection. LUS, on the other hand, is essentially without complication risk and unlike IOC can easily be performed multiple times during an operation to reassess the anatomy as dissection proceeds. In contrast, IOC generally affords a more comprehensive "road map" of biliary anat-

Table 5.1 Comparison between LUS and IOC of technique success rate and intraoperative time required to complete

		Success rate (%)		Time (min)	
Study	Number	LUS	IOC	LUS	IOC
Siperstein et al. [24]	300	100	94	–	–
Thompson et al. [17]	306	–	–	7	11
Machi et al. [14]	100	95	92	9	16
Birth et al. [12]	518	>99	92	7	16
Catheline et al. [16]	900	100	85	10	18
Tranter and Thompson [23]	135	98	90	–	–
Rijna et al. [19]	50	98	72	16	18
Greig [25]	48	100	78	13	–
Rothlin 1 [20]	100	100	93	5	16
Rothlin 2 [20]	100	100	90	5	14
Li [21]	103	100	91	9	14
Barteau [22]	125	91[a]	100	7	11
Falcone [18]	65	92	86	10	13

[a]9% of LUS did not visualize distal CBD
Abbreviations: *LUS* laparoscopic ultrasound, *IOC* intraoperative cholangiography

omy and is the first technical step in performing a laparoscopic common bile duct exploration.

In general, LUS has greater feasibility than IOC, with rates of scanning success approaching 100% with experience (Table 5.1) [12, 14, 16–25]. Reported failures are generally due to the initial learning curve or to malfunctioning equipment, whereas IOC has a defined failure rate of approximately 10% due to inability to cannulate small cystic ducts and obstruction of contrast passage due to cystic duct stones, valves, or tortuosity. In studies comparing the two modalities, LUS has been shown uniformly to have shorter completion times [12, 14, 16–23, 26].

Detection of Common Bile Duct Stones

A number of studies have evaluated the relative success of LUS and IOC for detecting CBD stones (Table 5.2) [12, 14, 16, 17, 20–25, 27]. In addition, two meta-analyses have been published comparing LUS with IOC [26, 28]. While both modalities were performed on each patient in these studies and the findings compared, there are several methodological issues that must be taken into account when evaluating their results. The most important is the absence of a gold-standard examination with which to compare the respective modalities and verify either the true presence or absence of stones. Since performing CBD exploration on all patients in this situation is ethically unjustified, a negative result on both LUS and IOC is uniformly assumed to be a true negative. This assumption has the potential to underestimate the number of false-negative exams, as missed stones can pass without

Table 5.2 Comparison between LUS and IOC of technique sensitivity and specificity

Study	Number	Sensitivity (%)		Specificity (%)	
		LUS	IOC	LUS	IOC
Siperstein et al. [24]	300	96	96	100	100
Thompson et al. [17]	360	90	98	100	98
Machi et al. [14]	100	89	88	100	98
Birth et al. [12]	518	83	100	100	99
Catheline et al. [16]	900	80	75	99	99
Tranter and Thompson [23]	135	96	86	100	99
Goletti [27]	45	88	100	100	97
Greig [25]	48/54[a]	71	83	96	95
Rothlin 1 [20]	100	100	75	98	99
Rothlin 2 [20]	100	91	64	100	100
Li [21]	103	82	75	99	99
Barteau [22]	125	71	93	100	76

[a]48 LUS, 54 IOC
Abbreviations: *LUS* laparoscopic ultrasound, *IOC* intraoperative cholangiography

causing symptoms. Likely, this is a small risk, as several studies have reported routine follow-up of patients (range 6–30 months) postoperatively, with no missed stones in the context of both tests being negative [26].

In most studies, a positive exam (on either LUS or IOC) was investigated via either surgical CBD exploration or ERCP, in order to confirm the result and clear the duct. This methodology, however, has the potential to overestimate the number of false positives, as CBD stones detected intraoperatively may have passed by the time of the CBD exploration or ERCP. Additionally, in the majority of studies, the surgeon viewed both exams without blinding, thus potentially influencing the performance and interpretation of the second test (in most cases IOC) in the instance of a positive initial result. One should evaluate the available data with these limitations in mind. Finally, ultrasonography is highly operator-dependent, making acquisition, sensitivity, specificity, and overall diagnostic accuracy variable between studies.

The two meta-analyses evaluating LUS compared with IOC determined similar sensitivity and specificity. Jamal et al. found 90% and 99% sensitivity and specificity for LUS compared to 87% and 98%, respectively, for IOC. Aziz et al. found 87% and 100% sensitivity and specificity for LUS compared to 87% and 99% for IOC. Individual studies have demonstrated sensitivity for detecting CBD stones ranges from 71% to 100% for LUS and 75% to 100% for IOC [12, 14, 16, 17, 20–25, 27]. It is instructive to take a closer look at several of the series that found LUS to be less sensitive than IOC. Thompson and colleagues found a cumulative sensitivity of 90% with LUS, as compared with 98% for IOC [17]. However, when the authors subdivided their series into three time periods, they found a sensitivity of 77% for LUS in the first cohort of 140 patients, as compared to 100% and 96% in the latter 78 and 142 patients. This improvement was primarily due to better detection of stones in the intrapancreatic portion of the distal CBD. During the second patient cohort, the authors routinely cannulated the cystic duct and injected saline in order to dilate the CBD. In the third group of patients, the authors performed this maneuver on a selective basis, only when the distal CBD could not be adequately visualized on initial examination. Similarly, Falcone et al. encountered LUS sensitivity improvement as their experience increased [18]. Surgeons with baseline experience of greater than ten LUS exams prior to the study were more likely than their less experienced colleagues to visualize the distal CBD: 73% vs 23%. When queried about the degree of difficulty in performing LUS, the more experienced cohort were more likely to consider the procedure "easy" (71% vs 24%) and less likely to consider it "difficult" (29% vs 60%).

Birth and colleagues found a sensitivity of 83% for LUS, as opposed to 100% for IOC [12]. Similar to the previously discussed studies, all four stones missed by LUS were in a pre-ampullary position in the distal CBD. Three of these missed stones were visualizable by LUS after instilling 400 ml of saline into the stomach and duodenum via a nasogastric tube. However, the authors still counted these as false negatives, as they were initially missed by LUS and only discovered after performing an IOC. The results of these two studies show that both increased operator experience and adjunct maneuvers to improve distal CBD imaging can increase LUS sensitivity to a level equal or superior to IOC. However, surgeons should keep in mind that imaging the distal CBD can be a challenging aspect of LUS. If the intrapancreatic portion of the duct cannot be clearly examined and there is suspicion of CBD stones, an IOC should be performed to confirm the absence of stones.

Although both modalities are highly specific in the detection of CBD stones, LUS is superior to IOC in this respect, with a nearly zero incidence of false positives. Although rare, false-positive results do occur during IOC, primarily due to the misinterpretation of air bubbles in the CBD as stones. For this reason, some authors have proposed using LUS as a confirmatory test when a CBD stone is detected on IOC [29].

Examination of Anatomy

In general, IOC provides a better delineation of biliary anatomy than LUS. This is because IOC allows the surgeon to simultaneously visualize the entire biliary tree, so that presumed relationship of the cystic duct with the hepatic and common bile ducts can be confirmed. In contrast, LUS is only able to visualize a single cross-sectional plane at a time. A complete view of the biliary anatomy must therefore be mentally constructed by correlating these 2D images with their position laparoscopically. This can be challenging, especially in cases with severe inflammation or aberrant anatomic configurations. One study found that LUS was only able to detect 82% of the anatomic anomalies found on IOC [30]. Another showed that IOC showed variant anatomy in 14% of cases, but LUS was unable to visualize any of these [31]. While most of these variants were in the proximal biliary tree, above the cystic duct-CBD junction, these findings caution the use of LUS for interpretation of unknown or confusing biliary anatomy. Our preference is to use IOC during cases in which a difficult dissection or unusual anatomy makes identification of the ductal relationships uncertain.

LUS does, however, provide several advantages over IOC with regard to anatomic examination. The ability to overlay color Doppler signaling on the sonographic image can be extremely helpful in delineating vascular from ductal structures. This can aid in confirming variations in arterial anatomy, such as a replaced right hepatic artery that could be potentially injured during dissection of the hepatocystic triangle. LUS also provides a more accurate measure of distance than IOC—important in reliably determining ductal diameters, stone size, and the interval between two anatomic structures. In general, IOC tends to overestimate the true diameter of the CBD due to dilation after contrast injection, blurring of duct edges, and the lack of a reliable reference length on the same plane as the duct [12]. Lastly, LUS does not require cystic duct cannulation and can be used multiple times throughout an operation. These characteristics often make its use advantageous to IOC during cases of severe cholecystitis, if the ductal structures cannot be easily identified early in the dissection [32].

Several studies have addressed the issue of whether the use of routine LUS for anatomic identification leads to a decrease in rates of CBD injury and other biliary complications.

Similar to IOC, there is only circumstantial evidence regarding this assertion, and the ability of either routine imaging modality to decrease CBD injury remains controversial even after 20 years of debate and study. Biffl and colleagues compared rates of biliary complications at a single institution in which two surgeons used LUS on a routine basis while the other three surgeons used IOC selectively [33]. The routine LUS group had no biliary complications, whereas the non-LUS surgeons had a 2.5% biliary complication rate, including a 0.8% rate of CBD injury and 0.7% rate of retained CBD stones. This disparity occurred despite the fact that the non-LUS surgeons performed more operations on average, with a lower percentage of patients operated on for acute cholecystitis. Another multicenter study showed that over a series of 1381 laparoscopic cholecystectomies with routine LUS, no CBD injuries occurred [34]. In these cases, use of LUS to delineate biliary anatomy was able to prevent conversion to open surgery in 6% of cases. Additionally, the authors found that supplementary IOC was only truly necessary in 2% of the cases.

Cost

While patient safety and the avoidance of biliary complications should be the primary concerns when evaluating the use of LUS or IOC, the cost associated with these modalities is an important secondary consideration, especially if they are to be employed on a routine basis. Although the initial purchase cost of an ultrasound scanner is substantial, it can be used during a multitude of operations across several surgical subspecialties. Several studies have shown LUS to be less expensive than IOC on a per-case basis, primarily due to the use of disposable catheters and the cost of a radiology technician during IOC. One study found that LUS cost on average $131, as opposed to $408 for IOC [35]. The authors calculated that even if IOC was used on a selective basis, its cost would average out to $157 per cholecystectomy performed and thus still be more expensive than routine LUS. Another study found a per-case cost of $362 and $665 for LUS and IOC, respectively, and that based on this differential, the cost of the ultrasound scanner itself would be recouped after 95 uses [27]. A recent study looking at cost-effectiveness of routine LUS compared to routine IOC and expectant management demonstrated LUS superiority in terms of both quality-adjusted life years (QALY) and cost per case [36]. An examination of our own data based on disposable equipment and additional operating time showed cost savings of $145 per case with LUS as compared with IOC [10].

Conclusion

LUS provides an excellent means of examining the biliary tree during laparoscopic cholecystectomy, with the primary goals of defining anatomic relationships and detecting choledocholithiasis. Beyond achieving these objectives, LUS allows the surgeon to look within the hepatocystic triangle and the hepatoduodenal ligament prior to and during the progression of surgical dissection. This allows for a more in-depth understanding of the often disorienting and potentially dangerous two-dimensional laparoscopic view of these complex anatomic structures. For this reason, we employ LUS in a routine fashion and make a point of incorporating its use into the curriculum for medical students and surgical residents. While LUS offers many advantages over IOC, the two modalities should be seen as complementary. Whether utilized in a routine or selective manner, it is essential for the modern laparoscopic surgeon to have a familiarity and facility with both techniques, in order to optimize patient safety and streamline the detection and treatment of CBD stones during laparoscopic cholecystectomy.

References

1. Lane RJ, Coupland GA. Ultrasonic indications to explore the common bile duct. Surgery. 1982;91(3):268–74.
2. Sigel B, Machi J, Beitler JC, Donahue PE, Bombeck CT, Baker RJ, et al. Comparative accuracy of operative ultrasonography and cholangiography in detecting common duct calculi. Surgery. 1983;94(4):715–20.
3. Jakimowicz JJ, Rutten H, Jurgens PJ, Carol EJ. Comparison of operative ultrasonography and radiography in screening of the common bile duct for calculi. World J Surg. 1987;11(5):628–34.
4. Strasberg SM, Hertl M, Soper NJ. An analysis of the problem of biliary injury during laparoscopic cholecystectomy. J Am Coll Surg. 1995;180(1):101–25.
5. Hakamada K, Narumi S, Toyoki Y, Nara M, Oohashi M, Miura T, et al. Intraoperative ultrasound as an educational guide for laparoscopic biliary surgery. World J Gastroenterol. 2008;14(15):2370–6.

6. Soper NJ. The utility of ultrasonography for screening the common bile duct during laparoscopic cholecystectomy. J Laparoendosc Adv Surg Tech A. 1997;7(5):271–6.
7. Strasberg SM, Brunt LM. Rationale and use of the critical view of safety in laparoscopic cholecystectomy. J Am Coll Surg. 2010;211(1):132–8.
8. Perry KA, Myers JA, Deziel DJ. Laparoscopic ultrasound as the primary method for bile duct imaging during cholecystectomy. Surg Endosc. 2008;22(1):208–13.
9. Santambrogio R, Bianchi P, Opocher E, Verga M, Montorsi M. Prevalence and laparoscopic ultrasound patterns of choledocholithiasis and biliary sludge during cholecystectomy. Surg Laparosc Endosc Percutan Tech. 1999;9(2):129–34.
10. Wu JS, Dunnegan DL, Soper NJ. The utility of intracorporeal ultrasonography for screening of the bile duct during laparoscopic cholecystectomy. J Gastrointest Surg. 1998;2(1):50–60.
11. Halpin VJ, Dunnegan D, Soper NJ. Laparoscopic intracorporeal ultrasound versus fluoroscopic intraoperative cholangiography: after the learning curve. Surg Endosc. 2002;16(2):336–41. Epub 2002/04/23
12. Birth M, Ehlers KU, Delinikolas K, Weiser HF. Prospective randomized comparison of laparoscopic ultrasonography using a flexible-tip ultrasound probe and intraoperative dynamic cholangiography during laparoscopic cholecystectomy. Surg Endosc. 1998;12(1):30–6.
13. Catheline JM, Turner R, Rizk N, Barrat C, Buenos P, Champault G. Evaluation of the biliary tree during laparoscopic cholecystectomy: laparoscopic ultrasound versus intraoperative cholangiography: a prospective study of 150 cases. Surg Laparosc Endosc. 1998;8(2):85–91.
14. Machi J, Tateishi T, Oishi AJ, Furumoto NL, Oishi RH, Uchida S, et al. Laparoscopic ultrasonography versus operative cholangiography during laparoscopic cholecystectomy: review of the literature and a comparison with open intraoperative ultrasonography. J Am Coll Surg. 1999;188(4):360–7.
15. Tomonaga T, Filipi CJ, Lowham A, Martinez T. Laparoscopic intracorporeal ultrasound cystic duct length measurement: a new technique to prevent common bile duct injuries. Surg Endosc. 1999;13(2):183–5.
16. Catheline JM, Turner R, Paries J. Laparoscopic ultrasonography is a complement to cholangiography for the detection of choledocholithiasis at laparoscopic cholecystectomy. Br J Surg. 2002;89(10):1235–9.
17. Thompson DM, Arregui ME, Tetik C, Madden MT, Wegener M. A comparison of laparoscopic ultrasound with digital fluorocholangiography for detecting choledocholithiasis during laparoscopic cholecystectomy. Surg Endosc. 1998;12(7):929–32.
18. Falcone RA Jr, Fegelman EJ, Nussbaum MS, Brown DL, Bebbe TM, Merhar GL, et al. A prospective comparison of laparoscopic ultrasound vs intraoperative cholangiogram during laparoscopic cholecystectomy. Surg Endosc. 1999;13(8):784–8.
19. Rijna H, Eijsbouts QA, Barkhof F, de Brauw LM, Cuesta MA. Assessment of the biliary tract by ultrasonography and cholangiography during laparoscopic cholecystectomy: a prospective study. Eur J Ultrasound. 1999;9(2):127–33.
20. Röthlin MA, Schöb O, Schlumpf R, Largiadèr F. Laparoscopic ultrasonography during cholecystectomy. Br J Surg. 1996;83:1512–6.
21. Li JW, Feng B, Wu L, Wang ML, Lu AG, Zang L, et al. Intraoperative cholangiography and laparoscopic ultrasonography are complementary in the detection of occult choledocholithiasis. Med Sci Monit. 2009;15(9):126–30.
22. Barteau JA, Castro D, Arregui ME, Tetik C. A comparison of intraoperative ultrasound versus cholangiography in the evaluation of the common bile duct during laparoscopic cholecystectomy. Surg Endosc. 1995;9(5):490–6.
23. Tranter SE, Thompson MH. A prospective single-blinded controlled study comparing laparoscopic ultrasound of the common bile duct with operative cholangiography. Surg Endosc. 2003;17(2):216–9.
24. Siperstein A, Pearl J, Macho J, Hansen P, Gitomirsky A, Rogers S. Comparison of laparoscopic ultrasonography and fluorocholangiography in 300 patients undergoing laparoscopic cholecystectomy. Surg Endosc. 1999;13(2):113–7.

25. Greig JD, John TG, Mahadaven M, Garden OJ. Laparoscopic ultrasonography in the evaluation of the biliary tree during laparoscopic cholecystectomy. Br J Surg. 1994;81:1202–6.
26. Jamal KN, Smith H, Ratnasingham K, Siddiqui MR, McLachlan G, Belgaumkar AP. Meta-analysis of the diagnostic accuracy of laparoscopic ultrasonography and intraoperative cholangiography in detection of common bile duct stones. Ann R Coll Surg Engl. 2016;98(4):244–9.
27. Goletti O, Buccianti P, Ferrari M, Celona G, Chiarugi M, Cavina E. Laparoscopic sonography: a real alternative to cholangiography during laparoscopic cholecystectomy? Hepato-Gastroenterology. 1995;42(5):612–8.
28. Aziz O, Ashrafian H, Jones C, Harling L, Kumar S, Garas G, Holme T, Darzi A, Zacharakis E, Athanasiou T. Laparoscopic ultrasonography versus intra-operative cholangiogram for the detection of common bile duct stones during laparoscopic cholecystectomy: a meta-analysis of diagnostic accuracy. Int J Surg. 2014;12(7):712–9.
29. Kimura T, Umehara Y, Yoshida M, Sakuramachi S, Kawabe A, Suzuki K. Laparoscopic ultrasonography and operative cholangiography prevent residual common bile duct stones in laparoscopic cholecystectomy. Surg Laparosc Endosc Percutan Tech. 1999;9(2):124–8.
30. Rothlin M, Largiader F. The anatomy of the hepatoduodenal ligament in laparoscopic sonography. Surg Endosc. 1994;8(3):173–80.
31. Teefey SA, Soper NJ, Middleton WD, Balfe DM, Brink JA, Strasberg SM, et al. Imaging of the common bile duct during laparoscopic cholecystectomy: sonography versus videofluoroscopic cholangiography. AJR Am J Roentgenol. 1995;165(4):847–51.
32. Pfluke JM, Bowers SP Jr. Laparoscopic intraoperative biliary ultrasonography: findings during laparoscopic cholecystectomy for acute disease. J Laparoendosc Adv Surg Tech A. 2011;21(6):505–9.
33. Biffl WL, Moore EE, Offner PJ, Franciose RJ, Burch JM. Routine intraoperative laparoscopic ultrasonography with selective cholangiography reduces bile duct complications during laparoscopic cholecystectomy. J Am Coll Surg. 2001;193(3):272–80.
34. Machi J, Johnson JO, Deziel DJ, Soper NJ, Berber E, Siperstein A, et al. The routine use of laparoscopic ultrasound decreases bile duct injury: a multicenter study. Surg Endosc. 2009;23(2):384–8.
35. Machi J, Oishi AJ, Tajiri T, Murayama KM, Furumoto NL, Oishi RH. Routine laparoscopic ultrasound can significantly reduce the need for selective intraoperative cholangiography during cholecystectomy. Surg Endosc. 2007;21(2):270–4.
36. Sun SX, Kulaylat AN, Hollenbeak CS, Soybel DI. Cost-effective decisions in detecting silent common bile duct gallstones during laparoscopic cholecystectomy. Ann Surg. 2016;263(6):1164–72.

Chapter 6
Laparoscopic Transcystic Common Bile Duct Exploration

Joseph B. Petelin and Timothy Mayfield

Overview

Choledocholithiasis is present in approximately 10% of those patients who have gallbladder stones [1, 2]. Surgeons have historically been expected to handle both of these problems in one setting [3]. Today many surgeons feel that laparoscopic common bile duct exploration (LCDE) is too time-consuming and difficult, especially considering the inadequate reimbursement associated with it. Nevertheless a number of techniques and instruments have been developed to facilitate LCDE [4–9]. Many of these maneuvers can be accomplished without the need to purchase expensive flexible choledochoscopic equipment. These techniques include flushing of the ductal system after administering glucagon, dilatation of the distal common bile duct/sphincter and flushing, balloon catheter manipulation, and basket manipulation—with or without fluoroscopic guidance. Choledochoscopic LCDE obviously requires investment in more expensive equipment, but the investment is very much worth the expense from a patient's perspective.

In general, less invasive techniques to common bile duct (CBD) stone removal via a transcystic duct approach are preferred over a transductal (choledochotomy) approach if possible because of lower morbidity, less operating time, and less stress on the surgeon (i.e., no need to suture the common bile duct and/or place a T-tube

Electronic supplementary material The online version of this chapter (doi: 10.1007/978-3-319-74503-9_6) contains supplementary material, which is available to authorized users.

J. B. Petelin, MD, FACS (✉)
Surgix™ Minimally Invasive Surgery Institute, Shawnee Mission, Kansas 66204, USA

Department of Surgery, Shawnee Mission Medical Center, Shawnee, KS, USA

T. Mayfield, MD
Department of General Surgery, UnityPoint Clinic Surgery, Des Moines, IA, USA

© Springer International Publishing AG, part of Springer Nature 2018

B. F. Santos, N. Soper (eds.), *Choledocholithiasis*,
https://doi.org/10.1007/978-3-319-74503-9_6

with the transcystic approach in most cases). The most important and fundamental requirement for the surgeon is to determine which approach is best for a given patient. What follows is a description of the preferred algorithm for decision-making, the necessary equipment, the room setup, and finally the technical maneuvers that are most likely to be successful.

Managing Patients with Common Bile Duct Stones

When CBD stones are identified preoperatively, endoscopic retrograde cholangiography and extraction with or without sphincterotomy (ERC +/− S) before operation are an option, but laparoscopic cholecystectomy (LC) and laparoscopic common duct exploration (LCDE) are a more efficient and less costly approach. Successful clearance of CBD stones and independent morbidity and mortality are equivalent with these two options. However, routine preoperative use of ERC +/− S for patients suspected of having CBD stones is associated with a normal exam in 40–60% of cases and subjects the patient to the added morbidity (~8 to 15%) of the ERC +/− S [10].

Common bile duct stones discovered during laparoscopic cholecystectomy are most cost-effectively and efficiently removed during the same operation, but simultaneous or subsequent ERC +/− S is an option, albeit a more expensive and inefficient one. Conversion of the procedure to an "open" common duct exploration or leaving the stones in place for postoperative ERC +/− S depends on the patient's status, the surgeon's ability, and the local availability of expert endoscopists.

When CBD stones are encountered postoperatively, they are best treated initially with ERC +/− S in most cases. If this is not successful, then repeat surgical intervention may be necessary (Fig. 6.1).

Equipment and Room Setup

The equipment that may be needed to perform LCDE is listed in Table 6.1. In most cases, only a handful of these items is required. LCDE equipment should be located in a central location near the operating room where biliary surgery is performed. This prevents physician and nurse frustration and delays when the nurse does not have to rummage through the entire supply room to find the needed items. In the operating room, LCDE equipment should be placed on a separate Mayo stand located near the surgeon if at all possible. I find it most convenient to stand in the same location on the patient's left side as for laparoscopic cholecystectomy (Fig. 6.2).

While these considerations might seem superfluous, most successful biliary tract surgeons would agree that proper preoperative organization significantly facilitates LCDE.

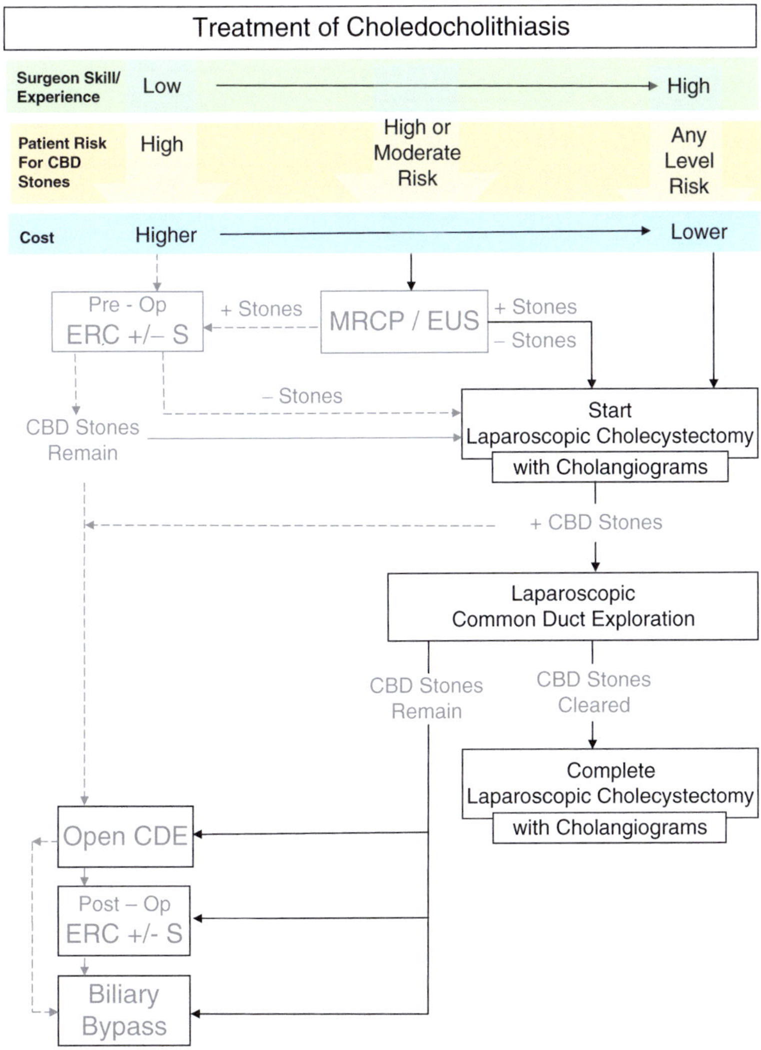

Fig. 6.1 Algorithm for surgical treatment of CBD stones

Access to the Common Duct

The least invasive approach for LCDE is via the cystic duct. Laparoscopic common bile duct exploration may be accomplished through a choledochotomy but is associated with increased morbidity, operative time, and length of stay—as documented in numerous studies. Conditions that may influence the best approach include the stone size and number of stones, the anatomy of the triangle of Calot,

Table 6.1 Equipment for LCDE

Items for transcystic approach to LCDE (some or all of this equipment may be needed)
14-gauge IV catheter, >2 in. in length
Fluoroscope (C-arm type)
Glucagon, 1–2 mg (given IV by the anesthetist)
Balloon-tipped catheters (4 French preferred over 3 French and 5 French)
Segura type baskets (4-wire, flat, straight, in-line configuration, <1 mm diameter total)
0.035 in. diameter long (>90 cm) guide wire
Mechanical "over-the-wire" dilators (7–12 French) (found in most urology departments)
High-pressure "over-the-wire" pneumatic dilator
IV tubing (for saline instillation through the choledochoscope)
Atraumatic grasping forceps (for choledochoscope manipulation)
Flexible choledochoscope with light source (smaller <3 mm diameter, with >1.1 mm working channel preferred)
Second camera
Second monitor (or second viewing area on the primary laparoscopic monitor)
Video switcher (for simultaneous same monitor display of laparoscopic and choledochoscopic or fluoroscopic images)
Waterpik™ (Teledyne, Fort Collins, CO)
Electrohydraulic or pulsed dye lithotripter

IV intravenous

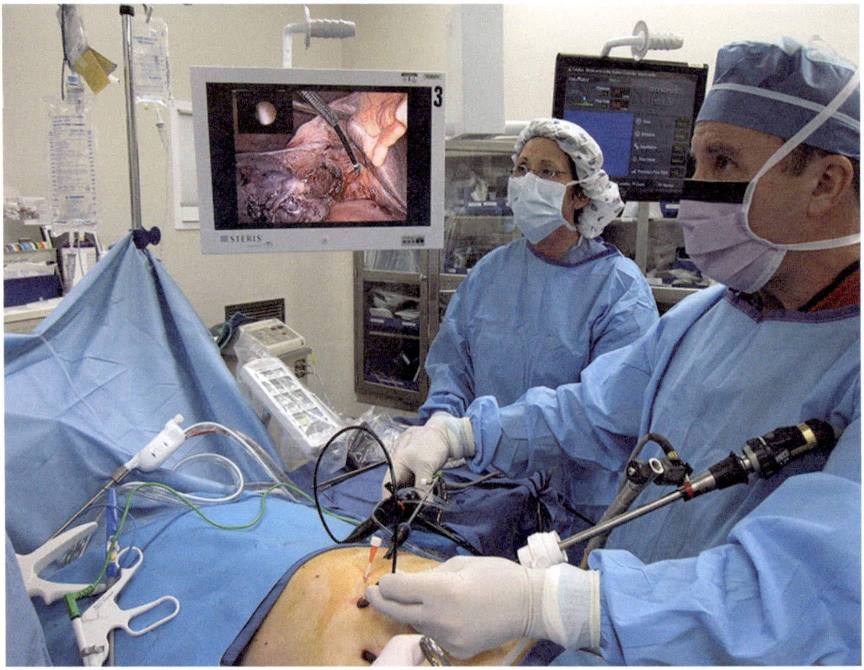

Fig. 6.2 Surgeon position for scope manipulation

the position of the cystic duct-common duct junction, the course of the cystic duct, the diameter of each of the ducts, the location of stones (e.g., hepatic ducts vs. CBD), and the degree of inflammation in the porta hepatis. Negative factors have more influence on the choice of access than positive ones. For example, stones >6 mm in diameter and intrahepatic stones are best approached through a choledochotomy. Similarly if the cystic duct is less than 4 mm in diameter, a choledochotomy is preferred. However if the common bile duct is <6 mm in diameter, then a transcystic approach would probably be safer. If the cystic duct joins the common duct medially, posteriorly, or distally, then a choledochotomy may be preferred. If there is tremendous inflammation in the porta hepatis, then accessing the common duct might be more difficult. Finally, if the surgeon's laparoscopic suturing skill is lacking, then a choledochotomy would likely be inadvisable (Table 6.2).

Table 6.2 Factors influencing LCDE approach

	Influence on approach	
Factor	Transcystic	Choledochotomy
Stone characteristics		
One stone	+	+
Multiple stones	+	+
Stones <6 mm diameter	+	+
Stones >6 mm diameter	–	Preferred approach
Intrahepatic stones	–	Preferred approach
Duct diameters		
Diameter of cystic duct <4 mm	–	Preferred approach
Diameter of cystic duct >4 mm	+	+
Diameter of common duct <6 mm	Preferred approach	–
Diameter of common duct >6 mm	+	+
Cystic duct location		
Cystic duct entrance-lateral	+	+
Cystic duct entrance-medial	–	Preferred approach
Cystic duct entrance-posterior	–	Preferred approach
Cystic duct entrance-distal	–	Preferred approach
Local conditions		
Inflammation-mild	+	+
Inflammation-marked	Preferred approach	–
Surgeon skill set		
Suturing ability-poor	Preferred approach	–
Suturing ability-good	+	+

+ *indicates a positive or neutral effect* on the approach
– *indicates a negative effect* on the approach
Negative factors have more influence on the approach than positive ones

Operative Details

Ductal Imaging: Defining the Anatomy and Finding the Stones

Fluoroscopic intraoperative cholangiography (IOC) allows real-time scanning of the ducts, provides a stable and accessible map of the anatomy, and is relatively easy to perform in most cases. It is the preferred method of imaging the ductal system for most surgeons. Some surgeons prefer laparoscopic ultrasonography (LUS), but LUS does not leave the surgeon with a ductal map and may be less effective in detecting intrahepatic stones than IOC. Delineation of the anatomy of the cystic duct and its relationship to the CBD is essential in determining whether a transcystic or a transductal approach is most appropriate (Fig. 6.3). For example, if the cystic duct is long and tortuous and enters the common bile duct quite distally, then access to common bile duct stones will be much more difficult if not impossible. Additionally, if the common bile duct diameter is less than 6 mm, then performing a choledochotomy and suturing it without creating a stricture would potentially present more room for error. The technical details for performing IOC are detailed in Chap. 4.

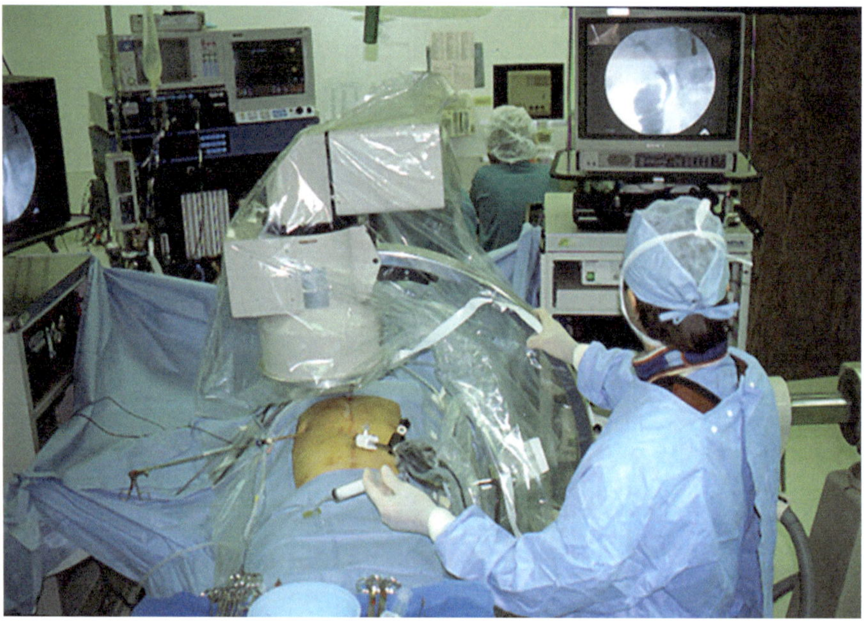

Fig. 6.3 Intraoperative cholangiograms

Preparing the Cystic Duct and/or Common Duct

When choledochoscopic maneuvers are attempted through the cystic duct, it will need to accept a 9 or 10 French diameter flexible scope. Over-the-wire mechanical graduated dilators or pneumatic dilators may be used to dilate the cystic duct if it is not already large enough to accept the scope (Figs. 6.4 and 6.5).

With either type of dilator, a guide wire (0.028 in. or 0.035 in. diameter) is first inserted through the midclavicular port, through the cystic duct, and into the common duct. When using graduated dilators, a 9 French size is usually the first to be advanced over the wire into the duct. Each successively larger dilator is advanced over the wire until the duct is patulous enough to accept the scope. I have found that if a 9 French over-the-wire dilator will not initially easily enter the cystic duct, then it is unlikely that safe dilatation to a large enough diameter to remove stones (11 or 12 French) will occur. Pneumatic dilators, which are much more costly and not reusable, may also be advanced over the wire into the cystic duct. The dilatation balloon is filled using a screw-type Levine syringe while observing both the ductal changes on the video monitor and the pressure changes on the gauge attached to the dilator syringe.

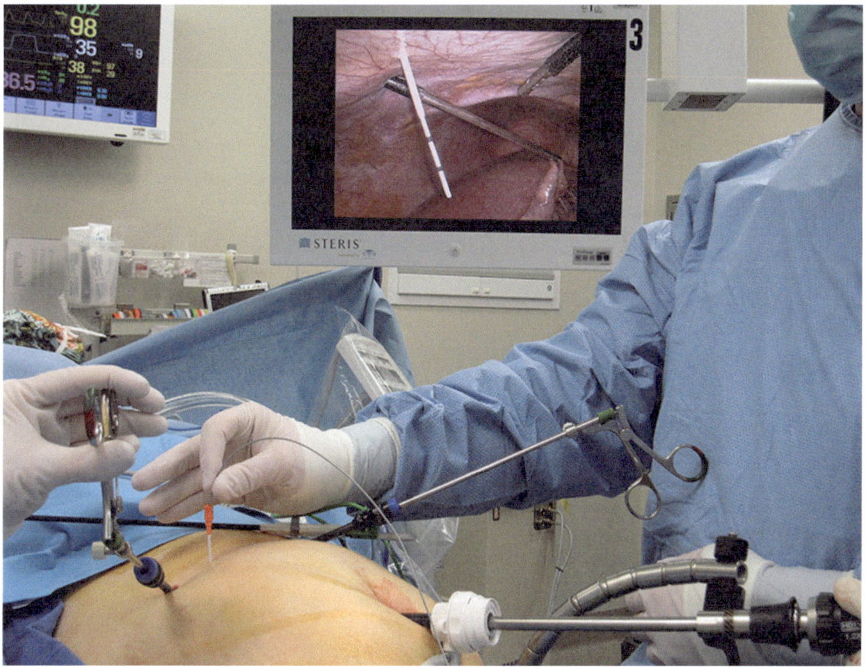

Fig. 6.4 Insertion of cholangiocath into 14-gauge angiocath

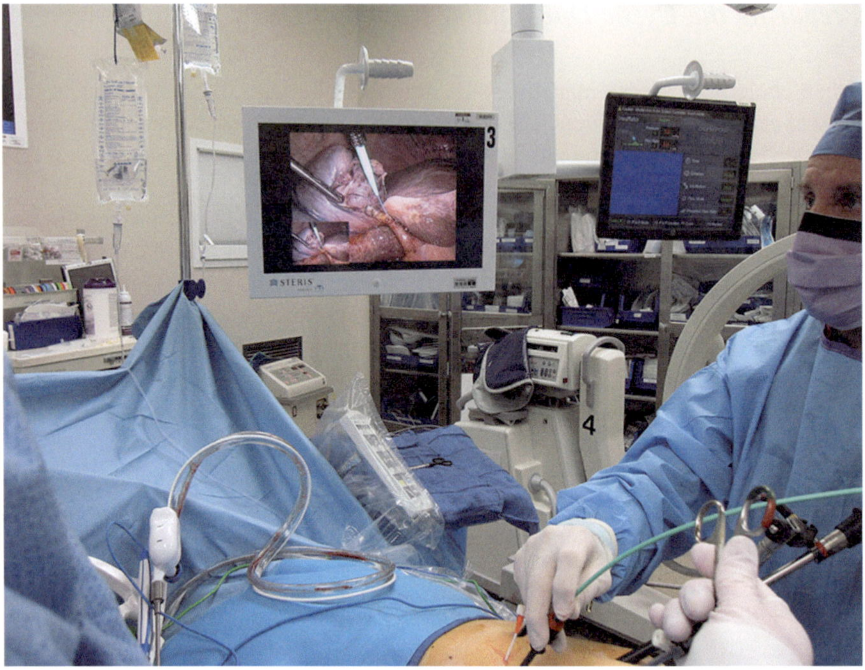

Fig. 6.5 Using over-the-wire dilators to dilate the cystic duct

Fig. 6.6 Wire insertion into scope working channel facilitates ductal entrance

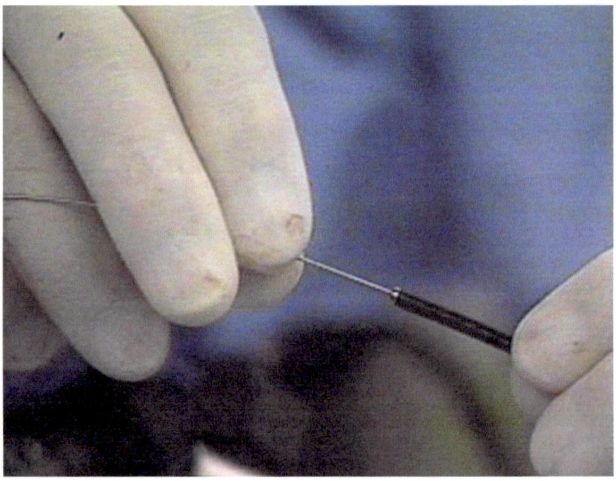

After dilatation, the guide wire may be removed or left in place for subsequent guidance of the choledochoscope into the ductal system. When it is used to guide the scope, the wire is loaded into the distal end of the working channel of the scope, which is then advanced into the ductal system over the wire (Fig. 6.6).

In difficult cases where the cystic duct pursues a circuitous course into the CBD, the lateral duodenal and ductal attachments may be released in order to "unwrap"

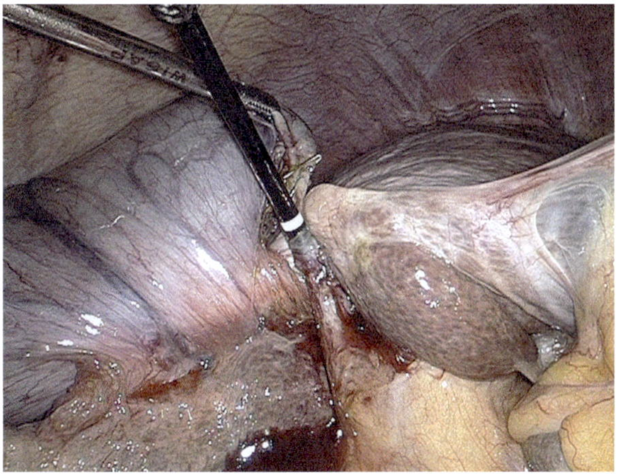

Fig. 6.7 Retraction of the gallbladder fundus toward the right diaphragm

the ductal system. It is also extremely important during transcystic choledochoscopy that proper retraction of the gallbladder and cystic duct be maintained in order keep the system as linear as possible. Usually this means that the gallbladder fundus is displaced toward the right hemidiaphragm by the assistant, while the operating surgeon performs the choledochoscopic and/or basket maneuvers. This not only straightens the extrahepatic ductal system but also displaces it anteriorly, bringing it into better view of the laparoscope. When this critical step is not followed, the cystic duct and the common duct collapse and wrinkle in an "accordion" fashion, thereby eliminating any possibility of efficient choledochoscopy. This is one of the added exigencies that the operating surgeon must deal with, and it is a very common source of frustration when an initial great choledochoscopic view of the CBD vanishes "for no apparent reason." So it is important to constantly check and recheck that the assistant is maintaining this retraction as he or she becomes mesmerized with the multitasking laparoscopic and choledochoscopic skills of the operating surgeon (Fig. 6.7).

Choledochotomy

Some authors prefer common duct access via a choledochotomy. Others use this approach when the cystic duct cannot be dilated enough to accept passage of the scope or the largest common duct stone or if intrahepatic pathology is suspected. A longitudinal incision, avoiding the CBD blood supply, approximately 1 cm in length, or as long as the diameter of the largest stone, is recommended by most authors (Fig. 6.8). This limits the amount of time that will be spent later in closing the choledochotomy. Stay sutures, which were commonly used in open common duct exploration, are not necessary and potentially harmful during LCDE because they can tear out of the duct during LCDE manipulations—making subsequent common bile duct closure much more difficult. Additionally, stay sutures would generally require extra ports and an assistant to carefully manage them.

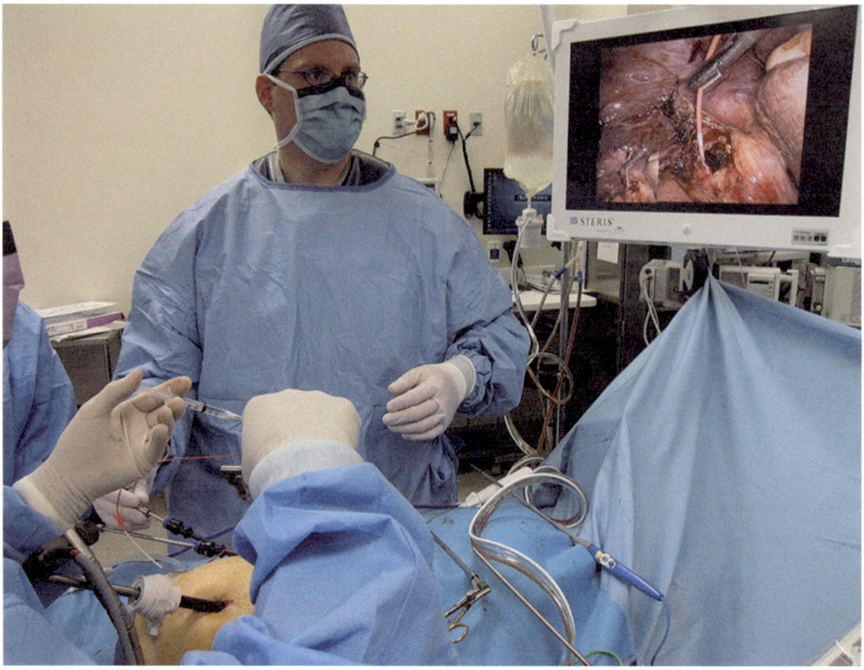

Fig. 6.8 Choledochotomy and stone capture with balloon catheter

Irrigation Techniques

When very small stones (< 3 mm diameter), sludge, or sphincter spasm is suspected to be responsible for lack of flow of contrast into the duodenum, glucagon (1–2 mg intravenous [IV]) may be administered by the anesthetist in order to relieve sphincter pressure. Transcystic flushing of the duct with saline or contrast material should be attempted after 30 s of administration in an attempt to gently force the debris into the duodenum. The process is monitored fluoroscopically. This technique often works well for 1–2 mm stones, but stones ≥4 mm are not likely to be flushed from the duct (Fig. 6.9).

Balloon Maneuvers

To employ this technique, a standard 4 French Fogarty balloon catheter is inserted into the abdomen through the 14-gauge sleeve that was used to perform the percutaneous cholangiograms. The catheter is guided into the common duct through the cystic duct with forceps introduced through the medial epigastric port in the same manner in which the cholangiogram catheter was introduced. The catheter is advanced all the way into the duodenum if possible. In my experience, when the

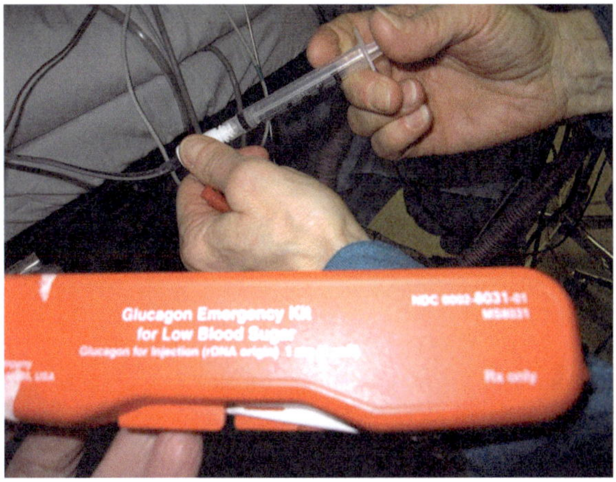

Fig. 6.9 Glucagon administration by the anesthetist

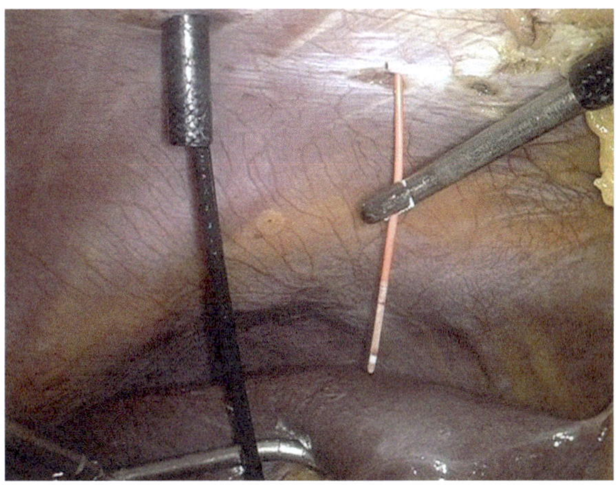

Fig. 6.10 Fogarty insertion through 14-gauge sleeve into the abdomen

10 cm mark on the catheter is visible at the cystic duct orifice through which it was inserted, the tip is generally in the duodenum. The balloon is inflated, and the catheter is gently withdrawn until resistance is met at the sphincter; the duodenum is observed to move with the catheter at this point. The balloon is deflated, the catheter is withdrawn 1 cm, and the balloon is reinflated. This should position it in the most distal portion of the duct, just proximal to the sphincter. The catheter is then withdrawn through the cystic duct using traction from the forceps via the medial epigastric port, keeping the catheter parallel to the duct. It is important to avoid simply pulling the catheter from its insertion at the skin level to avoid damage to the cystic duct. Stones expressed from the cystic duct are usually removed through one of the larger ports. In the uncommon event of displacement of the stone into the proximal hepatic duct, irrigation of the duct combined with changes in the operating table position will usually return the stone to the distal duct (Fig. 6.10).

When a choledochotomy is needed, the combined use of the choledochoscope and a balloon catheter is particularly useful for stones that defy capture with a basket, even under direct vision through the choledochoscope. The balloon is inserted alongside the scope (not in the scope channel). The balloon is advanced past the stone, inflated, and withdrawn to impact the stone against the scope. The entire scope-stone-balloon ensemble is then withdrawn through the ductal orifice. This technique is especially useful when dealing with intrahepatic stones. For intrahepatic stones, a 3 French Fogarty™ is usually employed because of the smaller diameter of the hepatic radicles.

Basket Maneuvers

Stone retrieval baskets may be used with or without a choledochoscope. When used independently the basket is inserted through the 14-gauge sleeve used for cholangiography. It is advanced into the common duct through the cystic duct, using forceps introduced through the medial epigastric port. The basket is opened immediately after it enters the proximal common bile duct. The deployed wires offer not only a "soft" distal end to the catheter but also provide increased resistance when the catheter reaches the distal end of the bile duct. When the basket is located in the distal common duct, it is moved back and forth in small increments while slowly withdrawing it as the wires of the basket are being closed. Stone capture is identified when the basket fails to close completely. The captured stone is removed through the cystic duct, and the stones are delivered from the abdomen as described previously. Great care must be exercised with this method so that accidental "capture" of the papilla of Vater does not occur.

A fluoroscope may be used to more accurately localize the stone(s) and basket tip (Fig. 6.11), but this technique requires positioning of the fluoroscope in such a

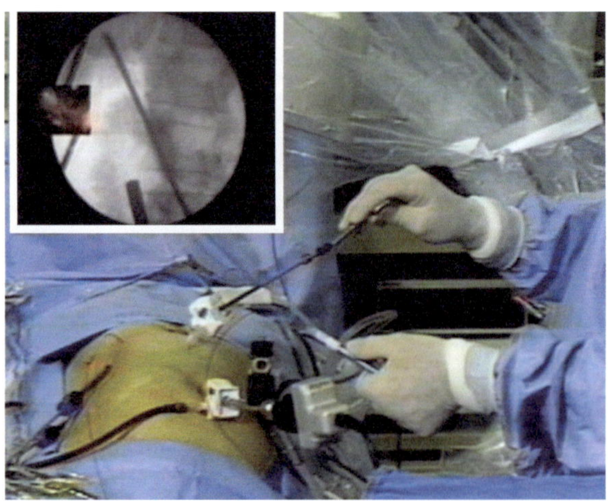

Fig. 6.11 Basket maneuvers with fluoroscopy. Note basket entry through the abdominal wall

way as to avoid interference with movements of the forceps in the medial epigastric port. This may be difficult to accomplish, especially in the obese patient.

Choledochoscopy

Choledochoscopic techniques are used when the conservative measures previously described fail to clear the common duct (Video 6.1). Interestingly, the aforementioned techniques are very often employed, while the nursing staff is preparing the choledochoscope and its accessories; and not infrequently, the common duct is cleared before the choledochoscope is even opened.

The choledochoscope is inserted in the most direct route to the triangle of Calot (usually via the midclavicular port) and, with or without wire guidance, into the cystic duct or the choledochotomy. It is very important to keep the port through which the scope is inserted oriented toward the cystic duct-common duct junction. In "the heat of the battle," it is common for the surgeon to unknowingly divert the tip of the scope insertion port away from this area toward the right lateral abdomen; this ensures that the choledochoscope must make at least two 90° turns before it enters the CBD, where it needs to usually make more turns, rendering the procedure nearly impossible (Fig. 6.12a, b).

When the transcystic duct approach is employed, if the scope will not traverse the cystic duct-common duct junction, further dissection along the lateral border of the cystic and common bile duct or a Kocher maneuver may provide a less convoluted path into the common duct. Note, however, that access to the proximal hepatic ductal system is usually not possible unless the cystic duct is very short or patulous and oriented at 90° to the common duct. When a choledochotomy is used, the scope may be directed either into the proximal system or the distal bile duct (Fig. 6.13).

Choledochoscope manipulations must be made accurately and extremely gently in order to accomplish the task at hand without destroying an expensive instrument. (When the latter happens, usually a third-tier hospital manager decides that LCDE is not worthwhile and refuses to provide new scopes.) At the level of the skin, the surgeon initially uses an atraumatic forceps inserted through the medial epigastric port to help guide the scope into the common duct. This is essentially the type of maneuver that is used to insert the cholangiogram catheter for cholangiography, hence the importance of performing routine cholangiography to practice this maneuver (Fig. 6.14). Saline instillation through the working channel of the scope is employed at this time in order to expand the common duct and provide better visualization. Further manipulations require the surgeon to use both hands on the scope in most cases. One hand controls the twisting maneuvers on the body of the scope at the port site, while the other holds the scope head and directs the tip of the scope with the deflection lever located there. Safe control of the scope as it enters the port is essential to avoid severely angulating and damaging the scope at that point (Fig. 6.15). The choledochoscopic and laparoscopic images must be kept in view,

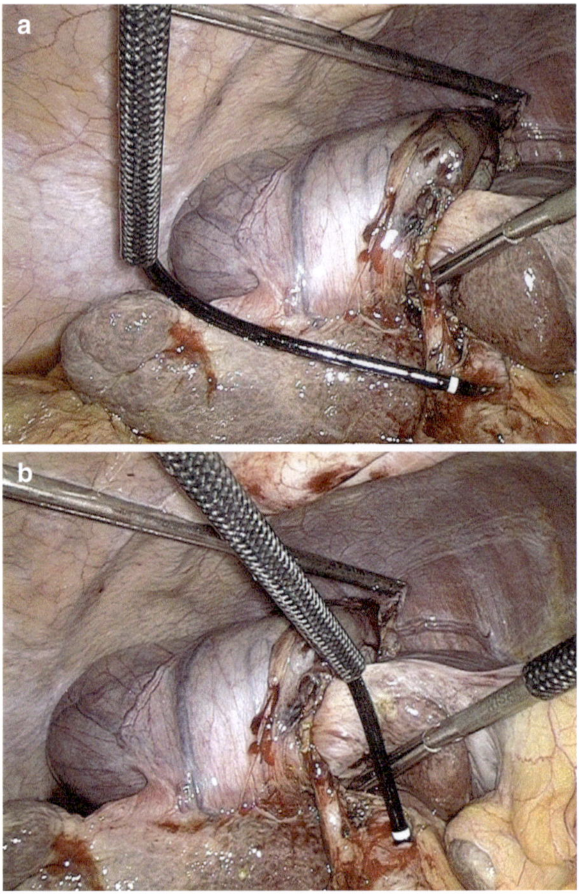

Fig. 6.12 (**a**) Incorrect scope port orientation. (**b**) The correct scope port orientation

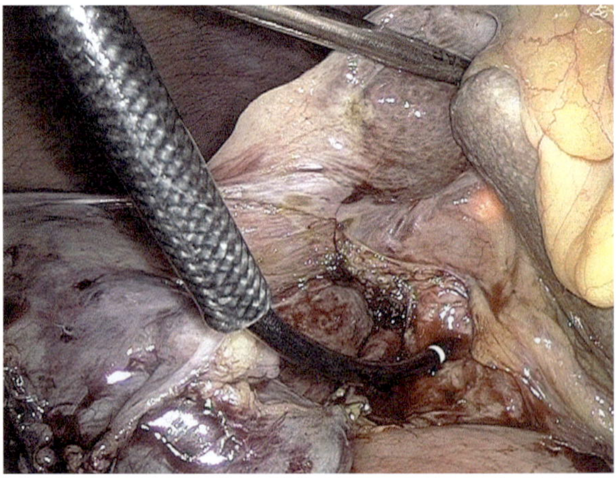

Fig. 6.13 Scope into choledochotomy; Choledochotomy facilitates intra-hepatic endoscopy as illustrated here

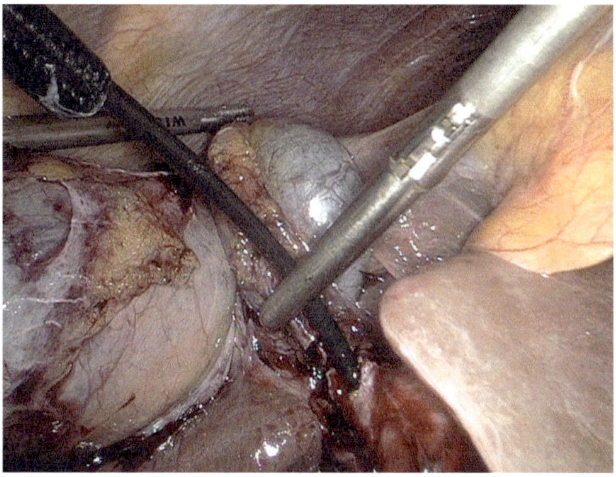

Fig. 6.14 Scope insertion into cystic duct

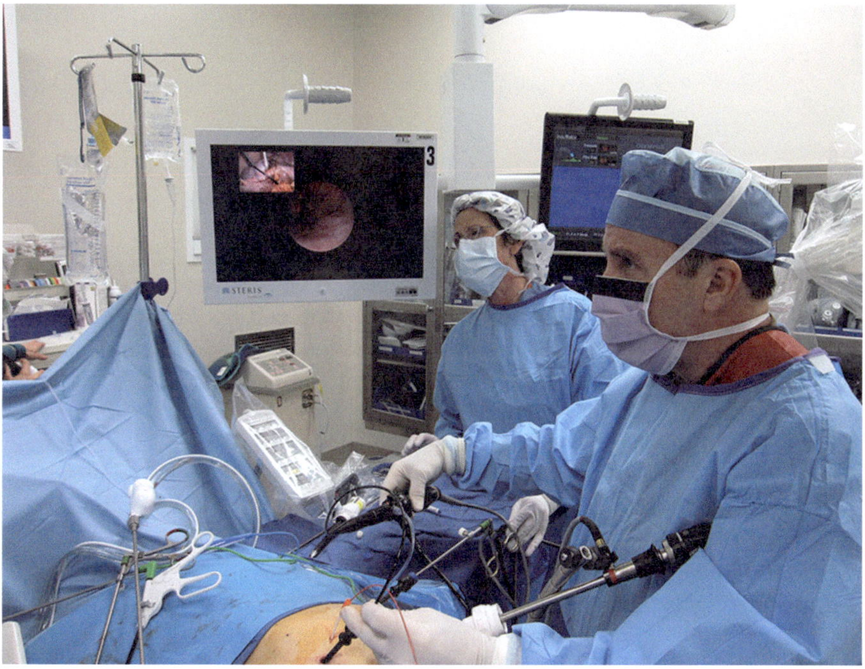

Fig. 6.15 Careful scope manipulations; Note: Gentle manipulations with the surgeon's right and left hand are extremely important to avoid scope damage

either on separate monitors or preferably on the same screen with a video switcher—a technological application we introduced in 1990 (Fig. 6.16).

There are at least two extremely essential considerations to facilitate successful choledochoscopy, as mentioned earlier: (1) the gallbladder fundus must be displaced toward the diaphragm, or the common bile duct collapses; and (2) the

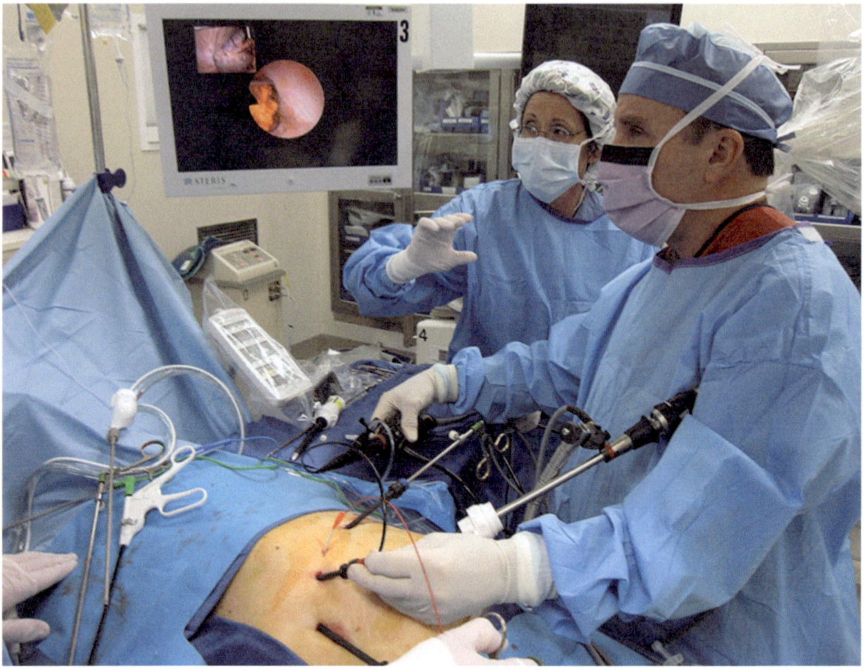

Fig. 6.16 Keeping both fields in view

choledochoscope should be inserted through the port with the most direct access to the common bile duct, and the surgeon must keep the port tip directed toward the common bile duct, not displaced laterally, as often happens with unsuccessful attempts to manipulate the choledochoscope in the common bile duct. While these concepts seem to make sense and are taken for granted, it is not uncommon for either or both of them to be violated during LCDE. So the take-home message for the surgeon is to constantly monitor both, especially when a "good" choledochoscopic view becomes "not good."

The surgeon manipulates the scope both at the head and at its insertion point at the scope port so that a stone is in direct view. The surgeon inserts the basket into the working channel of the scope and captures the stone(s) as described earlier. Sounds simple, but in reality this requires patience and diligence and constant and repeated monitoring of all the parameters mentioned previously: tissue retraction, picture-in-picture evaluation of both the laparoscopic and choledochoscopic images, scope maneuvers, and basket capture maneuvers (Fig. 6.17).

Lithotripsy

Intraoperative electrohydraulic or laser lithotripsy techniques have seen limited use since the introduction of laparoscopic common bile duct exploration (see Chap. 8) [11–14]. The primary indications for intraoperative lithotripsy continue to be an

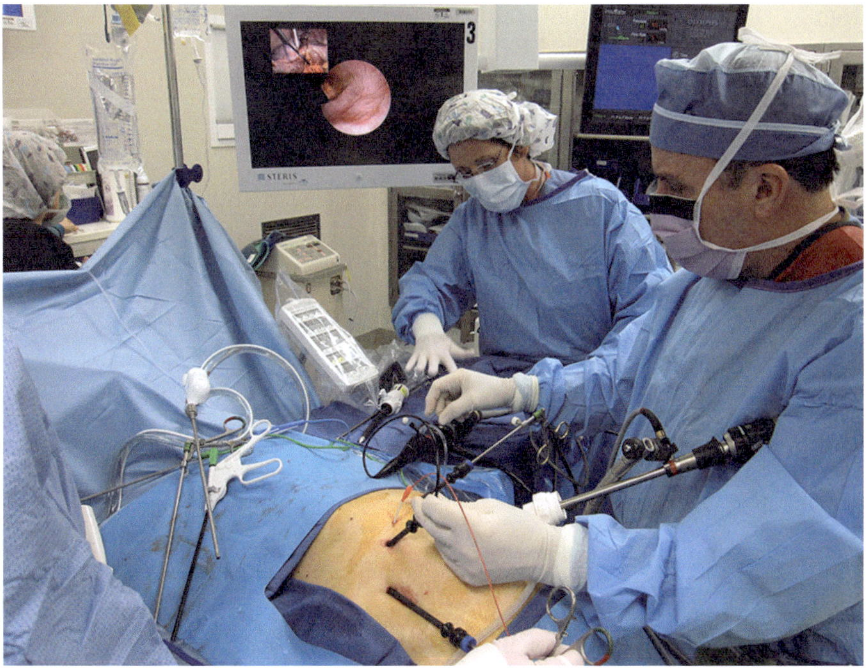

Fig. 6.17 Managing all aspects of stone capture: scope position with the left hand, basket insertion and stone capture with the right hand while keeping the stone in view

impacted stone that defies less aggressive removal techniques or a stone that is too large to be captured and removed through the cystic duct or the choledochotomy. Electrohydraulic lithotripters (EHL) are much less expensive than laser models and consequently have been used somewhat more frequently. EHL devices must be used with great caution because they may cause unwanted ductal damage if the tip of the EHL probe is not accurately applied to the stone. These devices are not used routinely for stones that are not impacted because they multiply the number of particles in the common bile duct, making stone and fragment capture much more complicated. This is unlike the process in urology where particles are flushed and more easily removed from the bladder.

Occasionally, the application of a Waterpik® (Teledyne, Fort Collins, CO)—a pulsatile saline jet stream—through the working channel of the scope may be useful in freeing stones or debris from the duct wall. The surgeon will have to configure his own adapter to connect the device to the scope because there are no ready-made adapters for this application.

Completion Cholangiography

Cholangiograms are repeated after the ductal exploration in order to ensure that ductal clearance had been accomplished and that ductal integrity is maintained. If cholangiograms reveal residual stones, the surgeon must decide whether to proceed with LCDE again, convert to open CDE, perform a biliary bypass, or leave the stones in place for subsequent ERC +/− S.

Complete the Cholecystectomy

Ligate the Cystic Duct

The cystic duct stump is secured either during the common duct exploration or after the completion cholangiograms (Fig. 6.18). If the cystic duct is dilated (>5 mm) or if subsequent ERC +/− S is planned, then ligatures (instead of or in addition to clips) should be considered to secure the duct, in order to prevent subsequent leak (Fig. 6.19).

Cholecystectomy

After completing the common bile duct exploration and subsequent cholangiography, the cystic duct is secured, and the cholecystectomy is performed. The gallbladder is removed through the umbilicus, and the umbilical wound closed at the fascial level.

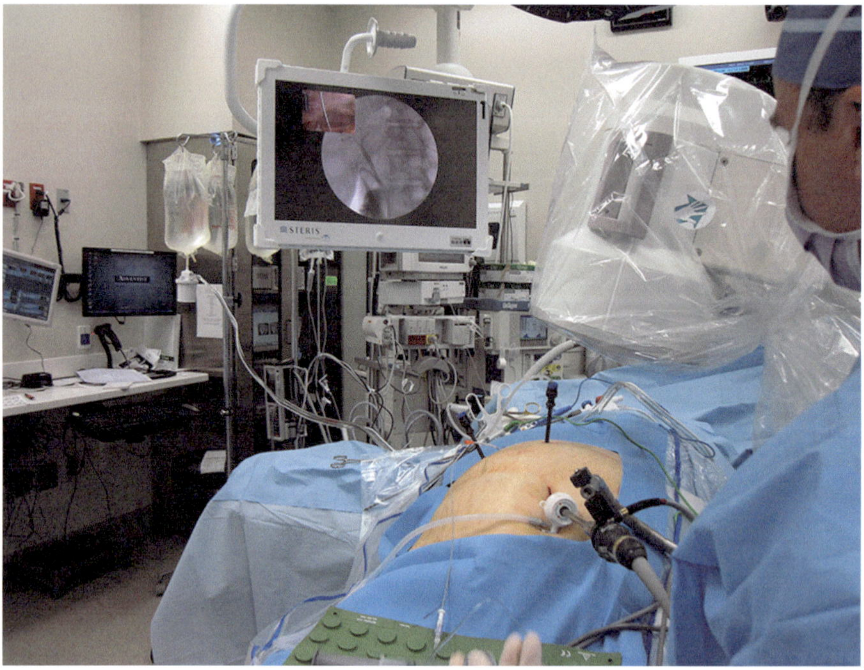

Fig. 6.18 Completion cholangiograms

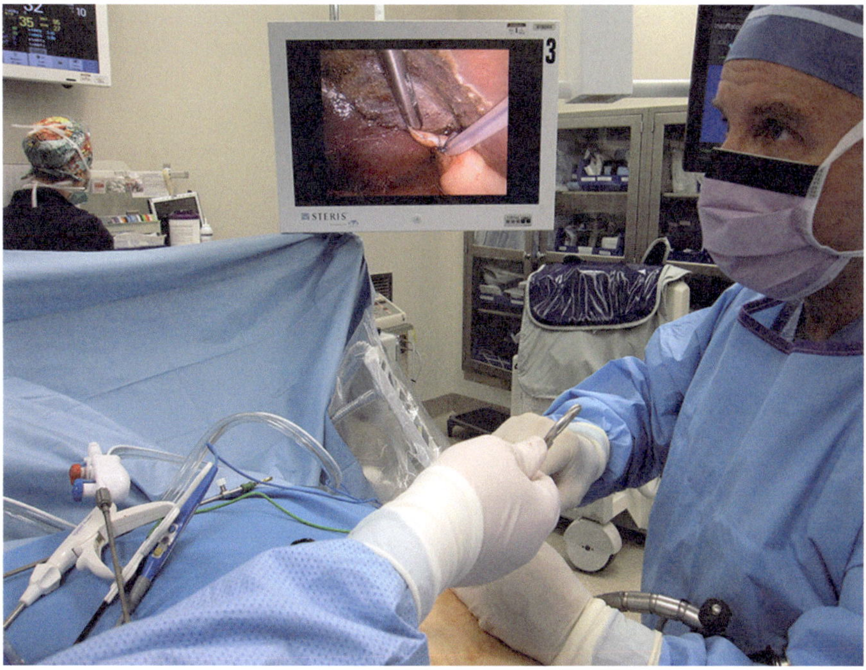

Fig. 6.19 Ligate cystic duct

Drain Placement

Drains are not routinely used after transcystic laparoscopic common bile duct exploration but are commonly used after trans-ductal exploration. A drain may be indicated in cases where intense inflammation, infection, or contamination is present, where a choledochotomy has been performed, or where tissue integrity may be questionable. If used, a closed system suction drain is inserted in its entirety through a 10 mm port into the abdomen. The proximal end is placed near the common duct, and the distal end is usually brought out through the abdominal wall through one of the most direct 5 mm port sites.

Results

General

As an individual surgeon's experience improves, one should expect successful ductal clearance in around 90% of cases of common bile duct stones. This is in contrast to a Cochrane review of a randomized study of only 104 patients where LCDE was only successful in 69% of patients compared to 97% success with ERC [15]. In this author's opinion with experience of more than 600 LCDEs and a 97% clearance rate, reviews such as that demonstrate a learning curve or lack of experience by those in the study and should not be emulated as an acceptable standard of care. Morbidity and mortality for LCDE in experienced hands have been demonstrated to be similar or better than that experienced in open surgery [14, 16–19].

Access Route

The transcystic route for ductal exploration is preferred when it is feasible, because of its associated lower morbidity, shorter length of stay, and better patient satisfaction. In cases where a choledochotomy is necessary, surgeon expertise in laparoscopic suturing is necessary.

Operative Time

Laparoscopic common bile duct exploration generally doubles or triples the time it usually takes to perform a laparoscopic cholecystectomy. In most cases in experienced hands, it adds around 60 min to a laparoscopic cholecystectomy.

Hospitalization

Whereas most patients can be discharged after laparoscopic cholecystectomy in less than 24 h, the length of stay for patients undergoing LCDE ranges from 1.3 to 7 days, depending on the severity of the disease, comorbid factors, access route, whether or not a T-tube was placed, and whether or not a biliary enteric anastomosis was created. For transcystic choledochoscopy the mean length of stay is 1.5 days. Length of stay for LCDE via choledochotomy is generally longer than that for the transcystic approach [4, 18].

Morbidity and Mortality

Morbidity and mortality after laparoscopic common bile duct exploration have been shown in a number of randomized trials to be equivalent to that experienced in open surgery, 10–15% and <1%, respectively.

The Future

Prior to the development of laparoscopic biliary surgery, surgeons performing cholecystectomy were expected to complete the entire job of removing the gallbladder and clearing the ductal system of stones 90% of the time. That mandate was largely ignored by most general surgeons who adopted laparoscopic cholecystectomy as the surgical procedure of choice for treating gallbladder disease. There are many reasons for this stance, but its validity is coming under increasing scrutiny since a one-stage procedure—laparoscopic cholecystectomy and laparoscopic common bile duct exploration with CBD stone extraction—has been shown to be superior to a two-stage procedure, ERCP +/− S and laparoscopic cholecystectomy, in terms of cost, length of hospitalization, and patient satisfaction.

Now, two decades have passed since the introduction of laparoscopic common bile duct exploration, and the technical aspects of the procedure have been widely published in a variety of formats, including this one, and have been validated through numerous clinical studies. It is incumbent upon biliary surgeons of the twenty-first century to develop the expertise to treat benign biliary tract disease resulting from gallstones in one setting, eliminating the need for a second operative procedure in 90% of cases, just as we did before the introduction of minimally invasive surgery.

References

1. Nahrwold D. The biliary system. In: Sabiston X, editor. Textbook of surgery. Philadelphia: WE Saunders; 1986.
2. Way LW, Admirand WJ, Dunphy JE. Management of choledocholithiasis. Ann Surg. 1972;176:347–59.
3. Beal J. Historical perspective of gallstone disease. Surg Gynecol Obstet. 1984;158:181–9.
4. Petelin J. Laparoscopic approach to common duct pathology. Surg Laparosc Endosc. 1991;1:33–41.
5. Hunter J. Laparoscopic transcystic common bile duct exploration. Am J Surg. 1992;163:53–8.
6. Carroll BJ, Phillips EH, Daykhovsky L, Grundfest WS, Gersham A, Fallas M, Chandra M. Laparoscopic choledochoscopy: an effective approach to the common duct. J Laparoendosc Surg. 1992;2:15–21.
7. Jacobs M, Verdeja JC, Goldstein HS. Laparoscopic choledocholithotomy. J Laparoendosc Surg. 1991;1(2):79–82.
8. Quattlebaum JK, Flanders HD. Laparoscopic treatment of common bile duct stones. Surg Laparosc Endosc. 1991;1(1):26–32.
9. Appel S, Krebs H, Fern D. Techniques for laparoscopic cholangiography and removal of common duct stones. Surg Endosc. 1992;6:134–7.
10. Fink AS. To ERCP or not to ERCP? That is the question. Surg Endosc. 1993;7:375–6.
11. Birkett D. Technique of cholangiography and cystic-duct choledochoscopy at the time of laparoscopic cholecystectomy for laser lithotripsy. Surg Endosc. 1992;6:252–4.

12. Fletcher D, Jones RM, O'Riordan B, Hardy KJ. Laparoscopic cholecystectomy for complicated gallstone disease. Surg Endosc. 1992;6:179–82.
13. Dion YM, Morin J, Dionne G, Dejoie C. Laparoscopic cholecystectomy and choledocholithiasis. Can J Surg. 1992;35:67–74.
14. Arregui M, Davis CJ, Arkush AM, Nagan RF. Laparoscopic cholecystectomy combined with endoscopic sphincterotomy and stone extraction or laparoscopic choledochoscopy and electrohydraulic lithotripsy for management of cholelithiasis with choledocholithiasis. Surg Endosc. 1992;6:10–5.
15. Dasari BV, Tan CJ, Gurusany KS, Martin DJ, Kirk G, McKie L, et al. Surgical versus endoscopic treatment of bile duct stones. Cochrane Database Syst Rev. 2013;(9):CD003327.
16. Rhodes M, Sussman L, Cohen L, Lewis MP. Randomised trial of laparoscopic exploration of common bile duct versus postoperative endoscopic retrograde cholangiography for common bile duct stones. Lancet. 1998;351:159–61.
17. Petelin J. Surgical management of common bile duct stones. Gastrointest Endosc. 2002;56(6):S183–9.
18. Petelin JB. Laparoscopic common bile duct exploration—lessons learned from >12 years' experience. Surg Endosc. 2003;17:1705–15.
19. Phillips EH. Laparoscopic transcystic duct common bile duct exploration—outcome and costs. Surg Endosc. 1995;9:1240–2.

Chapter 7
Laparoscopic Transcholedochal Exploration

Miguel A. Hernández, B. Fernando Santos, and Morris E. Franklin Jr

Introduction

Laparoscopic transcholedochal common bile duct exploration (LTCD) represents the most versatile surgical approach for the treatment of choledocholithiasis. The transcholedochal approach was originally based on the gold standard technique of open common bile duct exploration and in the laparoscopic era has continued to evolve into an effective and safe option for treating the patient with choledocholithiasis. Compared with transcystic access, LTCD provides potential access to the entire proximal and distal biliary tree, obviates the need for devices necessary to cannulate and dilate the cystic duct, and may be utilized for removal of stones of any size or occasionally entrapped devices from prior failed endoscopic or percutaneous procedures. LTCD, however, is more technically challenging than transcystic exploration and has a higher risk profile, making proper patient selection and attention to technical detail important in order to ensure optimal outcomes.

Electronic supplementary material The online version of this chapter (doi: 10.1007/978-3-319-74503-9_7) contains supplementary material, which is available to authorized users.

M. A. Hernández, MD · M. E. Franklin Jr, MD, FACS (✉)
Department of Minimally Invasive Surgery, Texas Endosurgery Institute,
San Antonio, TX, USA
e-mail: fellow@texasendosurgery.com; franklin@texasendosurgery.com

B. F. Santos, MD
Department of Surgery, Geisel School of Medicine, Dartmouth College, Hanover, NH, USA

Veterans Affairs Medical Center, White River Junction, Hartford, VT, USA

© Springer International Publishing AG, part of Springer Nature 2018

B. F. Santos, N. Soper (eds.), *Choledocholithiasis*,
https://doi.org/10.1007/978-3-319-74503-9_7

Patient Selection and Indications

The indications for LTCD are similar to those for transcystic exploration and include patients in whom choledocholithiasis is confirmed preoperatively or intraoperatively (Table 7.1). LTCD may be used as the primary strategy for laparoscopic common duct clearance or for patients in whom a transcystic approach has failed or is not feasible (Fig. 7.1). LTCD is ideally suited to patients undergoing concurrent cholecystectomy but may in certain situations be performed even after prior cholecystectomy (unlike transcystic exploration). LTCD in patients with a prior cholecystectomy is indicated when either endoscopic retrograde cholangiopancreatography (ERCP) is not available or most commonly for patients in whom ERCP is difficult or has failed (such as those with a history of a prior Billroth II or Roux-en-Y gastric bypass). The surgeon performing LTCD should have a high degree of confidence in the diagnosis of choledocholithiasis compared to when performing transcystic exploration, however, as LTCD represents a more technically challenging operation requiring laparoscopic suturing skills and with a higher risk profile.

It is advisable to avoid a choledochotomy in patients with a small-diameter bile duct (<7 mm) to reduce the risk of a biliary stricture, even when T-tubes are used. Patients with small-diameter bile ducts may be better approached with either transcystic exploration if the bile duct is larger than 3 mm or with endoscopic stone clearance.

Table 7.1 Indications and contraindications for laparoscopic transcholedochal exploration

Indications for laparoscopic transcholedochal exploration
Contraindicated or failed transcystic approach • Large bile duct stones (>6–8 mm diameter) • Multiple bile duct stones • Proximal ductal stones • Small or tortuous cystic duct • Severe inflammation of the cystic duct (not including common bile duct) • Prior cholecystectomy
Failure of endoscopic stone extraction • Large or obstructing stones • Retained devices (e.g., entrapped stone baskets) • Altered anatomy precluding endoscopic approach (e.g., prior gastric bypass or Billroth II) • ERCP unavailable
Contraindications to laparoscopic transcholedochal exploration
Technical factors • Inability to suture laparoscopically
Unfavorable anatomy • Small common bile duct (<7 mm diameter) predisposing to stricture • Severe inflammation in the porta hepatis precluding safe dissection of the common bile duct
Patient factors • Severe cholangitis (better served with initial endoscopic drainage) • Long-standing jaundice (prompting suspicion for malignancy) • Active chemotherapy or impaired wound healing (may be better served with endoscopic clearance)

ERCP endoscopic retrograde cholangiopancreatography

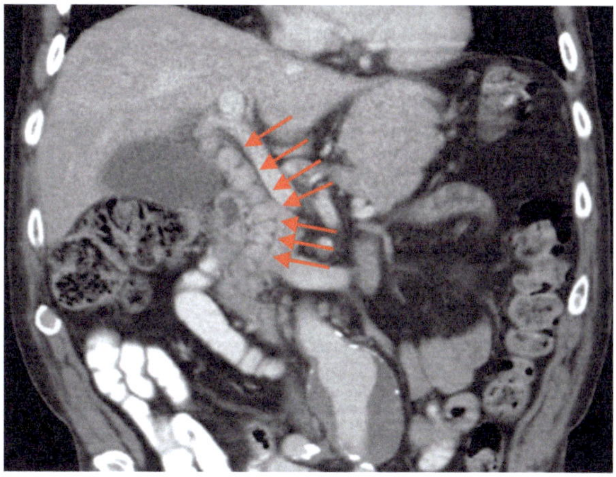

Fig. 7.1 Computed tomography (CT) scan with large stones. The CT scan shows a patient with a dilated common bile duct containing multiple large stones (red arrows). This patient is not appropriate for a transcystic approach. A transcholedochal approach was chosen instead

Informed consent prior to any cholecystectomy should include the possibility of requiring laparoscopic common bile duct exploration. If transcholedochal exploration is a possibility, the risk of bile leak, bile duct injury, and bile duct stricture should be discussed, as well as the possibility that the patient may require either internal (biliary stent) or external drainage (T-tube or closed suction drain) or secondary procedures such as ERCP or follow-up esophagogastroduodenoscopy (EGD) for stent removal if a biliary stent is used.

Patient Positioning and Setup

The best situation is when the surgeon knows prior to the operation that a transcholedochal exploration will be required so that all the instruments are set up ahead of time (Table 7.2). Regardless, certain considerations can make biliary exploration easier such as having a C-arm set up in the room and routinely using an operating room table capable of cholangiography. Generally, it may be helpful to tuck the patient's arm on the side from which the C-arm approaches to facilitate cholangiography. Initial trocar placement is the same as for a four-port cholecystectomy. The initial exposure and dissection to a critical view of safety are done identical to a conventional laparoscopic cholecystectomy.

Cholangiography

Routine intraoperative cholangiography through the cystic duct is strongly recommended for most cases, as it will delineate the biliary anatomy and the location of stones and provide a roadmap for the exploration (Fig. 7.2). When there is clear confirmation of large stones on preoperative imaging, however, the preoperative

Table 7.2 List of equipment for transcholedochal exploration

Equipment for transcholedochal exploration		
Item	Manufacturer	Product no.
Core equipment		
• C-arm		
• Operating room table compatible with cholangiography		
• Liver retractor (in cases of prior cholecystectomy)		
• Choledochoscope (video scope preferable to fiber-optic scope to eliminate the need for extra light cord and camera)	Karl Storz	11292 VSUK
• Alton Dean irrigation pump (optional) with saline bag		
• Extension tubing for continuous irrigation		
Choledochotomy		
• Laparoscopic Berci micro-knife	Karl Storz	26169DO
• Laparoscopic scissors		
Ductal clearance		
• Laparoscopic suction irrigator		
• 14 French red rubber catheter		
• Assortment of wire baskets		
- Nitinol wire basket	Cook	G31027
- Segura hemisphere basket	Boston Scientific	380106
• Assortment of balloon catheters		
- 4F Fogarty balloon	Edwards Lifesciences	120804F
- Biliary extraction balloon plus wire guide	Olympus	B-230Q-A, G-240-2545S
Choledochotomy closure		
• Fine absorbable suture (4-0 Vicryl on RB-1 needle)		
• T-tube (optional, 8-14 French)		
• Biliary stent (optional)		
• 7F laparoscopic biliary stent	Cook	G36251
• 8.5F biliary stent	Boston Scientific	M00534630
• Closed suction drain	Cook	G31027

Note: Manufacturer and product numbers listed are examples—other suppliers may be available

cholangiogram is not mandatory. Likewise, in cases where purulent debris is noted to emanate from the cystic ductotomy, or in cases of cholangitis, an initial cholangiogram should be deferred in order to reduce the risk of bacteremia from pressurizing the biliary tree. Antibiotic prophylaxis preoperatively is recommended, especially for patients with prior biliary manipulation or suspected cholangitis.

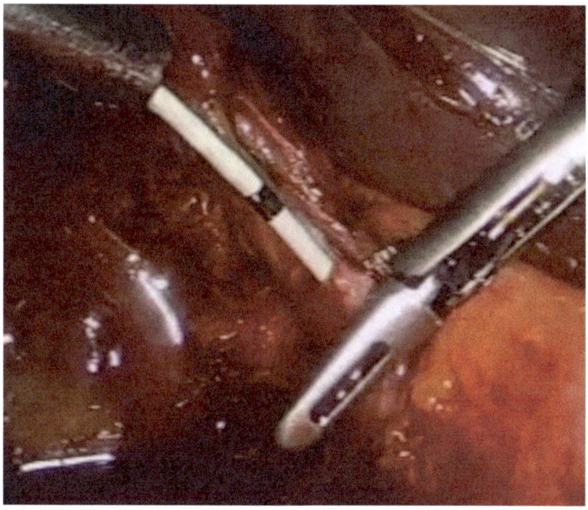

Fig. 7.2 Intraoperative cholangiography. A catheter is inserted into the cystic duct and secured with a locking instrument for cholangiography

Choledochotomy

Once the decision has been made to proceed with transcholedochal exploration, the surgeon may remain on the left side of the patient or move to the right side of the patient with placement of an additional trocar in the right lower quadrant between the most lateral trocar and the camera to facilitate the dissection. Working from the right side allows for a comfortable angle for making the ductotomy and for suturing. With the surgeon on the right side, the surgeon uses the lateral-most trocar plus the extra right lower quadrant trocar, while the assistant moves to the left of the patient and retracts the gallbladder cephalad using the subxiphoid trocar. The supraduodenal common bile duct may be seen as a bluish green tubular structure in the right anterior aspect of the porta hepatis (Fig. 7.3). The peritoneum covering of the hepatoduodenal ligament should be incised over the anterior aspect of the bile duct, and gentle blunt dissection should be used to expose the bile duct. Dissection along its lateral and medial aspects as well as any attempt to encircle the bile duct should be avoided to avoid injury to the "3 o'clock" and "9 o'clock" arteries supplying and running parallel to the bile duct. Exposure should be just enough to allow a 1–2 cm longitudinal incision over the duct. If the location of the bile duct is in doubt, a fine needle may be used to aspirate the bile, confirming the location of the bile duct. A longitudinal incision is preferred so as to not disrupt the blood supply to the common bile duct. The incision may be made with a laparoscopic knife or with fine scissors (Fig. 7.4a–d). Stay sutures are generally unnecessary and are at risk of being pulled through, tearing the duct. The incision length should generally remain less than 1.5 cm due to the ability of the CBD to distend and stretch. Care should be

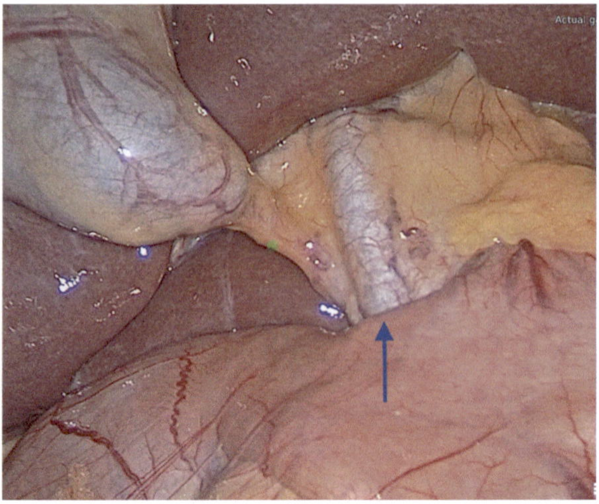

Fig. 7.3 Supraduodenal common bile duct. The common bile duct can usually be seen as a bluish green tubular structure in the right anterior aspect of the porta hepatis

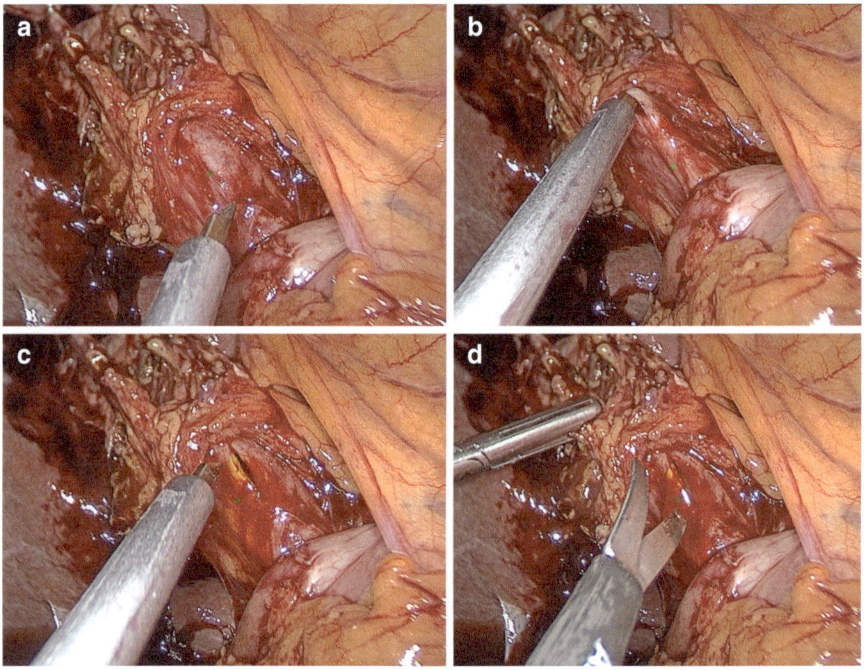

Fig. 7.4 Choledochotomy. The choledochotomy may be created with a laparoscopic knife (**a**) or with scissors. The knife is gently inserted into the common bile duct, with care not to injure the back wall of the duct (**b**). Once the initial incision has been made (**c**), it is extended further longitudinally with the knife or with scissors (**d**)

taken to not make the incision to the right of the midplane of the duct, so that the incision is not made into a cystic duct-common duct septum that is present in about 20% of patients when the cystic duct runs parallel to the common duct.

Stone Extraction

Extraction of stones through the choledochotomy may be accomplished with a variety of ways. In general it is recommended to begin with the simplest maneuver, proceeding to more complex maneuvers if necessary:

1. *Irrigation*: The surgeon places the tip of the suction irrigator into the choledochotomy to irrigate the duct. Small stones and debris are easily cleared with this simple maneuver, and larger, free-floating stones may be drawn toward the choledochotomy by following the flow of saline. Once seen at the choledochotomy site, these larger stones can be grasped and removed. A 14F red rubber catheter may also be inserted through a 5 mm trocar and passed distally or proximally and flushed vigorously as it is withdrawn to dislodge more distant stones (Fig. 7.5a–d).
2. *Balloon extraction*: A Fogarty balloon catheter or an ERCP stone extraction balloon passed over a wire (positioned across the papilla) is passed through the choledochotomy and guided distally. The balloon is guided just past resistance, and then slowly withdrawn and inflated, then gradually withdrawn through the

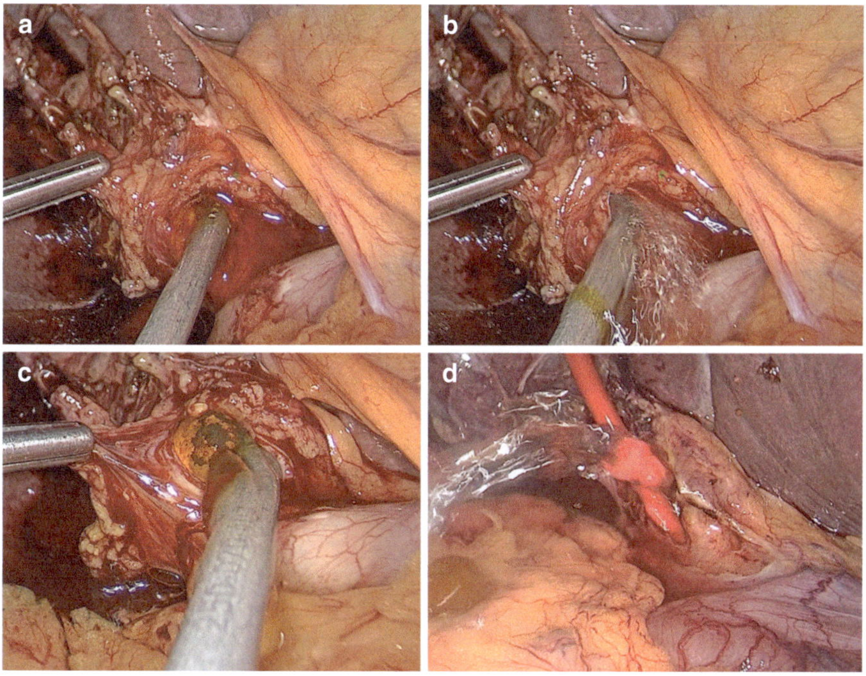

Fig. 7.5 Irrigation. The suction irrigator is placed at the ductotomy (**a**) and vigorous flushing is performed (**b**). The flow of water clears debris and brings a stones to the ductotomy (**c**). More distal or proximal flushing can be performed by passing a 14F red rubber catheter and vigorously flushing as the catheter is withdrawn. A stone that has been flushed out this way is seen on the left side of the image (**d**)

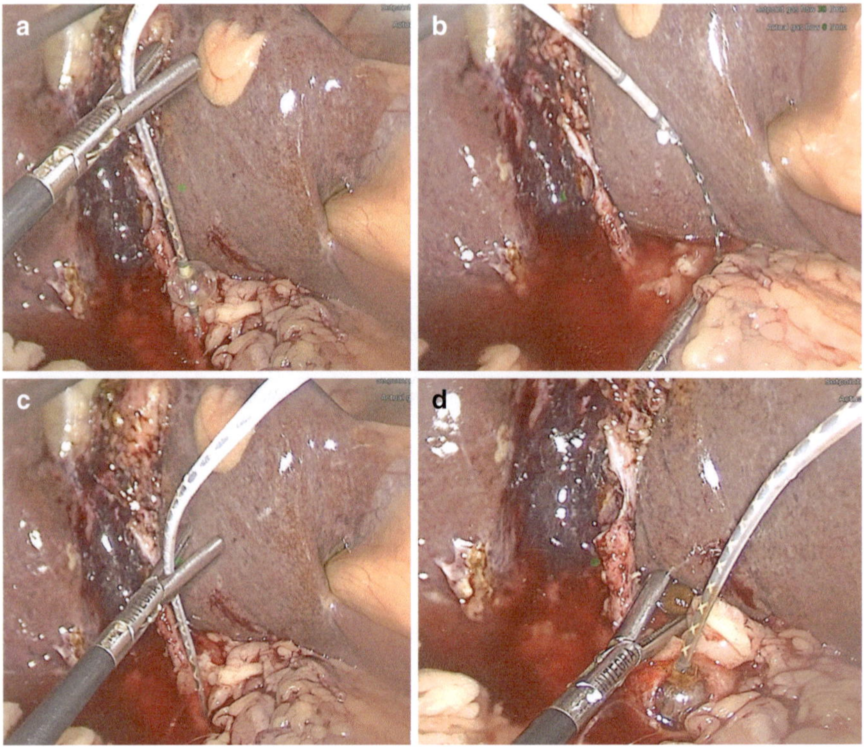

Fig. 7.6 Balloon extractor. An embolectomy catheter or balloon extraction device passed over a wire (**a** and **b**) is inserted distally past the papilla (**c**). The balloon is withdrawn until resistance is felt at the papilla, then the balloon is let down, slightly withdrawn, and reinflated to sweep stones out of the choledochotomy (**d**)

choledochotomy to remove debris. This technique may require several passes of the balloon to remove all the debris (Fig. 7.6a–d).

3. *Choledochoscopy*: If the aforementioned attempts at clearing the duct are unsuccessful or if there appear to be no more stones to remove, then direct visualization of the duct via choledochoscopy should be done to confirm stone clearance. The irrigation is connected to the scope and tested. A bag of saline may be pressurized using an arterial line cuff, or alternatively an Alton Dean irrigation pump may be used to more reliably pressurize a larger saline bag. The scope is placed through an introducer sheath (to prevent leakage of pneumoperitoneum) and inserted into a 5 mm trocar (right upper quadrant trocar at the midclavicular line). The saline should be turned on to clear debris and distend the ducts during choledochoscopy. The scope should be directed proximally (Fig. 7.7a–e) and distally to visualize the entire biliary tree to confirm ductal clearance. If stones are found, a wire basket through the scope, or a balloon extractor passed beside the scope, is used to remove stones. The closed basket or balloon is passed beyond the stone and then opened or inflated and withdrawn to capture the stone. Slight back and forth manipulation with an open wire basket may be necessary

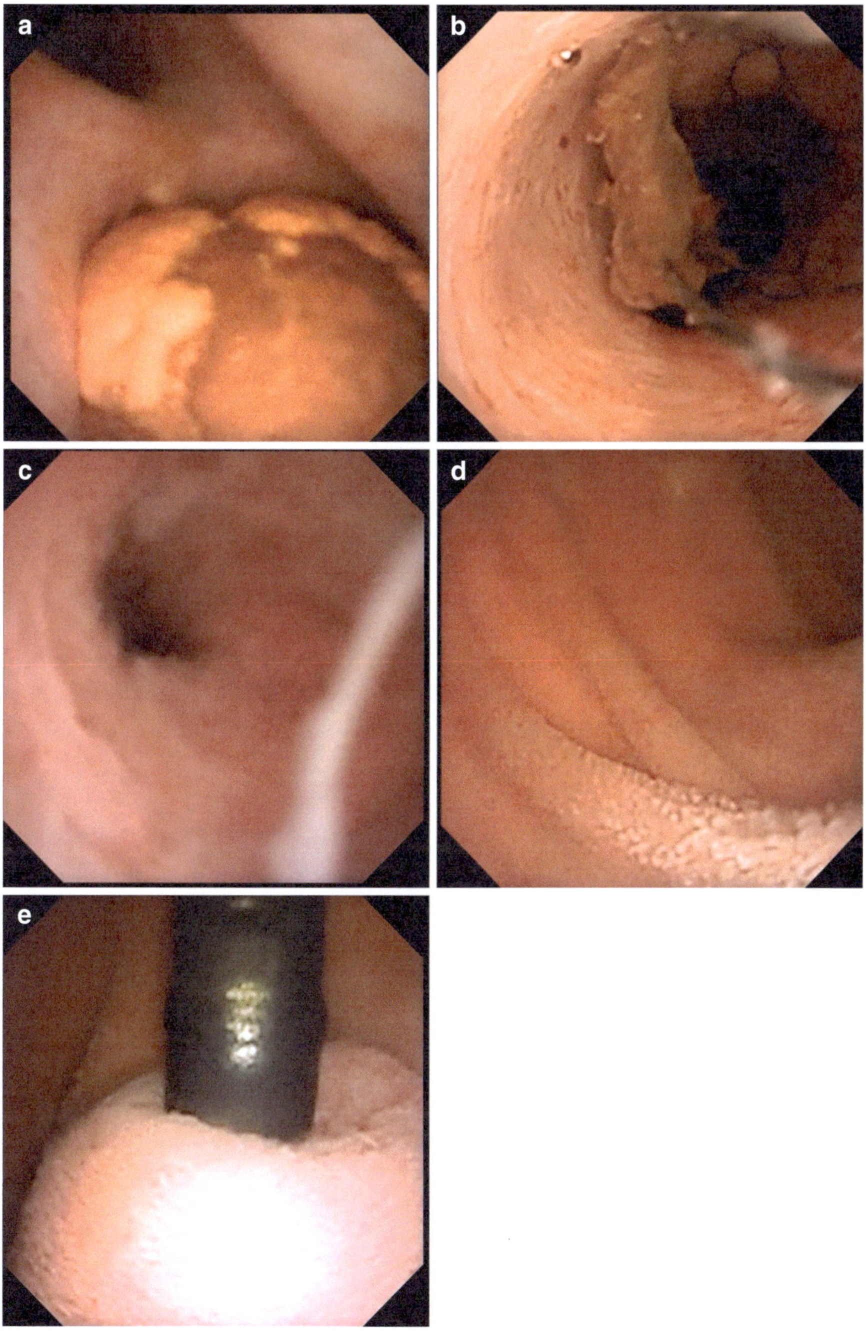

Fig. 7.7 Choledochoscope views. An intrahepatic stone is visible (**a**). A distal stone is captured using a wire basket through the scope (**b**). The papilla is seen from the common duct side (**c**). The scope is gently advanced through the papilla into the duodenum to confirm no stones remain (**d**). Some scopes with high degrees of flexion allow retroflexion in the duodenum to examine the duodenal aspect of the papilla (**e**)

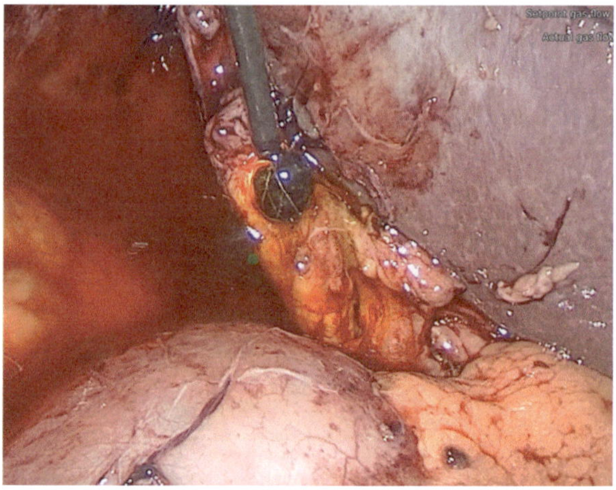

Fig. 7.8 Stone basket. The stone basket and choledochoscope are withdrawn as a unit through the choledochotomy

to capture the stone prior to closing the basket around the stone. The scope and captured stone are then withdrawn together out of the choledochotomy (Fig. 7.8) and retrieved with a laparoscopic instrument. A small-diameter choledochoscope can usually be gently guided past the papilla into the duodenum, confirming that no distal stones are left. Retroflexion to view the papilla may sometimes be performed with the newer, video scopes capable of 270° flexion. Likewise, the scope should be directed proximally to visualize the proximal hepatic ducts to confirm no stones remain.

Choledochotomy Closure

The choledochotomy closure may be accomplished in several ways including primary closure, closure over a T-tube, and primary closure plus internal drainage with a biliary stent. A closed suction drain should be placed adjacent to the repair in case of an early bile leak, regardless of the closure technique. While closure over a T-tube was commonly performed in the "open" era, there has been a trend away from T-tube closure in the literature, with some studies showing an advantage for primary closure compared to T-tube closure in terms of reducing operative time, decreased hospital length of stay, and possibly even a decreased risk of bile leak. Likewise, biliary stents have emerged as an option to provide postoperative internal drainage without the use of a T-tube. Selection of the proper closure technique for each patient should be individualized and depends on surgeon experience, patient factors, and technical considerations.

Primary Closure

Primary closure alone may be adequate in straightforward cases, in which there has been minimal to no manipulation of the papilla, where there is no purulence in the bile duct, and where there is a low concern for retained stones and in relatively fit patients. The duct may be closed in an interrupted or running fashion using fine absorbable 4-0 sutures such as Vicryl (polyglactin 910) or PDS (polydioxanone). The running technique has the advantage of greater expediency compared with the interrupted technique. The suture bites should be full thickness, about 1–2 mm from the cut edge of the duct, and be spaced about every 2 mm (Fig. 7.9a–d; Video 7.1). The suture line should be tested by flushing saline through the cystic duct using a cholangiogram catheter, while observing for leakage of saline. Additional interrupted sutures are placed at the site of any leaks, and the closure is rechecked. A closing cholangiogram should also be performed to check for extravasation of contrast and confirm ductal patency and the absence of filling defects. The main advantage of primary closure is that the patient does not need an extended period of T-tube drainage and avoids the potential discomfort and potential complications associated with having a T-tube. One of the downsides of primary closure, though, is that there is a potentially greater risk of bile leak should pressurization of the bile duct occur

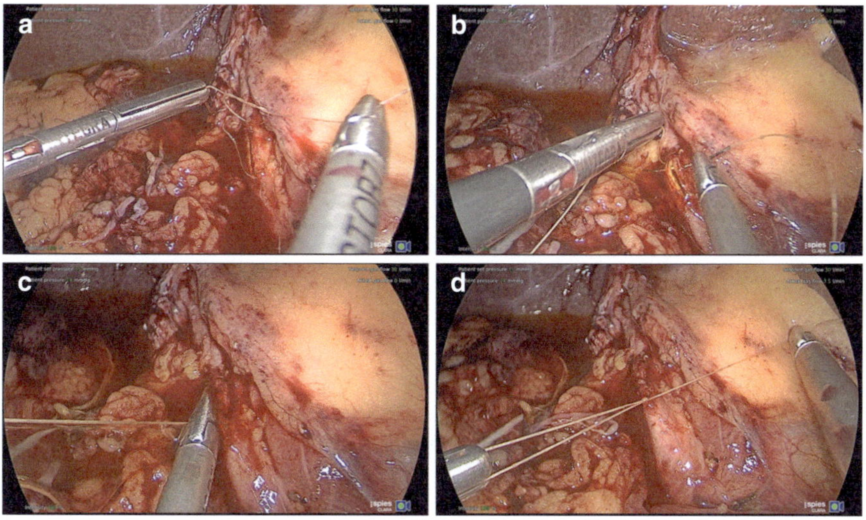

Fig. 7.9 Primary closure. The suture line is begun at the apex of the incision using 4-0 Vicryl on an RB-1 needle (**a**). A running suture line is performed taking 1–2 mm bites in each side of the incision (**b**). It is important to cinch after each bite to prevent the suture line from loosening (**c**). The suture line is completed and tied (**d**)

postoperatively as in cases with extensive papillary manipulation or in cases with a high risk of retained stones. There is also the possibility of impaired biliary drainage in cases of ampullary edema or cholangitis. Nevertheless, for the well-selected patient, there is evidence that this technique reduces operative time, shortens hospital length of stay, and may actually have lower complication rates than T-tube closure.

T-Tube Closure

T-tubes are the traditional adjunct to choledochotomy closure and are routinely used by some surgeons, including the senior author. Routine users argue that instrumentation of the common bile duct and the maneuvers used for stone removal may result in edema of the papilla and elevated pressures in the biliary tree, creating an environment that places the closure at risk for biliary leak. Placement of a T-tube allows for resolution of edema and spasm while preventing biliary stasis. In patients with cholangitis, ensuring this continued drainage of bile is especially important to prevent recurrent cholangitis and ensure resolution of sepsis. The T-tube also provides continued access to the biliary tree for interval cholangiography, stone extraction for any retained stones, or to facilitate wire access for subsequent ERCP. The T-tube technique has an advantage over the use of an internal biliary stent in that the biliary prosthesis is removed by simply pulling the T-tube at the bedside, without the need for an additional endoscopic procedure as in the case of a biliary stent. Although transcystic drainage can also be achieved in some patients (as an alternative to a T-tube), the placement of a T-tube in the common bile duct is more widely applicable and will be the only technique described. There is variation in the size of T-tubes used by surgeons, with some surgeons advocating the use of a 14F T-tube to allow easier access for percutaneous interventions should these be necessary. The senior author prefers the use of an 8F tube, as it reduces patient discomfort and requires a smaller opening in the bile duct. The T-tube is prepared by trimming the crossbar of the T to approximately twice the size of the choledochotomy with one short and one long limb. The crossbar segment is then incised longitudinally to open the back wall, and the tube is inserted into the duct with the long limb in the distal duct (Fig. 7.10). A 4-0 Vicryl running suture is used to close the choledochotomy in a continuous manner. The first bite is the most important and is taken close to the tube with care to not incorporate the tube. This first bite should snug up the tube to the duct and is crucial in terms of anchoring the tube and preventing migration or leaking. Subsequent bites are placed moving in a caudal direction until the duct is completely closed (Video 7.2). The T-tube is then exteriorized at the end of the surgical procedure through one of the right upper quadrant 5 mm trocar sites. It is important to allow for a small amount of laxity in the tube so that postoperative abdominal distention does not create tension on the tube and cause it to become dislodged. Even with placement of a T-tube, placement of a closed suction drain adjacent to the T-tube is recommended to help detect and control a possible

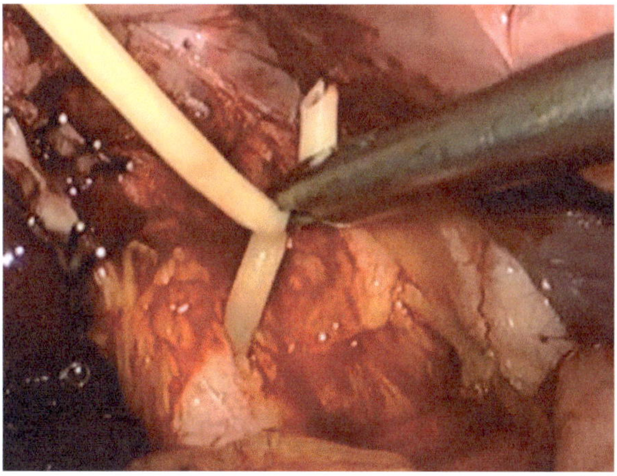

Fig. 7.10 T-tube. The T-tube is inserted with the long limb in the distal duct

postoperative bile leak. Although postoperative T-tube management is highly variable among surgeons, most surgeons keep the tube in for at least 2–6 weeks.

The technique of the senior author using 8F T-tubes will be described. After the operation, the surgeon places the drainage bag at the level of the floor for approximately 12 h, while the closed suction drain is checked for any evidence of bile leak. If the drainage is not bilious, the T-tube is repositioned at the level of the bed for another 12 h. After this time period, the bag is placed at the head of the bed. If the bile is not seen in the closed suction drain, the T-tube is clamped. It is thought that this method, with its various positional changes, may allow testing of the integrity of the repaired choledochotomy by sequentially varying the intraductal pressure. The closed suction drain is then removed prior to discharge, and the patient is scheduled for a cholangiogram 10–15 days postoperatively. If there are no retained stones or bile leak, the T-tube is removed. Should retained stones be present, they are removed endoscopically.

Primary Closure with Biliary Stent

Primary closure with a biliary stent is a newer technique that combines the ease of a primary closure with the internal drainage provided by a transampullary stent. Prior to choledochotomy closure, the surgeon inserts a biliary stent through the choledochotomy. Either a laparoscopic 7F biliary stent may be used (Fanelli stent, Cook Medical) (Video 7.3) or an 8.5F biliary stent designed for ERCP deployment may be used. If using an ERCP-type stent, a preloaded 5–7 cm stent that is fixed to the delivery catheter with a suture (Fig. 7.11) and is able to be repositioned by withdrawing the catheter is recommended (e.g., Advanix™ stent, Boston Scientific) (Video 7.4). The surgeon obtains wire access across the papilla and then backloads the stent delivery system onto the wire. The stent delivery system generally has fluoroscopic markers that are positioned across the papilla, and, once in position, the

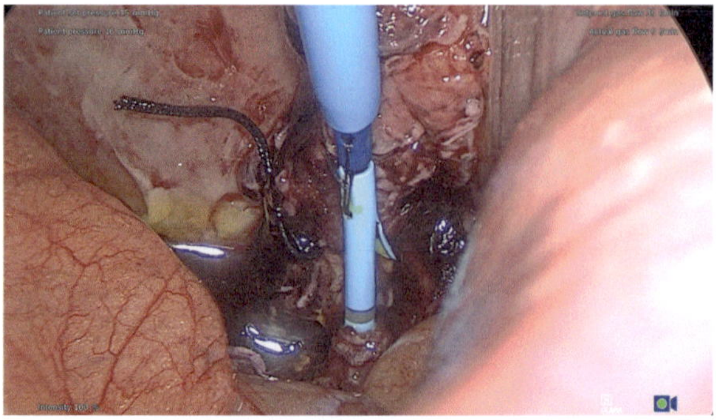

Fig. 7.11 Biliary stent with suture fixation. A biliary stent delivery system with fixation of the stent to the delivery catheter allows the surgeon to withdraw the stent if necessary, unlike delivery systems with a push catheter mechanism only

stent is deployed. The choledochoscope can be used to confirm the position of the stent across the papilla from the common bile duct side (Fig. 7.12a, b). The stent does not need to lie across the choledochotomy closure site but rather functions to ensure continued internal drainage once the choledochotomy is closed, to prevent pressurization of the bile duct and the possibility of a bile leak as a result. Once the stent is in place and the choledochotomy is closed, the surgeon performs a closing cholangiogram to confirm a watertight closure of the choledochotomy and that no filling defects remain. A closed suction drain is placed adjacent to the choledochotomy closure to monitor for postoperative bile leak. The drain is generally removed prior to the patient's discharge from the hospital. An EGD is scheduled as an outpatient to remove the biliary stent after 2–4 weeks. The stent is removed using either foreign body forceps or a snare, using a standard gastroscope. A clear cap may be fitted to the end of the gastroscope to facilitate visualization of the papilla and grasping of the stent if necessary (Fig. 7.13).

Outcomes

The clinical experience at the Texas Endosurgery Institute from 1991 to 2016 includes a total of 8591 patients having undergone laparoscopic cholecystectomy with intraoperative cholangiography. Of these patients, 626 (7.2%) were diagnosed with choledocholithiasis, of which 400 (64%) patients were women. Of the 626 patients with choledocholithiasis, 150 (24%) underwent successful laparoscopic transcystic common bile duct exploration, with the remaining 476 (76%) patients undergoing transcholedochal bile duct exploration. The choledochotomy was closed using a T-tube in 457 (96%) patients. Postoperative complications included four (0.6%) patients with bleeding that was controlled nonoperatively, two (0.3%) patients with jaundice, six (0.9%) patients with pancreatitis, six (0.9%) patients with wound infections, four (0.6%) patients with a biloma, and two (0.3%) patients with cholangitis. Retained stones were found in 11 (1.7%) patients with those

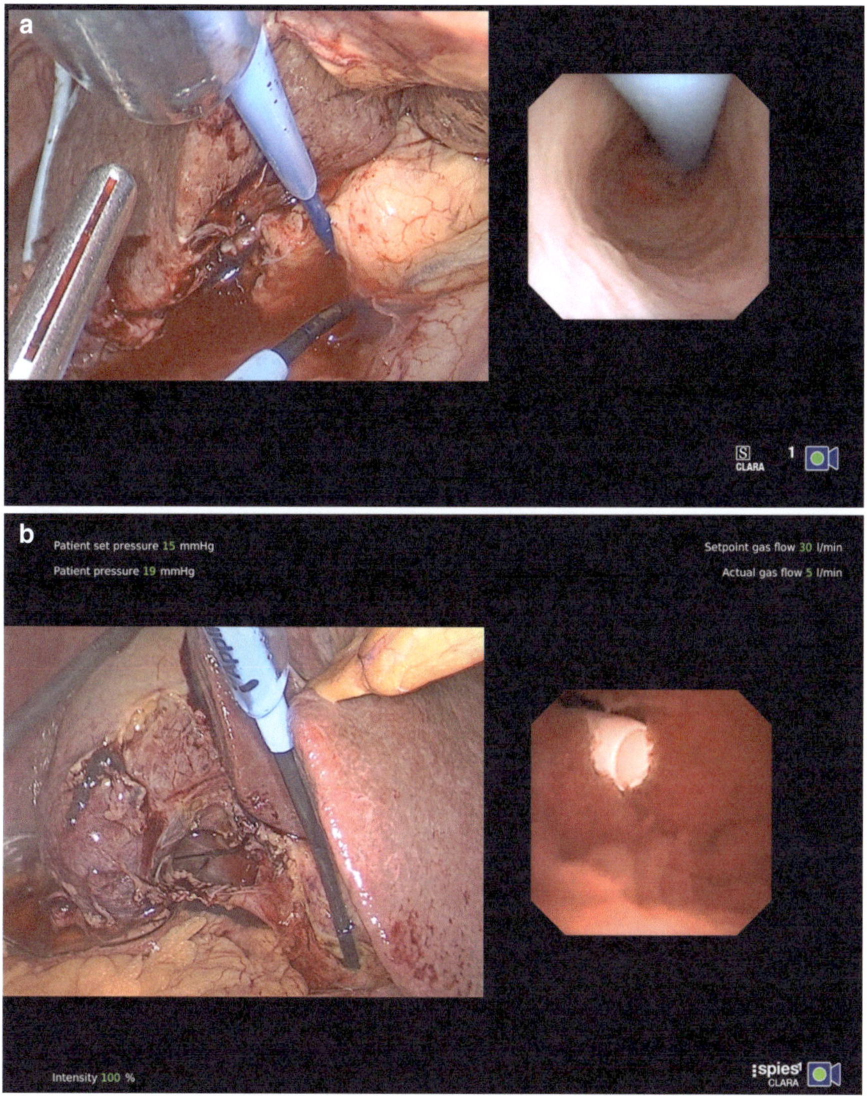

Fig. 7.12 Biliary stent seen from choledochoscope. The stent may either be positioned across the papilla by fluoroscopy or it may be guided across the papilla by the choledochoscope (**a**). Once deployed, the proximal side of the stent can be seen by the choledochoscope (**b**)

patients requiring ERCP for stone clearance. Bile leaks from the T-tube closure occurred in 27 (4.3%) patients, of whom 11 (1.7%) required re-exploration. Other T-tube complications occurred in five patients (0.8%).

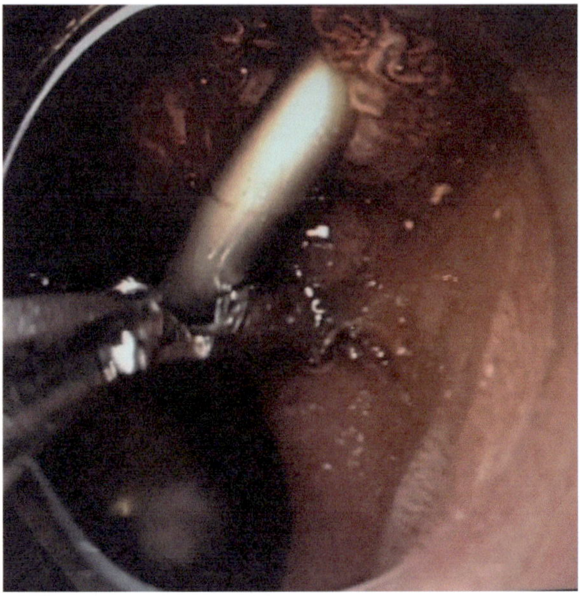

Fig. 7.13 Stent removal with esophagogastroduodenoscopy (EGD). The stent may be removed 2–4 weeks after the operation using foreign body forceps or a snare. A clear cap placed on the end of the scope facilitates visualization of the papilla and removal of the stent

Conclusion

Laparoscopic transcholedochal common bile duct exploration represents a versatile and well-established technique for the clearance of common bile duct stones. This technique does require advanced laparoscopic skills including suturing, but allows the surgeon to safely and effectively manage the vast majority of patients with choledocholithiasis, even in the setting of large stones.

References

1. Dorman JP, Franklin ME Jr. Laparoscopic common bile duct exploration by choledochotomy. Semin Laparosc Surg. 1997;4:34–41.
2. Petelin JB. Laparoscopic common bile duct exploration. Surg Endosc. 2003;17:1705–15.
3. Trazuma S. Epidemiology, pathogenesis, and classification of biliary stones (common bile duct and intrahepatic). Best Pract Res Clin Gastroenterol. 2006;20:1075–83.
4. Phillips EH. Laparoscopic common bile duct exploration: long-term outcome. Arch Surg. 1999;134:839–43.
5. Varban O, Assimos D, Passman C, Westcott C. Laparoscopic common bile exploration and holmium laser lithotripsy: a novel approach to the management of common bile duct stones. Surg Endosc. 2010;24:1759–64.
6. Rogers SJ, Cello JP, Horn JK, Siperstein AE, Schecter WP, Campbell AR, et al. Prospective Randomized Trial of LC+LCBDE vs ERCP/S+LC for common bile duct stone disease. Arch Surg. 2010;145(1):28–33.

7. Campagnacci R, Baldoni A, Baldarelli M, Rimini M, De Sanctis A, Di Emiddio M, et al. Is laparoscopic fiberoptic choledochoscopy for common bile duct stones a fine option or a mandatory step? Surg Endosc. 2010;24:547–53.
8. Hanif F, Ahmed Z, Abdel Sanie M, Nassar AHM. Laparoscopic transcystic bile duct exploration: the treatment of first choice for common bile duct stones. Surg Endosc. 2010;24:1552–6.
9. El-Geidle AAR. Is the use of T-tube necessary after laparoscopic choledochotomy? J Gastrointest Surg. 2010;144:844–8.

Chapter 8
Stone Fragmentation Technologies and the Approach to Impacted Stones

Leslie K. Nathanson

Introduction

Pure cholesterol and pure pigment stones account for only 20% of gallstones, and mixed stones are considered as variants of cholesterol stones as they usually contain over 50% cholesterol and account for about 80% of gallstones in Western countries. Chemical analysis shows a continuous spectrum of stone composition rather than three mutually exclusive stone types, and 10–20% contain enough calcium to be rendered radiopaque. Pigment, cholesterol, and mixed gallstones are more dense than secondary brown stones formed within the bile ducts.

Pigmented gallstones are composed mainly of calcium hydrogen bilirubinate, in a polymerized and oxidized form in "black" stones and in unpolymerized form in "brown" stones. Black stones form in sterile gallbladder bile, but brown stones form secondary to stasis and anaerobic infection in any part of the biliary tree. Oriental hepatolithiasis syndrome is the most serious manifestation of brown pigment stone disease [1].

Stone fragmentation technology has been developed primarily for the more common presentation of obstructing renal calculi, which are denser than gallstones, and so techniques that evolved over time to solve renal calculi fragmentation work well in the biliary tree.

The evolution of biliary stone fragmentation techniques over the last 30 years has ranged widely, originating from the pioneering days of open surgery using tactile finger compression fragmentation with high probability of bile duct and ampullary dam-

Electronic supplementary material The online version of this chapter (doi: 10.1007/978-3-319-74503-9_8) contains supplementary material, which is available to authorized users.

L. K. Nathanson, FRACS, FRCS Ed(Hon)
Wesley Hospital, Brisbane, QLD, Australia

© Springer International Publishing AG, part of Springer Nature 2018

B. F. Santos, N. Soper (eds.), *Choledocholithiasis*,
https://doi.org/10.1007/978-3-319-74503-9_8

age, Desjardins forceps tactile-guided crush, or angled rigid choledochoscope-guided forceps fragmentation to the introduction of visually ("scope") guided pneumatic, electrohydraulic, and laser fragmentation. These techniques have been complemented by occasional use of extracorporeal shock wave lithotripsy (ESWL) [2].

Stone Fragmentation Technologies

Instrument Fragmentation

Desjardins forceps insertion via a choledochotomy during open exploration of the bile duct allow experienced surgeons to grasp impacted distal stones and retrieve them (Fig. 8.1). This is often unsuccessful as the Desjardins forceps is relatively bulky within the confines of the bile duct, and insufficient space is present to get a purchase on the impacted stone. Clumsy persistence can perforate the bile duct. Current technologies with visual guidance of rapidly effective, safe, and cheap lithotripsy techniques such as pneumatic fragmentation are not overly difficult to use and should be part of the biliary surgeon's skills.

An endoscopic retrograde cholangiopancreatography (ERCP)-guided crushing basket in a coil spring catheter was also part of the early ERCP approach to large and impacted stones (mechanical lithotripsy). The coil spring catheter and strong basket are advanced into the bile duct, the stone engaged under fluoroscopic control, and then a crank handle winds the basket back against the coil spring catheter, fragmenting the stone. Fragments are removed and the process repeated until duct clearance is achieved (see Chap. 12).

Pneumatic Lithotripsy

Ballistic force in a handpiece is created from compressed air, which induces rapid small forward and backward movement of a 0.8–1 mm diameter solid rod placed in the operating channel of a semirigid ureteroscope (Fig. 8.2) or semirigid choledochoscope (Fig. 8.3). The device can be set to single- or multi-fire mode with activation by a foot pedal (Fig. 8.4). Contact with the bile duct wall does *not* easily lead to bile duct wall perforation, and activation within the choledochoscope does *not*

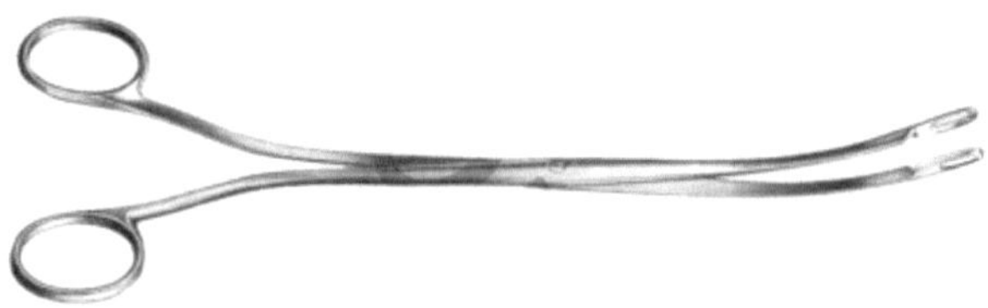

Fig. 8.1 Desjardins forceps for open CBD exploration

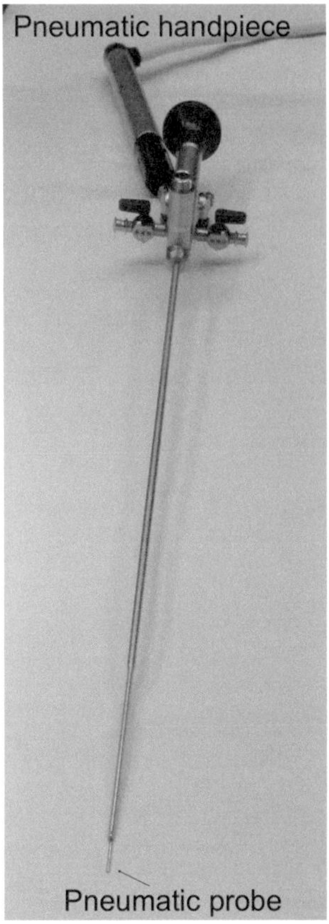

Fig. 8.2 Semirigid short ureteroscope with pneumatic probe in the operating channel. The handpiece must be held in line with the operating channel during use

damage it. The device is widely available in most hospitals and poses no risk to the operator, with added benefits of relatively cheap reusable components.

This is in marked contrast to the risks associated with electrohydraulic and laser lithotripsy.

The choledochoscope requires a second instrument stack, camera, light source, and warm saline irrigation. It is inserted via the most lateral subcostal or epigastric port and is surprisingly easy to use. The technique is easily learned, and most hospitals carry the equipment.

Electrohydraulic Lithotripsy

Electrohydraulic lithotripsy (EHL) systems consist of a bipolar probe and a charge generator. When a charge is transmitted across the electrodes at the tip of the probe, a spark is created. This induces expansion of the surrounding fluid and pressure shock wave to fragment the stone [3]. Saline irrigation provides a media for shock

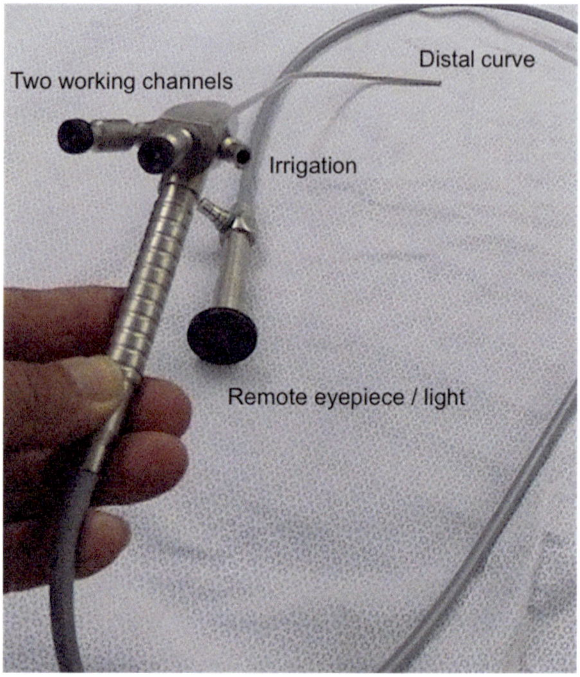

Fig. 8.3 Semirigid choledochoscope (Storz, Germany). Note dual operating channel and eyepiece and light source connections away from the operating channels to facilitate ease of use. The curve distally requires insertion directly through the skin, a short 12 mm port, or through a flexible port

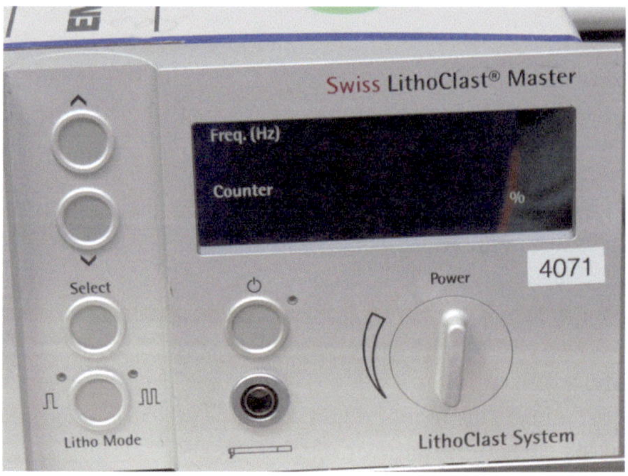

Fig. 8.4 The pneumatic shock wave generator. Single- or multi-fire modes are set, and activation is by foot pedal

wave energy transmission and assures visualization by flushing away debris. The procedure is done under direct flexible choledochoscopic guidance to avoid errant application of shock waves that *easily* cause ductal trauma and perforation. The probe is aimed directly at the stone and is optimally positioned 5 mm from the tip of the endoscope and 1–2 mm from the stone. Activation is performed using a foot switch. Activation of the probe within the operating channel will immediately *destroy* the choledochoscope.

Laser Lithotripsy

Several endoscopic laser lithotripsy systems have been used for biliary applications [3]. Focusing laser light of a high-power density on the surface of a stone creates a plasma bubble with cavitation that shatters the stone surface.

Holmium: yttrium aluminum garnet (YAG) lasers are widely used for urologic indications and are very effective for biliary stones. The laser-light wavelength is in the near-infrared spectrum, at 2100 nm, and delivers comparatively high-energy pulses of about 500–1000 mJ. As with EHL, direct visualization of the stones is generally recommended to prevent ductal trauma.

The frequency-doubled, double-pulse neodymium:YAG (FREDDY) laser uses wavelengths of 532 and 1064 nm and generates up to 120–160 mJ of energy (approximately 24 mJ at 532 nm). Laser-pulse duration is 1.2 ms at 160 mJ, with single or dual pulse at adjustable rates of 1, 3, 5, or 10 Hz. The recommended settings to start are 120 mJ single pulse and 3–5 Hz repetition rate, which can be increased to 160 mJ and 10 Hz. Double pulse at 120 or 160 mJ will cause the fiber to burn back into the buffer more readily than single-pulse settings.

Lasers are currently not familiar or frequently used technology for general surgeons and require an operator's license and use in a laser-safe operating theater with laser-trained nursing staff available. Eye protection for the patient and operating room staff is of paramount importance. In addition, great care must be taken to avoid misdirecting the laser onto the bile duct wall as this will result in *bile duct perforation*. The expensive choledochoscope will also be *destroyed* if the laser is activated while the tip of the delivery fiber is close to or within the choledochoscope operating channel.

Stone fragmentation is only done enough to crack the stone into large fragments with speedy stone fragment retrieval using a Dormia basket.

Extracorporeal Shock Wave Lithotripsy

ESWL uses shock wave generation with an external source focused on the stone within the duct, with either nasobiliary, transhepatic, or very occasionally a T-tube drain access allowing fluoroscopic stone identification, fragmentation, and then removal. Design of devices has evolved since the 1980s with first-generation water-bath electrohydraulic (HM3, Dornier, discharge limit 2000), second-generation (HM4 Dornier), and third-generation electromagnetic (Dornier, discharge limit 3000) using fluoroscope stone identification and targeting. The Dornier MPL 9000 uses an ultrasound targeting system.

The Approach to Impacted Stones

Cystic Duct Stone Impaction

This is often suspected during dissection of the distal gallbladder to define the cystic duct and critical view of safety during cholecystectomy. A bulge of the cystic duct may be found with tissue induration around that region. Once the critical view is defined, the clipping of the cystic duct proximally allows an incision for the cholangiogram. Failure of bile flashback will confirm the impression of a transiting stone obstructing the cystic duct. To massage the stone back up the cystic duct, atraumatic bowel grasping forceps can gently be applied to the cystic duct beyond the stone, milking it out of the cystic ductotomy, with bile flashback confirming clearance. The cholangiogram can now proceed as usual.

Stones impacted lower down the cystic duct, sometimes with a very low entry to the bile duct, may only be apparent on cholangiography. Awareness of the following techniques will save time by moving steadily from one to the next as required:

For an *apparently* impacted stone, the *first* step is to pass a 4F or 5F Fogarty balloon catheter up to, but not past, the stone. Using fluoroscopic guidance, inflate the balloon to just more than the duct diameter. A sharp retraction of the inflated balloon will often dislodge an apparently impacted stone, illustrated by contrast flow distally, allowing basket retrieval. Only *after* this maneuver has failed should attempts be made to push a guide wire, Fogarty balloon, or basket around the impacted stone. This is because these steps all run the risk of aggravating impaction rather than succeeding.

If fluoroscopic clearance of the cystic duct stone fails, the next step is to use a choledochoscope. This situation is ideally suited for a semirigid choledochoscope or ureteroscope [4, 5] because it is very likely that the access to the point of obstruction along the cystic duct will be quite direct (Figs. 8.2 and 8.3). The stone is cracked quickly and easily with the pneumatic lithoclast and fragments removed with a Dormia basket (Fig. 8.5a–c).

The alternative is to use 3 mm flexible choledochoscope with laser or EHL fragmentation (see later).

The other situation that may arise during Dormia basket removal of bile duct stones via the cystic duct is impaction of the stone in the basket at the cystic duct-common hepatic duct junction. This is easily dealt with if the semirigid choledochoscope is being used with its second operating channel allowing insertion of pneumatic probe and fragmentation of the stone within the basket (Fig. 8.6).

Bile Duct Stones

During cholecystectomy, fluoroscopic C-arm cholangiography remains the intraoperative tool of choice to outline the bile ducts and to assess stone load and the site of stone impaction. The goal is to clear the mobile stones completely and then remove

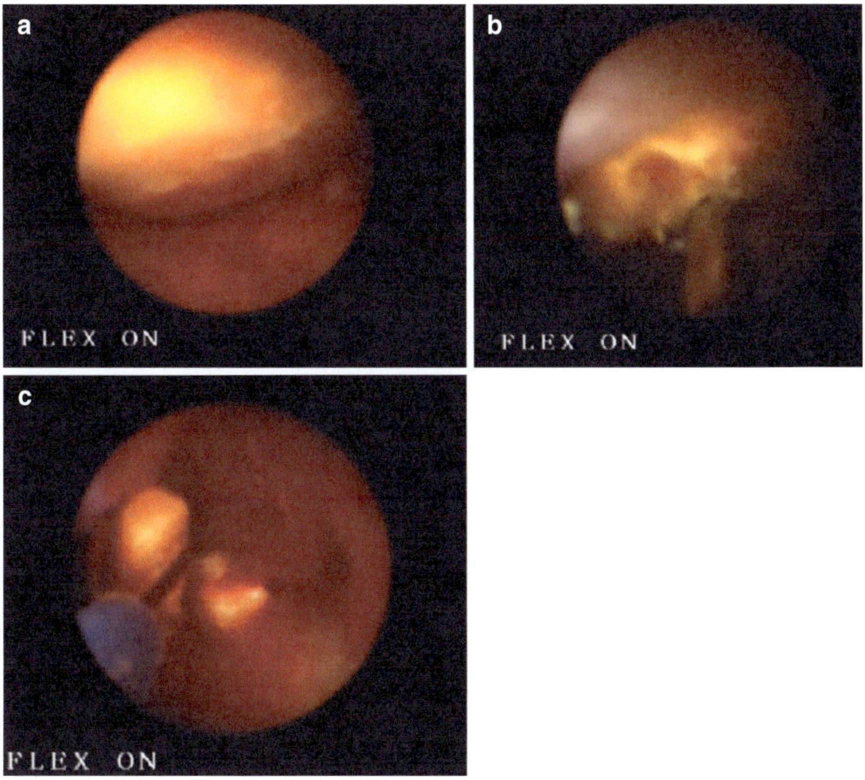

Fig. 8.5 (**a**) Semirigid choledochoscope view of impacted stone. (**b**) Pneumatic probe stone fragmentation by submillimeter movements backward and forward from the handpiece. (**c**) Once disimpacted, fragments are removed by Dormia basket. This is quicker than complete fragmentation and washing into the duodenum. It also decreases the chance of fragments being displaced into the proximal biliary tree

the impacted stone (Fig. 8.7a–c). This can be achieved via the trans-cystic or choledochotomy route, depending on the diameter of the bile duct, size, and number of stones.

For an *apparently* impacted stone, the *first* step is to pass a 4F or 5F Fogarty balloon catheter up to, but not past, the stone. Using fluoroscopic guidance, inflate the balloon to just more than the duct diameter. A sharp retraction of the inflated balloon will often dislodge an apparently impacted stone, illustrated by contrast flow distally, allowing basket retrieval. Only *after* this maneuver has failed should attempts be made to push a guide wire, Fogarty balloon, or basket around the impacted stone. This is because these steps run the risk of aggravating impaction rather than succeeding.

The fastest technique for cracking impacted calculi is using pneumatic lithotripsy. It does require delivery through a semirigid choledochoscope or short ureteroscope and does not work down flexible choledochoscopes (Videos 8.1a and 8.1b).

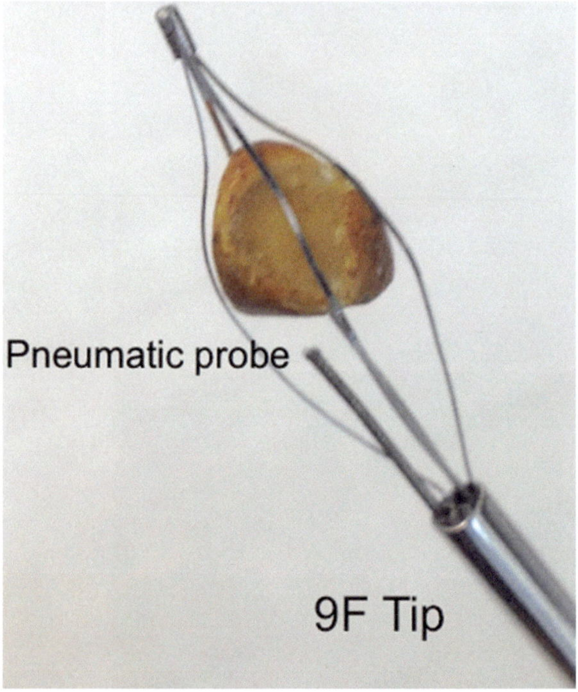

Fig. 8.6 Fragmentation of stone entrapped within Dormia basket by insertion of pneumatic probe through the second operating channel

A second light source, camera, and screen are set up, irrigation connected, and choledochoscope inserted via the right subcostal or epigastric port, depending on the patient body habitus and direction of bile duct [4, 5]. A nasogastric tube is passed to avoid gastric distension of refluxed irrigation fluid, which can occur with a long procedure. The trans-cystic technique is facilitated by cystic duct transection and then endo-looping it as a tether to guide intubation. The pneumatic handpiece requires assembly and activation pedal placed conveniently. Intermittent or multi-fire modes are available (Fig. 8.4). Poor fragmentation performance will be due to incorrect assembly of the probe to the handpiece. Once fragmented and dis-impacted, the stones are removed with a Dormia basket (Fig. 8.5a–c).

Where flexible cholechoscopy is used, the setup with light source, camera, and irrigation is then followed by setting up the EHL probe or laser. For trans-cystic 3 mm choledochoscopes, a long shaft "bariatric" 5 mm port acts as an oversleeve to deliver the choledochoscope close to the cystic duct to minimize looping of the scope (Fig. 8.8). The EHL and laser fiber tip must be clear of the end of the operating channel, in view, and then aimed correctly before considering firing. Saline irrigation will keep the view clear. Once dis-impacted, fragments are removed with a Dormia basket (Fig. 8.9).

ERCP currently is by far the most commonly used approach to impacted stones and will not be addressed in detail in this chapter [6]. Approaches vary from direct

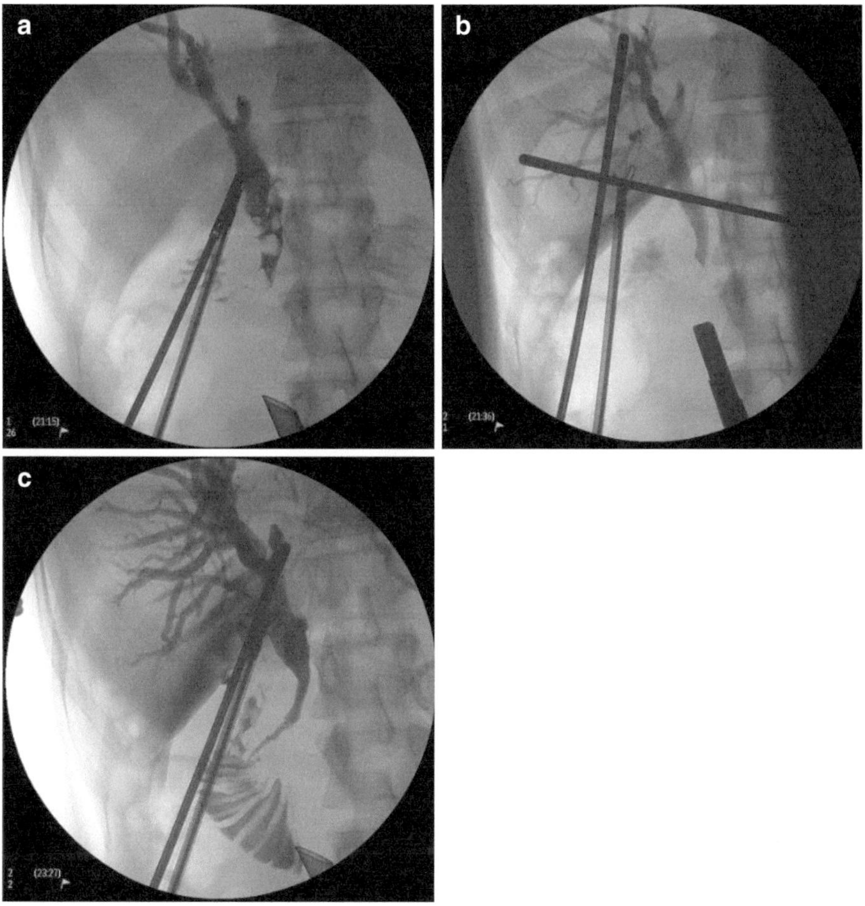

Fig. 8.7 (**a**) Cholangiogram outline of multiple stones within the bile duct above an impacted distal stone. (**b**) Proximal stones removed in sequence from those closest to the cystic duct, using a Dormia basket. The impacted stone was not able to be shifted with a balloon or traversed by guide wire. (**c**) Completion cholangiogram after pneumatic fragmentation and removal (see Fig. 8.5)

precut onto bulging ampullary stones, mechanical basket lithotripsy, to inserting a cholangioscope via the operating channel and performing laser lithotripsy. Difficult ERCP is associated with acute angulation bile duct, short distal bile duct, large stones, duodenal diverticulum, and the use of fragmentation [7].

When using EHL and laser lithotripsy delivered with flexible scopes, while they are the most elegant techniques, caution must be exercised to prevent injury to theater staff. In addition, keep in mind that activation within the operating channel of the choledochoscope will damage it. Accidental poor aim and activation onto the bile duct will lead to perforation.

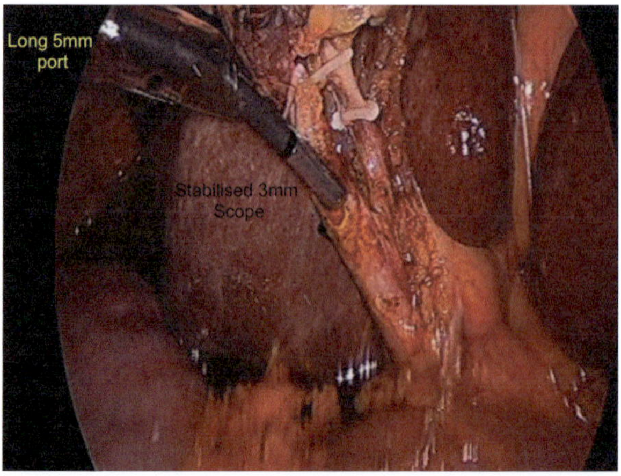

Fig. 8.8 Stabilization of the 3 mm flexible choledochoscope by the use of a long bariatric 5 mm port to act as an oversheath controlled by the surgical assistant. This facilitates intubation of the cystic duct and minimizes uncontrolled looping

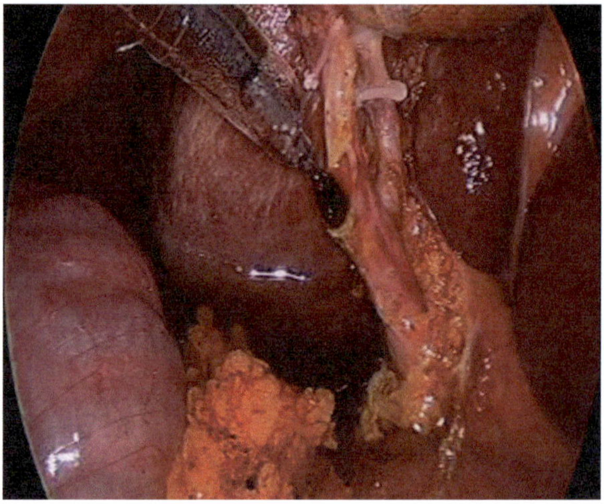

Fig. 8.9 Trans-cystic removal of fragmented stone using a 3 mm flexible choledochoscope

Intrahepatic Stones

Preoperative imaging with contrasted computed tomography (CT) scanning and magnetic resonance imaging (MRI) allows mapping of the position of impacted stones and strictures. A classification (Table 8.1 [8]) based on the distribution of hepatolithiasis and the presence of strictures is useful [9]. Biliary access with percutaneous transhepatic drainage, nasobiliary drain, or T-tube provides access for contrast imaging of the impacted stone. The access tracts need to mature for 4–6 weeks, a guide wire passed, and the drain removed and replaced with a suitable caliber access sheath. An appropriate size cholangioscopic access with saline irrigation allows pneumatic, laser, or EHL stone fragmentation and extraction with subsequent balloon dilation of strictures.

Table 8.1 Tsunoda classification of intrahepatic stones [8]

Intrahepatic anatomical findings	Class
No marked dilatation or strictures of intrahepatic ducts	I
Diffuse dilatation of intrahepatic ducts without strictures	II
Unilateral solitary or multiple cystic dilatation of intrahepatic ducts with strictures	III
Bilateral intrahepatic stones	IV

Outcomes over 25 years have reported clearance of 99% of cases with low stone load requiring 1 intervention, while complex cases with multiple stones sometimes have required up to 15 interventions [8]. This Japanese series using laser fragmentation has been mirrored by a more recent European experience using EHL [9]. Complications of cholangitis and bleeding are rare. Cases with malignant strictures often go on to have stents placed permanently. Recurrent stone formation is a long-term problem experienced in 15% patients after 2 years follow-up and has been successfully treated with re-intervention [9].

T-Tube Tract Stone Extraction

Although used far less frequently in this era, T-tube drain decompression can still selectively provide drainage and subsequent access to the bile duct. For patients with previous gastric bypass where ERCP has not been feasible, after choledochotomy and a complex exploration of the bile duct, then inserting a T-tube can be very useful. If residual stones are present, the T-tube tract is left to mature for 6 weeks and allows quite simple access using a rigid ureteroscope or flexible choledochoscope.

Extracorporeal Shock Wave Lithotripsy

Patients usually are positioned supine with the shock waves entering posteriorly. In patients with intrahepatic stones, a left oblique or right oblique position may improve stone identification during lithotripsy. Also, if fluoroscopy revealed the spinal column to be close to the target area, a left or right oblique position moves the spinal cord outside the target area. Prophylactic antibiotics are routinely used.

For stone identification and control of disintegration, contrast medium via the nasobiliary tube, percutaneous drain, or T-tube with fluoroscopy allows targeting and monitors stone fragmentation every 200 discharges. With all lithotripters used, the discharge energy is set at the upper range: lithotripter HM3, 23 kV; lithotripter HM4, 23 kV; lithotripter Dornier, 90%; and lithotripter MPL9000, 23 kV. Shock wave application continues until sufficient stone fragmentation is observed or until the upper limit of discharges of the respective lithotripter is reached. In the latter case, retreatment is possible within 1 week. Relief of pain during shock wave delivery can be in conjunction with deep sedation or general anesthesia. Bile is aspirated via the nasobiliary tube or percutaneous drain at intervals of about 200 shock wave discharges and inspected for hemobilia.

Large and impacted stones with biliary strictures are common indications where ESWL has been used after failed ERCP [10]. In this report with a median stone size of 20 mm, subsequent ERCP extraction of fragments or spontaneous passage resulted in 90% clearance of stones. Success was not influenced by the presence of strictures or if the stones were intrahepatic or extrahepatic. Morbidity included arrhythmia in 11%, hemobilia in 4.4%, cholangitis in 1.3%, ERCP perforation in 1.9%, and severe cholecystitis in 0.9%.

Conclusion

This overview covers a wide range of equipment and approaches to impacted stones and their management. Most surgeons will not have all these tools available for managing their patients. With careful imaging and planning, individualized treatment allows the optimal use of the equipment that is available. By familiarity with equipment, knowledge of how to progress from one technique to the next, rehearsal, and then more regular use, surgeons will be rewarded with single-stage management and happy patients [6].

References

1. Nagaraja V, Cox MR, Eslick GD. Systematic review and meta-analysis of the minimally invasive techniques for the management of cholecysto-choledocholithiasis. J Hepatobil Pancreat Sci. 2014;21:896–901.
2. Moody F, Amerson J, Berci G, Bland KL, Cotton PB, Graham JB, et al. Lithotripsy for bile duct stones. Am J Surg. 1989;158:241–7.
3. Blind PJ, Lundmark M. Management of bile duct stones: lithotripsy by laser, electrohydraulic, and ultrasonic techniques. Eur J Surg. 1998;164:403–9.
4. Quadri S, Khan M, Khan N. Use of pneumatic lithotripsy for managing difficult CBD calculi. Int J Surg. 2011;9:59–62.
5. Chander J, Vindal A, Lal P, Gupta N, Ramteke VK. Laparoscopic management of CBD stones: an Indian experience. Surg Endosc. 2011;25:172–81.
6. Sandzén B, Haapamäki MM, Nilsson E, Stenlund HC, Oman M. Treatment of common bile duct stones in Sweden 1989-2006: an observational nationwide study of a paradigm shift. World J Surg. 2012;36(9):2146–53.
7. Kim HJ, Choi HS, Park JH, Park DI, Cho YK, Sohn CI, et al. Factors influencing the technical difficulty of endoscopic clearance of bile duct stones. Gastrointest Endosc. 2007;66:1154–60.
8. Watanabe Y, Sato M, Tokui K, Nezu K, Shiraishi S, Sato K, et al. Painless lithotripsy by flashlamp-excited dye laser for impacted biliary stones: an experimental and clinical study. Eur J Surg. 2000;166:455–8.

9. Cannavale A, Bezzi M, Ceratti F, Lucatelli P, Fanello G, Salvatori FM, et al. Combined radiological-endoscopic management of difficult bile duct stones: 18-year single center experience. Ther Adv Gastroenterol. 2015;8(6):340–51.
10. Sackman M, Holl J, Sauter GH, Pauletzki J, von Ritter C, Paumgartner G. Extracorporeal shock wave lithotripsy for clearance of duct stones resistant to endoscopic extraction. Gastrointest Endosc. 2001;53(1):27–32.

Chapter 9
Adjuncts to Common Bile Duct Exploration

Vimal K. Narula and Mazen R. Al-Mansour

Introduction

Up to 5–20% of patients with gallstone disease have common bile duct (CBD) stones. With more than 20 million people having gallstone disease in the United States alone, choledocholithiasis represents a significant global healthcare problem [1]. Choledocholithiasis was traditionally a condition managed almost exclusively by surgeons via open common bile duct exploration (CBDE) during the "open" surgical era. Advances in radiology, endoscopy, and laparoscopic surgery have increased the options for removal of CBD stones while avoiding the morbidity of an open surgical procedure [2, 3]. While the success rate of CBDE (whether open or laparoscopic) exceeds 90% in the average patient, factors including the stone size, bile duct diameter, number of stones, and the presence of altered anatomy (periampullary diverticulum, Billroth II gastrojejunostomy, and Roux-en-Y configuration) make stone removal more challenging in some patients. This chapter discusses adjuncts to CBDE, including biliary drains, biliary stents, balloon papillary dilation, and antegrade sphincterotomy. These techniques can be of great value in managing more challenging cases of choledocholithiasis.

Biliary Drains

Biliary drains allow external drainage of the biliary tree and provide access for the bile duct, allowing subsequent cholangiography and in some cases percutaneous biliary interventions.

V. K. Narula, MD (✉) · M. R. Al-Mansour, MD
Department of General and Gastrointestinal Surgery, The Ohio State University/Wexner Medical Center, Columbus, OH, USA
e-mail: Raaja.narula@osumc.ed; Mazen.almansour@osumc.edu

© Springer International Publishing AG, part of Springer Nature 2018

B. F. Santos, N. Soper (eds.), *Choledocholithiasis*,
https://doi.org/10.1007/978-3-319-74503-9_9

T-Tubes

T-tubes are long rubber tubes with a horizontal short limb at the end that sit in the bile duct and allow drainage. T-tube placement requires either open or laparoscopic choledochotomy. After stones are cleared from the bile duct, the horizontal bar is placed inside the bile duct through the choledochotomy. Care needs to be exercised to make sure that the diameter of the horizontal bar is appropriate for the size of the bile duct and that the length of the proximal (cephalad) limb is appropriate. An inappropriately large horizontal bar or a long proximal limb may result in biliary obstruction. The distal limb is usually made longer than the proximal limb, with some surgeons even preferring to leave it long enough to stent open the sphincter of Oddi as it passes into the duodenum. The back wall of the horizontal bar can be trimmed to facilitate tube placement and removal and and to improve drainage (Fig. 9.1a–e). The choledochotomy should be closed with fine absorbable sutures snugly around the tube (to prevent bile leak), paying attention to avoid inadvertently catching the

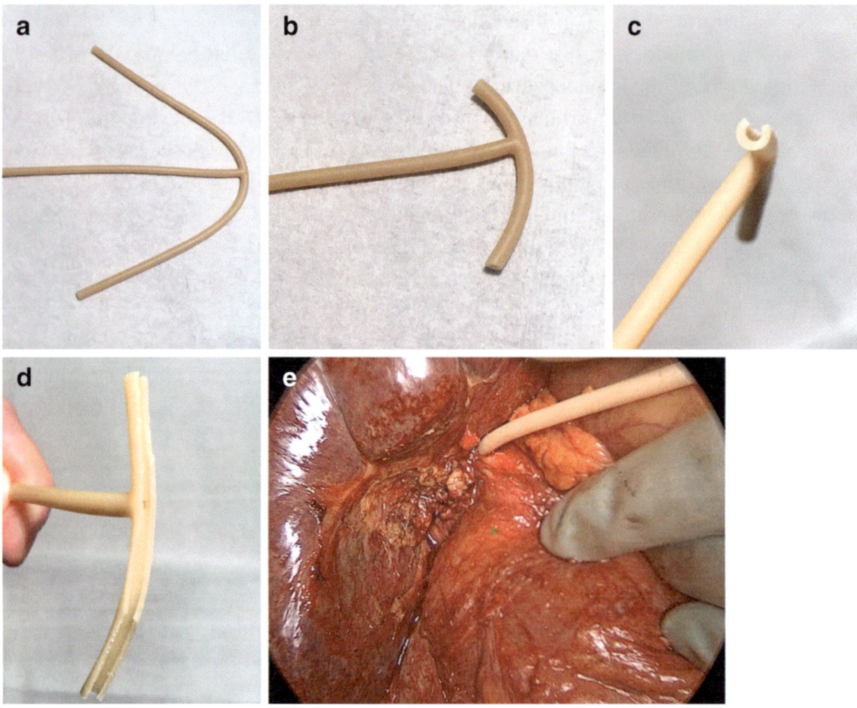

Fig. 9.1 The intact T-tube (**a**) is fashioned by trimming the horizontal limb to a short proximal segment and long distal segment (**b**). The back wall of the horizontal bar can be trimmed (**c**, **d**) to facilitate tube placement and removal and to improve drainage. The T-tube can either be secured through the choledochotomy or alternatively exteriorized through a separate ductotomy as in this case of Mirizzi's syndrome (**e**) requiring closure of a cholecystocholedochal fistula using a remnant gallbladder flap

T-tube during closure. The T-tube should be left in place for at least 2 weeks to allow the tract around the tube to mature. A T-tube cholangiogram is performed to confirm ductal clearance prior to T-tube removal. If stones are seen on the cholangiogram, the T-tube tract allows percutaneous instrumentation of the bile duct for stone clearance. T-tubes can be placed to allow biliary drainage in patients when impacted CBD stones cannot be cleared with common duct exploration as a bailout maneuver. This allows biliary decompression and provides percutaneous access for subsequent lithotripsy and passage of dilating and extracting balloons and baskets or until endoscopic clearance can be attempted. Alternatively, the surgeon may drain the bile duct using a straight drain placed via the cystic duct into the common bile duct (C-tube) and secured in place with a tie around the cystic duct [4, 5].

Although T-tubes are a valuable adjunct to common duct exploration, primary choledochotomy closure has also been shown to be safe and effective [6–15]. Routine choledochotomy closure over T-tube has come under scrutiny in recent years due to concerns of complications including bile leak, bile peritonitis, fluid and electrolyte imbalances, and tube dislodgment. Three meta-analyses of studies comparing primary ductal closure and ductal closure over T-tubes after laparoscopic transductal CBDE have shown that primary ductal closure was associated with fewer complications, shorter operative times, shorter hospital length of stay, and decreased costs when compared to ductal closure over T-tubes [16–18]. A Cochrane systematic review, including 6 trials and 359 patients, found similar mortality and serious morbidity rates between primary ductal closure and closure over T-tube after open CBDE. However, the T-tube group had longer operative times and hospital length of stay. Although routine T-tube use may not confer an advantage over primary closure for straightforward cases, it remains a valuable adjunct for difficult cases, impacted stones, cases of sepsis where biliary drainage postoperatively is paramount, or in patients with altered anatomy where postoperative access and biliary drainage would otherwise be difficult.

Internal-External Biliary Drains

Another option for biliary drainage includes percutaneously placed internal-external biliary drains (Figs. 9.2 and 9.3). These pigtail catheters are placed percutaneously into the liver parenchyma and guided through the intrahepatic biliary tree to the extrahepatic biliary tree into the duodenum where the pigtail portion prevents proximal migration into the bile duct. These drains have an intra-biliary segment with side holes for bile to enter the catheter, as well as side holes on the pigtail portion. Bile enters the side holes in the intra-biliary segment and then drains either to the external bag or into the duodenum through the pigtail segment. Clamping the tube externally preferentially allows drainage of bile into the duodenum through the pigtail section. These drains may be used for drainage of an obstructed bile duct secondary to choledocholithiasis or for drainage of a bile duct injury/leak in patients with altered anatomy or who have failed endoscopic therapy.

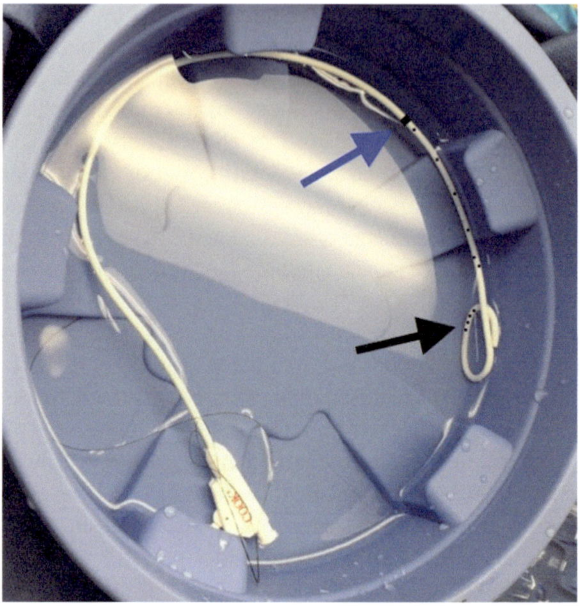

Fig. 9.2 Internal-external biliary drain. The catheter has a proximal radiopaque marker (blue arrow), which marks the most proximal portion of the intra-biliary drainage segment (side holes visible). The distal portion of the catheter has a pigtail shape with side holes (black arrow) that sits within the duodenum, preventing proximal migration and allowing drainage of bile into the duodenum

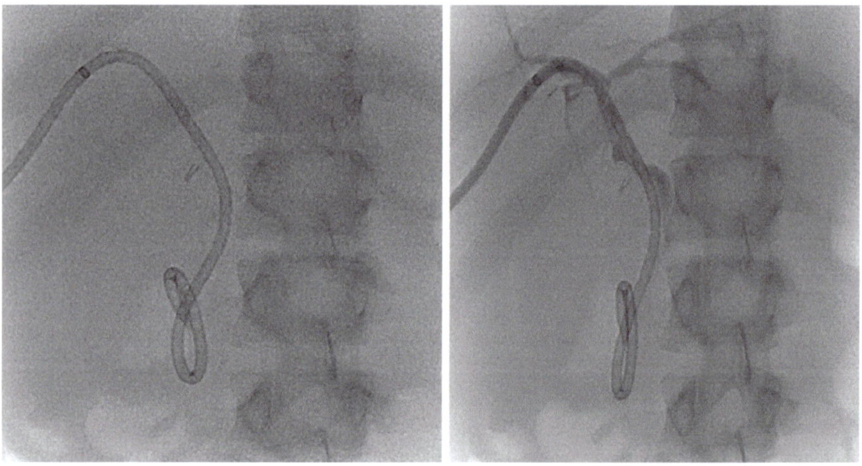

Fig. 9.3 Internal-external biliary drain. The drain was placed in this case to manage a stricture resulting from iatrogenic common bile duct injury (at the site of the surgical clips)

A surgical technique for retrograde placement of an internal-external biliary drain at the time of open CBDE has also been described as an alternative to T-tube use [4, 19]. A catheter is advanced through a choledochotomy after open CBDE retrograde into the hepatic ducts until it can be palpated through the liver parenchyma. It is then advanced further puncturing the liver parenchyma under ultrasound guidance to avoid any major vessels. The catheter is then extracted through the abdominal wall. This technique is rarely used nowadays.

Nasobiliary Drains

Nasobiliary drains are another form of external biliary drain. The distal part of the drain is typically placed into the bile duct in a retrograde fashion during endoscopic retrograde cholangiopancreatography (ERCP). The proximal portion of the drain is then brought out through the nose and is connected to gravity drainage. Nasobiliary drains are used more frequently in Asia than in the United States and play a role in specific clinical situations. In cases of severe cholangitis requiring emergent ERCP, for example, they allow temporary biliary decompression as an alternative to the use of more expensive plastic biliary stents, to avoid prolonged attempts at endoscopic stone clearance when difficult stones are encountered in unstable patients, or as a safer alternative to sphincterotomy in coagulopathic patients. Nasobiliary drainage is usually adequate to provide biliary drainage while the patient is stabilized, prior to definitive therapy. An interval cholangiogram using contrast media or even air may be performed to check for stone size and tube position and plan further therapy such as endoscopic stone clearance, common duct exploration, or in some situations extracorporeal shock wave lithotripsy (ESWL) prior to definitive endoscopic clearance (Fig. 9.4). Maintaining the drain in place during laparoscopic or open transductal CBDE allows closure of the choledochotomy over the endonasobiliary drain. When used in this setting, endonasobiliary drains have been shown to be safe and effective compared to T-tube use. Like the T-tube, the nasobiliary drain allows the surgeon to perform postoperative cholangiography to confirm stone clearance prior to tube removal. The nasobiliary tube is best used to provide short-term drainage (to reduce patient discomfort from a nasal tube) and unlike a T-tube eliminates the need to wait for tract maturation prior to tube removal, resulting in shorter tube duration for the patient [7, 20–22]. A downside of nasobiliary drains, however, is that they do not allow for percutaneous stone removal, unlike the use of a T-tube tract, and also require endoscopy for placement.

Biliary Stents

Biliary stents allow internal drainage of bile into the digestive tract. The stent is positioned across the papilla with the proximal portion in the bile duct and the distal portion in the duodenum. Biliary stents are most commonly placed endoscopically during ERCP and are indicated for temporary drainage prior to definitive CBD stone clearance, post-cholecystectomy bile leaks, iatrogenic bile duct injuries, and for benign and malignant biliary strictures [23]. Biliary stents may also be surgically placed through a transcystic approach for temporary internal drainage, through

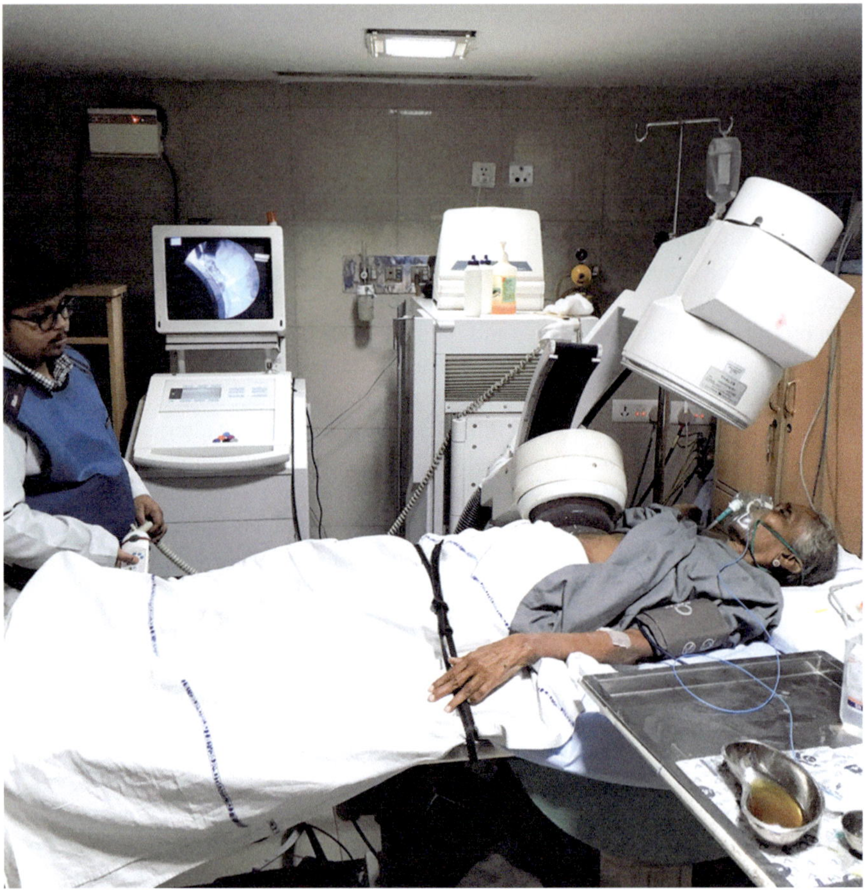

Fig. 9.4 Nasobiliary drainage is useful for temporary drainage of the biliary tree. In this photograph, a patient with a nasobiliary drain in place undergoes external shock wave lithotripsy to break up massive common duct stones to make subsequent endoscopic stone clearance feasible. The nasobiliary drain ensures continued biliary drainage and allows interval cholangiography to assess the progress of stone fragmentation prior to definitive stone clearance

a choledochotomy as an adjunct to ductal closure, or as an alternative to common duct exploration that facilitates postoperative ERCP. Different types of biliary stents exist and will be discussed.

Endoscopic Stent Placement

Endoscopic stents can be placed during ERCP in the setting of CBD stones for a variety of reasons. In the emergency setting, stents may be placed in cases of cholangitis as an alternative to sphincterotomy (in coagulopathic patients) or stone clearance in unstable patients, to allow continued biliary drainage and stabilization of the patient. Once the patient has recovered, repeat ERCP may be performed to complete stone clearance.

The use of biliary stents in the management of difficult to clear CBD stones (such as large and multiple stones) is also well described, as a temporary drainage option that prevents jaundice or cholangitis until all the stones can be cleared with subsequent interventions including repeat endoscopic, percutaneous, or surgical stone extraction. Repeat ERCP for stone removal 3–6 months after stent placement is successful in 63–96% of patients who fail initial endoscopic stone removal. The presence of a biliary stent itself is believed to lead to a reduction in stone size and can result in stone fragmentation or softening, which can facilitate lithotripsy and stone extraction with a balloon [24–27]. In contrast, the addition of a pharmacologic choleretic agent (such as ursodeoxycholic acid) does not seem to reduce stone size, increase stone fragmentation, or facilitate subsequent stone extraction [28, 29]. Stents are also helpful to the endoscopist as their presence facilitates repeat cannulation of the papilla and also in cases of difficult deep biliary cannulation (e.g., when a biliary stricture is present).

In contrast to temporary use, stents have also been proposed as a long-term adjunct to sphincterotomy in patients with CBD stones who carry high surgical risk, such as the elderly or patients with multiple comorbidities and in whom complete endoscopic ductal clearance is difficult or fails [30–36]. The stent allows decompression of the biliary tree, which addresses jaundice and prevents cholangitis, and may serve as a definitive measure in frail patients or those with a limited life expectancy. A study of 201 patients with stones not amenable to endoscopic removal who underwent sphincterotomy and 7 F double-pigtail stent placement found a median stent patency of almost 5 years with a 7.4% rate of recurrent cholangitis and 18.5% rate of recurrent jaundice [36]. When choosing a strategy of long-term stent therapy, some endoscopists prefer routine exchanges of the stents to prevent occlusion and cholangitis, while others cite safe long-term outcomes without the need for routine stent exchanges. The use of two or more plastic stents as definitive therapy for choledocholithiasis may help mitigate the risk of stent occlusion [28, 36–39].

Plastic Biliary Stents

Temporary plastic stents are the most commonly used stents for the management of choledocholithiasis. These stents use different fixation systems to prevent stent migration including flaps and pigtail ends. The flap-equipped stents are straight plastic tubes that utilize flaps to secure the stent in place proximally and distally to prevent inadvertent retrograde or antegrade migration, respectively. The stents vary in size from 7 F to 12 F and vary in length from 5 to 15 cm. The stent is placed into the bile duct with the flap-containing distal end protruding into the duodenum (Fig. 9.5). Pigtail stents utilize looping flexible ends to anchor the stent in place (Fig. 9.6) [40]. Bile flows through the stent as well as around the stent by capillary action. Plastic stents can remain in place for up to 3 months before the risk of occlusion and subsequent cholangitis increases [23].

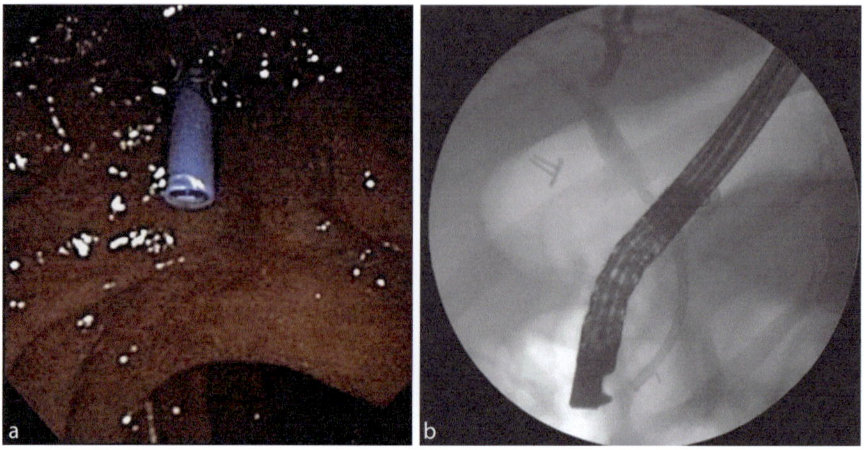

Fig. 9.5 (**a**) Endoscopic view of flap-anchored plastic stent. (**b**) Fluoroscopic view of flap-anchored plastic stent

Fig. 9.6 Plastic biliary stents (Bruno MJ. Ch 51. Palliation of Malignant Pancreaticobiliary Obstruction. In: Ginsberg GG, Gostout CJ, Kochman ML, Norton ID, editors. Clinical Gastrointestinal Endoscopy, 2nd ed. Elsevier Saunders. 2011; p. 706–20)

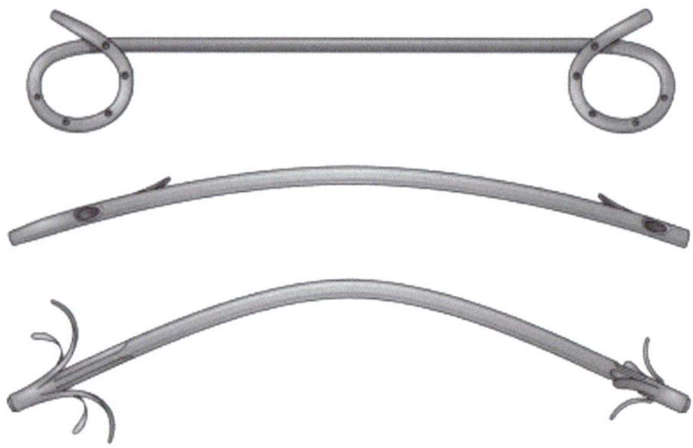

Metal Biliary Stents

Metal stents are composed of a metal alloy that expands to a predetermined shape once deployed in the biliary tree. Metal stent types include uncovered self-expanding metallic stents (SEMS), partially covered SEMS, and fully covered SEMS. Uncovered SEMS are not removable, and therefore their use should be limited to the palliation of malignant biliary strictures since tissue in-growth prevents safe removal. Covered stents are composed of a metallic lattice that is covered with various types of materials to prevent tissue or tumor in-growth. These covered stents are removable and thus may be used for benign strictures or in cases of difficult common duct stones. The use of these stents for the management of CBD stones has been described with outcomes similar to those of plastic stents, with complications including stent migration either into or out of the bile duct, pancreatitis, perforation, and bleeding [41, 42]. It is unclear whether the use of the more expensive covered SEMS for difficult choledocholithiasis cases confers any benefit compared to the use of cheaper plastic stents in terms of stone removal rates or complications. Table 9.1 compares the different types of biliary stents.

Table 9.1 Biliary stents

Stent	Description	Indication	Complications
Flap-anchored plastic stents	• Removable • Different materials (polyethylene, polyurethane, polytef [Teflon]) • Sizes (7 F to 12 F) • Length (5–15 cm) • Flaps at both ends anchor stent in place • Radiopaque	• Biliary stricture • Bile leak • Iatrogenic biliary injury • Choledocholithiasis	Migration Occlusion Cholangitis
Pigtail (Double J) plastic stents	• Removable • Pigtail ends anchor stent in place • Radiopaque	• Biliary stricture • Bile leak • Iatrogenic biliary injury • Choledocholithiasis	Migration Occlusion Cholangitis
Fully covered SEMS Examples: Viabil (Conmed, Utica, NY, USA), WallFlex (Boston Scientific, Natick, MA, USA), Niti-S (Taewoong Medical Co., Ltd., Gyeonggi-do, South Korea)	• Removal • Metal frame with full polyurethane or silicone cover • Radiopaque	• Biliary stricture • Biliary leak • Iatrogenic biliary injury • Choledocholithiasis	Migration Occlusion Cholangitis
Partially covered SEMS Example: Wallstent (Boston Scientific, Natick, MA, USA)	• Removal (but extraction can be challenging) • Metal frame with polyurethane or silicone cover except at ends • Radiopaque	• Biliary stricture • Biliary leak • Iatrogenic biliary injury • Choledocholithiasis	Occlusion Tissue in-growth Migration Cholangitis
Uncovered SEMS Example: Wallstent (Boston Scientific, Natick, MA, USA)	• Permanent • Metal frame (stainless steel alloy, nitinol) • Radiopaque	• Malignant biliary stricture	Occlusion Tissue in-growth Cholangitis

SEMS self-expanding metal stent

Surgical Stent Placement

Biliary stents can also be placed operatively during open or laparoscopic CBDE. Closure of the choledochotomy over plastic biliary stents (both pigtail-type and straight flap-anchored stents) is well described. The stent can be placed via the choledochotomy or antegrade through the cystic duct over a guidewire, followed by closure of the choledochotomy [7, 43–50]. When compared to choledochotomy closure over T-tube, stent placement is associated with shorter operative times and shorter length of stay [51–54]. A disadvantage of using stents for this purpose is the need for postoperative upper endoscopy for stent retrieval. Some surgeons modify the stents by removing the proximal anchor (flap or pigtail loop) and replacing it with a rapidly absorbable suture material to allow spontaneous and intentional distal migration of the stent through the digestive tract, obviating the need for postoperative endoscopy [54–57]. In patients with altered anatomy (Billroth II or Roux-en-Y gastrojejunostomy), ERCP can be extremely challenging, and primary closure of the choledochotomy or closure over a biliary drain (T-tube or C-tube) may be more appropriate than a stent in this setting. Ductal closure over biliary stents might be a better option than T-tube placement or ductal closure without a stent in patients with small-caliber bile ducts in order to avoid stricture formation; however, strong data to support this practice is lacking. Table 9.2 compares the different methods of closing the choledochotomy during CBDE.

Stent-Related Complications

The use of biliary stents is safe but complications may arise. The most common include stent occlusion with resulting jaundice, elevated liver function enzymes, and cholangitis. Stent migration (proximal or distal) of plastic stents may occur at a

Table 9.2 Common techniques for closure of choledochotomy after transductal CBDE

Technique	Allows cholangiogram	Advantages	Disadvantages
Primary closure	No	• Short operative time • Reduced costs • Improved patient satisfaction	• Concerns for stricture formation in small bile ducts
Closure over T-tube	Yes	• External biliary drainage • Allows percutaneous instrumentation	• Longer operative times • Longer hospital stay • Complications (bile leak, bile peritonitis, tube dislodgement) • Higher cost
Closure over nasobiliary tube	Yes	• External biliary drainage	• Requires preoperative ERCP
Closure over biliary stent	No	• Internal biliary drainage	• Most require postoperative upper endoscopy for stent removal

CBDE common bile duct exploration, *ERCP* endoscopic retrograde cholangiopancreatography rate between 3% and 10%. Proximal migration into the biliary tree makes endoscopic removal challenging. Distal migration into the gastrointestinal tract usually results in complete stent passage without any problems [58, 59]. Rarely, intestinal perforation can result from migration of biliary stents [60–62] or erosion of the stent through the biliary tree [63, 64].

Balloon Papillary Dilation

First described in 1982, endoscopic balloon papillary dilation (EBPD) has been utilized as both an alternative and an adjunct to endoscopic sphincterotomy to facilitate removal of CBD stones [65–70]. Compared to sphincterotomy, EBPD (at least in theory) maintains the integrity of the sphincter of Oddi and may prevent long-term complications resulting from reflux of duodenal contents into the biliary tree. Endoscopic balloon dilation has a particularly useful role in patients with challenging anatomy such as Billroth II gastrojejunostomy as well as in coagulopathic patients [23, 71–73].

EBPD is performed by passing a large, radially dilating balloon into the bile duct after deep cannulation. The balloon is inflated (to a diameter of up to 20 mm) for a period of time (30 s to 5 min) resulting in stretching of the sphincter of Oddi. The dilating balloon reliably inflates to predetermined diameters based on the atmospheric pressure applied. The use of a manual pressure pump allows controlled inflation and deflation of the balloon to the desired diameter (Fig. 9.7). If the initial endoscopic sphincterotomy is not adequate for the retrieval of large stones, the additional stretching from EBPD can facilitate stone removal [74]. Despite initial hesitation, multiple studies have shown that EBPD after endoscopic sphincterotomy is safe, including in certain high-risk patients (e.g., those with a periampullary diverticulum) [75–77].

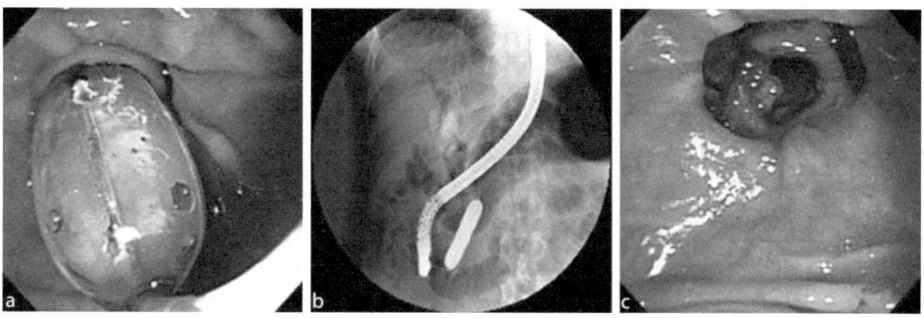

Fig. 9.7 Endoscopic balloon papillary dilation. (**a**) Endoscopic view of the inflated balloon. (**b**) Fluoroscopic view of the inflated balloon. (**c**) Endoscopic view of the dilated papilla after successful dilation (Reprinted under the terms of Creative Commons Attribution Non-Commercial License (http://creativecommons.org/licenses/by-nc/4.0) from Chung JW, Chung JB. Endoscopic papillary balloon dilation for removal of choledocholithiasis: indications, advantages, complications, and long-term follow-up results. Gut Liver. 2011 Mar;5(1):1–14)

This technique has been borrowed from the endoscopic realm and used as an adjunct to percutaneous and surgical CBDE (either laparoscopic or open) [78–80]. The dilation balloon is passed antegrade via a transcystic or transductal approach across the sphincter of Oddi using fluoroscopic guidance. After the dilation is completed, the use of pressure washing (flushing) is more likely to result in dislodgement of the stones into the duodenum. Alternatively, stones can be pushed distally into the duodenum via the dilated sphincter using extraction balloons or the choledochoscope. When the balloon is positioned at the sphincter distal to the stone, care should be exercised while withdrawing the deflated balloon to prevent proximal dislodgement of the stones into the hepatic ducts [81].

The success rate of EBPD for stone clearance exceeds 90% and is comparable to endoscopic sphincterotomy in removal of large stones. The 10% complication rate of this technique is also similar to endoscopic sphincterotomy. However, bleeding is more common after endoscopic sphincterotomy, while pancreatitis seems to be more frequent after balloon dilation [72]. The mechanism behind the increased rate of post-ERCP pancreatitis in patients undergoing EBPD is unknown. A retrospective study showed that the rate of hyperamylasemia was 30% when balloon papillary dilation was performed endoscopically compared to 7% when it was performed percutaneously. The duration of balloon inflation may play a role in the rate of pancreatitis. It has been shown that a shorter duration of balloon inflation (<5 min versus ≥5 min) when EBPD is performed without sphincterotomy results in higher rates of pancreatitis (18% versus 0%). It is hypothesized that a shorter duration of balloon dilation may result in less complete disruption of the sphincter of Oddi fibers, leading to swelling, spasm, and post-procedure obstruction of the pancreatic duct that leads to pancreatitis [82]. Higher rates of pancreatitis seen with endoscopic EBPD rather than percutaneous EBPD suggests that other factors, such as the passage of larger instruments including lithotripsy catheters and baskets, rather than the balloon dilation itself, may lead to the higher incidence of pancreatitis [83]. Another complication of EBPD includes injury to the bile duct; therefore, the size of the balloon used should not exceed the diameter of the bile duct.

Antegrade Sphincterotomy

Antegrade sphincterotomy is an intraoperative option that can be used to facilitate deep biliary cannulation during intraoperative ERCP or as an adjunct to common duct exploration. The surgeon passes a guidewire in antegrade fashion through the cystic duct across the papilla and into the duodenum. A sphincterotome is then passed over the wire and used to create the sphincterotomy. This should be performed under the endoscopic guidance of a side-viewing duodenoscope. An appropriately sized sphincterotomy is performed at the 11 or 12 o'clock position of the papilla opposite to the location of the pancreatic duct. The common duct stones are then either flushed or pushed into the duodenum from above (Fig. 9.8a–c). This technique has been described both percutaneously and laparoscopically [5, 84–86]. This technique is similar to a rendezvous procedure in which the surgeon passes a wire antegrade

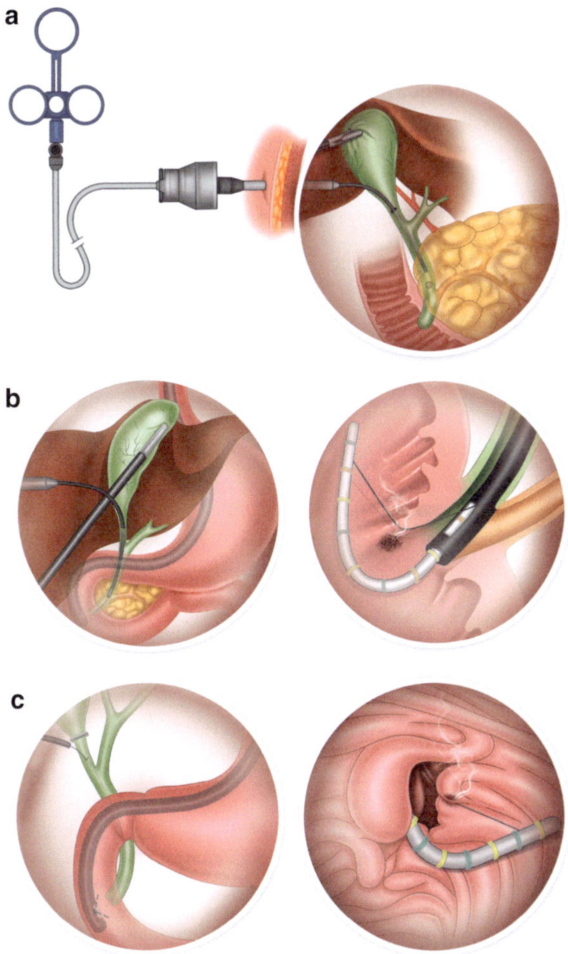

Fig. 9.8 Laparoscopic antegrade sphincterotomy. (**a**) A standard endoscopic sphincterotome is inserted through the right upper quadrant 5.0 mm cannula using an introducer sheath to minimize gas leakage. (**b**) Left: The side-viewing duodenoscope is positioned directly opposite the ampulla so that the sphincterotome may be guided into proper position under direct vision. Right: The sphincterotome is bowed, which exposes the cutting wire, and maneuvered until it is at the 12 o'clock position. (**c**) Left: A guidewire may be used to facilitate passage of the sphincterotome across the ampulla. Right: A blend of coagulation and cutting current is used to divide the sphincter up to the first transverse fold of the duodenum (Reprinted with permission from Zucker KA, Curet MJ. Laparoscopic Antegrade Transcystic Sphincterotomy. In: Phillips EH, Rosenthal RJ (eds). Operative Strategies in Laparoscopic Surgery. Berlin, Heidelberg: Springer-Verlag. 1995: 54-58)

through the cystic duct and through the papilla so that an ERCP operator can snare the wire and obtain wire access for retrograde sphincterotomy. The ERCP operator then performs stone extraction in a conventional fashion. Compared to the rendezvous procedure, antegrade sphincterotomy has been found to be associated with shorter operative times and equivalent stone extraction and complication rates [87].

Conclusion

The management of difficult cases of choledocholithiasis requires adequate knowledge of different approaches and their advantages and disadvantages. Patients with high surgical risk and altered anatomy and those with impacted stones benefit from adjuncts to common bile duct exploration including biliary drains, biliary stents, balloon papillary dilation, and antegrade sphincterotomy. Appropriate use of these different approaches—whether they be endoscopic, percutaneous, surgical, or a combination of approaches—leads to the optimal management of choledocholithiasis while minimizing complications.

References

1. Everhart JE, Khare M, Hill M, Maurer KR. Prevalence and ethnic differences in gallbladder disease in the United States. Gastroenterology. 1999;117(3):632–9.
2. Hazey JW. Historical perspective and treatments for common bile duct stones. In: Hazey JW, Conwell DL, Guy GE, editors. Multidisciplinary management of common bile duct stones. Cham: Springer International Publishing; 2016. p. 1–4.
3. Khadra H, Jackson T, Marks J. Management of surgical complications. In: Hazey JW, Conwell DL, Guy GE, editors. Multidisciplinary management of common bile duct stones. Cham: Springer International Publishing; 2016. p. 129–44.
4. Hotta T, Taniguchi K, Kobayashi Y, Johata K, Sahara M, Naka T, et al. Biliary drainage tube evaluation after common bile duct exploration for choledocholithiasis. Hepatogastroenterology. 2003;50(50):315–21.
5. Ponsky JL, Heniford BT, Gersin K. Choledocholithiasis: evolving intraoperative strategies. Am Surg. 2000;66(3):262–8.
6. Ambreen M, Shaikh AR, Jamal A, Qureshi JN, Dalwani AG, Memon MM. Primary closure versus T-tube drainage after open choledochotomy. Asian J Surg. 2009;32(1):21–5.
7. Chen C-C, Wu S-D, Tian Y, Zeng X-T, Siwo EA, Xian G-Z. The fading role of T-tube in laparoscopic choledochotomy: primary choledochorrhaphy and over pigtail j and endonasobiliary drainage tubes. J Laparoendosc Adv Surg Tech A. 2010;20(10):807–11.
8. Decker G, Borie F, Millat B, Berthou JC, Deleuze A, Drouard F, et al. One hundred laparoscopic choledochotomies with primary closure of the common bile duct. Surg Endosc. 2003;17(1):12–8.
9. El-Geidie AAR. Is the use of T-tube necessary after laparoscopic choledochotomy? J Gastrointest Surg. 2010;14(5):844–8.
10. Gurusamy KS, Samraj K. Primary closure versus T-tube drainage after open common bile duct exploration. Cochrane Database Syst Rev. 2007;(1):CD005640.
11. Saeed N, Nasir MT, Khan MI, Channa GA. Choledochorraphy (primary repair) versus t-tube drainage after open choledochotomy. J Ayub Med Coll Abbottabad JAMC. 2012;24(1):18–20.
12. Sorensen VJ, Buck JR, Chung SK, Fath JJ, Horst HM, Obeid FN. Primary common bile duct closure following exploration: an effective alternative to routine biliary drainage. Am Surg. 1994;60(6):451–4.
13. Zhu QD, Tao CL, Zhou MT, Yu ZP, Shi HQ, Zhang QY. Primary closure versus T-tube drainage after common bile duct exploration for choledocholithiasis. Langenbecks Arch Surg. 2011;396(1):53–62.
14. Zhang H-W, Chen Y-J, Wu C-H, Li W-D. Laparoscopic common bile duct exploration with primary closure for management of choledocholithiasis: a retrospective analysis and comparison with conventional T-tube drainage. Am Surg. 2014;80(2):178–81.

15. Ahmed I, Pradhan C, Beckingham IJ, Brooks AJ, Rowlands BJ, Lobo DN. Is a T-tube necessary after common bile duct exploration? World J Surg. 2008;32(7):1485–8.
16. Podda M, Polignano FM, Luhmann A, Wilson MSJ, Kulli C, Tait IS. Systematic review with meta-analysis of studies comparing primary duct closure and T-tube drainage after laparoscopic common bile duct exploration for choledocholithiasis. Surg Endosc. 2016;30(3):845–61.
17. Wu X, Yang Y, Dong P, Gu J, Lu J, Li M, et al. Primary closure versus T-tube drainage in laparoscopic common bile duct exploration: a meta-analysis of randomized clinical trials. Langenbecks Arch Surg. 2012;397(6):909–16.
18. Yin Z, Xu K, Sun J, Zhang J, Xiao Z, Wang J, et al. Is the end of the T-tube drainage era in laparoscopic choledochotomy for common bile duct stones is coming? A systematic review and meta-analysis. Ann Surg. 2013;257(1):54–66.
19. Kusano T, Isa T, Shimoji H, Miyazato H, Muto Y, Furukawa M. Results of retrograde transhepatic biliary drainage after a common bile duct exploration for choledocholithiasis. Hepatogastroenterology. 1999;46(29):2776–80.
20. Otani K, Ueki T, Matsumura K, Maruo T, Minoda R, Otsuka Y, et al. Comparison between endoscopic biliary stenting and nasobiliary drainage in patients with acute cholangitis due to choledocholithiasis: is endoscopic biliary stenting useful? Hepatogastroenterology. 2015;62(139):558–63.
21. Wani MA, Chowdri NA, Naqash SH, Parray FQ, Wani RA, Wani NA. Closure of the common duct-endonasobiliary drainage tubes vs. t tube: a comparative study. Indian J Surg. 2010;72(5):367–72.
22. Zhang H-F, Hu S-Y, Zhang G-Y, Wang K-X, Chen B, Li B. Laparoscopic primary choledochorrhaphy over endonasobiliary drainage tubes. Surg Endosc. 2007;21(11):2115–7.
23. Pearl J. Techniques of endoscopic retrograde cholangiopancreatography. In: Marks JM, Dunkin BJ, editors. Principles of flexible endoscopy for surgeons. New York: Springer; 2013. p. 215–26.
24. Aslan F, Arabul M, Celik M, Alper E, Unsal B. The effect of biliary stenting on difficult common bile duct stones. Przeglad Gastroenterol. 2014;9(2):109–15.
25. Horiuchi A, Nakayama Y, Kajiyama M, Kato N, Kamijima T, Graham DY, et al. Biliary stenting in the management of large or multiple common bile duct stones. Gastrointest Endosc. 2010;71(7):1200–3.e2.
26. Fan Z, Hawes R, Lawrence C, Zhang X, Zhang X, Lv W. Analysis of plastic stents in the treatment of large common bile duct stones in 45 patients. Dig Endosc. 2011;23(1):86–90.
27. Sharma SS, Jhajharia A, Maharshi S. Short-term biliary stenting before mechanical lithotripsy for difficult bile duct stones. Indian J Gastroenterol. 2014;33(3):237–40.
28. Lee TH, Han J-H, Kim HJ, Park SM, Park S-H, Kim S-J. Is the addition of choleretic agents in multiple double-pigtail biliary stents effective for difficult common bile duct stones in elderly patients? A prospective, multicenter study. Gastrointest Endosc. 2011;74(1):96–102.
29. Katsinelos P, Kountouras J, Paroutoglou G, Chatzimavroudis G, Zavos C. Combination of endoprostheses and oral ursodeoxycholic acid or placebo in the treatment of difficult to extract common bile duct stones. Dig Liver Dis. 2008;40(6):453–9.
30. Ang TL, Fock KM, Teo EK, Chua TS, Tan J. An audit of the outcome of long-term biliary stenting in the treatment of common bile duct stones in a general hospital. J Gastroenterol. 2006;41(8):765–71.
31. Hong W, Zhu Q, Huang Q. Endoscopic sphincterotomy plus endoprostheses in the treatment of large or multiple common bile duct stones. Dig Endosc. 2011;23(3):240–3.
32. Horiuchi A, Kajiyama M, Ichise Y, Tada H, Fujiwara N, Tanaka N. Biliary stenting as alternative therapy to stone clearance in elderly patients with bile duct stones. Acta Gastro-Enterol Belg. 2014;77(3):297–301.
33. Li KW, Zhang XW, Ding J, Chen T, Wang J, Shi WJ. A prospective study of the efficacy of endoscopic biliary stenting on common bile duct stones. J Dig Dis. 2009;10(4):328–31.
34. Peters R, Macmathuna P, Lombard M, Karani J, Westaby D. Management of common bile duct stones with a biliary endoprosthesis. Report on 40 cases. Gut. 1992;33(10):1412–5.

35. Yang J, Peng J, Chen W. Endoscopic biliary stenting for irretrievable common bile duct stones: indications, advantages, disadvantages, and follow-up results. Surg J R Coll Surg Edinb Irel. 2012;10(4):211–7.
36. Slattery E, Kale V, Anwar W, Courtney G, Aftab AR. Role of long-term biliary stenting in choledocholithiasis. Dig Endosc. 2013;25(4):440–3.
37. Di Giorgio P, Manes G, Grimaldi E, Schettino M, D'Alessandro A, Di Giorgio A, et al. Endoscopic plastic stenting for bile duct stones: stent changing on demand or every 3 months. A prospective comparison study. Endoscopy. 2013;45(12):1014–7.
38. Maxton DG, Tweedle DE, Martin DF. Stenting for choledocholithiasis: temporizing or therapeutic? Am J Gastroenterol. 1996;91(3):615–6.
39. Ye X, Huai J, Sun X. Effectiveness and safety of biliary stenting in the management of difficult common bile duct stones in elderly patients. Turk J Gastroenterol. 2016;27(1):30–6.
40. Bruno MJ. Palliation of malignant pancreaticobiliary obstruction. In: Ginsberg GG, Gostout CJ, Kochman ML, Norton ID, editors. Clinical gastrointestinal endoscopy. St. Louis: Elsevier Saunders; 2011. p. 706–20.
41. Bakhru MR, Kahaleh M. Expandable metal stents for benign biliary disease. Gastrointest Endosc Clin N Am. 2011;21(3):447–62, viii.
42. Cerefice M, Sauer B, Javaid M, Smith LA, Gosain S, Argo CK, et al. Complex biliary stones: treatment with removable self-expandable metal stents: a new approach (with videos). Gastrointest Endosc. 2011;74(3):520–6.
43. Dietrich A, Alvarez F, Resio N, Mazza O, de Santibañes E, Pekolj J, et al. Laparoscopic management of common bile duct stones: transpapillary stenting or external biliary drainage? JSLS. 2014;18(4):pii: e2014.00277.
44. Fujii M, Okino M, Fujioka K, Yamashita K, Hamano K. Placement of a double-pigtail ERBD tube after primary closure of the common bile duct in three patients with choledocholithiasis. J Hepatobiliary Pancreat Surg. 2005;12(5):386–90.
45. Isla AM, Griniatsos J, Karvounis E, Arbuckle JD. Advantages of laparoscopic stented choledochorrhaphy over T-tube placement. Br J Surg. 2004;91(7):862–6.
46. Kuroki T, Tajima Y, Tsuneoka N, Kitasato A, Adachi T, Kosaka T, et al. Placement of a plastic biliary stent tube with primary closure of the common bile duct after laparoscopic common bile duct exploration. Hepatogastroenterology. 2010;57(102–103):1034–6.
47. Lee JS, Yoon YC. Laparoscopic common bile duct exploration using V-Loc suture with insertion of endobiliary stent. Surg Endosc. 2016;30(6):2530–4.
48. Wei Q, Hu H-J, Cai X-Y, Li L-B, Wang G-Y. Biliary drainage after laparoscopic choledochotomy. World J Gastroenterol. 2004;10(21):3175–8.
49. Bandyopadhyay SK, Khanna S, Sen B, Tantia O. Antegrade common bile duct (CBD) stenting after laparoscopic CBD exploration. J Minimal Access Surg. 2007;3(1):19–25.
50. Pérez G, Escalona A, Jarufe N, Ibáñez L, Viviani P, García C, et al. Prospective randomized study of T-tube versus biliary stent for common bile duct decompression after open choledocotomy. World J Surg. 2005;29(7):869–72.
51. Lyon M, Menon S, Jain A, Kumar H. Use of biliary stent in laparoscopic common bile duct exploration. Surg Endosc. 2015;29(5):1094–8.
52. Tang CN, Tai CK, Ha JPY, Tsui KK, Wong DCT, Li MKW. Antegrade biliary stenting versus T-tube drainage after laparoscopic choledochotomy – a comparative cohort study. Hepatogastroenterology. 2006;53(69):330–4.
53. Xin Y, Zhu X, Wei Q, Cai X, Wang X, Huang D. Comparison of quality of life between two biliary drainage procedures in laparoscopic common bile duct exploration. Hepatogastroenterology. 2007;54(74):331–3.
54. Xu Y, Dong C, Ma K, Long F, Jiang K, Shao P, et al. Spontaneously removed biliary stent drainage versus T-tube drainage after laparoscopic common bile duct exploration. Medicine (Baltimore). 2016;95(39):e5011.
55. Huang J, Zhu J. Spontaneously removed endobiliary J stent drainage after laparoscopic common bile duct exploration. Surg Endosc. 2009;23(6):1398–402.

56. Kim EK, Lee SK. Laparoscopic treatment of choledocholithiasis using modified biliary stents. Surg Endosc. 2004;18(2):303–6.
57. Tian MG, Shi WJ, Zhong CJ, Zhang XW, Chen TM. Laparoscopic treatment of choledocholithiasis with novel self-releasing biliary stent. J Laparoendosc Adv Surg Tech A. 2009;19(3):405–8.
58. Cerisoli C, Diez J, Giménez M, Oria M, Pardo R, Pujato M. Implantation of migrated biliary stents in the digestive tract. HPB. 2003;5(3):180–2.
59. Katsinelos P, Kountouras J, Paroutoglou G, Chatzimavroudis G, Paikos D, Zavos C, et al. Migration of plastic biliary stents and endoscopic retrieval: an experience of three referral centers. Surg Laparosc Endosc Percutan Tech. 2009;19(3):217–21.
60. Chittleborough TJ, Mgaieth S, Kirkby B, Zakon J. Remove the migrated stent: sigmoid colon perforation from migrated biliary stent. ANZ J Surg. 2016;86(11):947–8.
61. El Zein MH, Kumbhari V, Tieu A, Saxena P, Messallam AA, Azola A, et al. Duodenal perforation as a consequence of biliary stent migration can occur regardless of stent type or duration. Endoscopy. 2014;46(Suppl 1):E281–2.
62. Zeb F, Kevans D, Muir K, Courtney G, Tadros E, Aftab A. Duodenal impaction/perforation of a biliary stent – a rare complication in the management of choledocholithiasis. J Gastrointest Liver Dis JGLD. 2009;18(3):391–2.
63. Dundee PE, Franzi SJ, Thomas PR. Unique complication of a biliary stent: erosion through the common hepatic duct wall. ANZ J Surg. 2007;77(3):194.
64. Sinha S, Wardle A, Kalidindi V, Banga N, Stoker DL. Erosion and perforation of the biliary tree by plastic biliary endoprostheses. Endoscopy. 2010;42(9):760–3.
65. Chung JW, Chung JB. Endoscopic papillary balloon dilation for removal of choledocholithiasis: indications, advantages, complications, and long-term follow-up results. Gut Liver. 2011;5(1):1–14.
66. Nagashima I, Takada T, Shiratori M, Inaba T, Okinaga K. Percutaneous transhepatic papillary balloon dilation as a therapeutic option for choledocholithiasis. J Hepatobiliary Pancreat Surg. 2004;11(4):252–4.
67. Tsai T-J, Lai K-H, Lin C-K, Chan H-H, Wang E-M, Tsai W-L, et al. Role of endoscopic papillary balloon dilation in patients with recurrent bile duct stones after endoscopic sphincterotomy. J Chin Med Assoc JCMA. 2015;78(1):56–61.
68. Watanabe H, Hiraishi H, Koitabashi A, Sasai T, Kanke K, Oinuma T, et al. Endoscopic papillary balloon dilation for treatment of common bile duct stones. Hepatogastroenterology. 2004;51(57):652–7.
69. Zippi M, De Felici I, Pica R, Traversa G, Occhigrossi G. Endoscopic papillary balloon dilation for difficult common bile duct stones: our experience. World J Clin Cases. 2013;1(1):19–24.
70. Testoni PA, Mariani A, Aabakken L, Arvanitakis M, Bories E, Costamagna G, et al. Papillary cannulation and sphincterotomy techniques at ERCP: European Society of Gastrointestinal Endoscopy (ESGE) Clinical Guideline. Endoscopy. 2016;48(7):657–83.
71. Shakhatreh MH, Groce JR. Gastroenterologic treatment and outcomes. In: Hazey JW, Conwell DL, Guy GE, editors. Multidisciplinary management of common bile duct stones. Cham: Springer International Publishing; 2016. p. 85–91.
72. Baron TH, Harewood GC. Endoscopic balloon dilation of the biliary sphincter compared to endoscopic biliary sphincterotomy for removal of common bile duct stones during ERCP: a metaanalysis of randomized, controlled trials. Am J Gastroenterol. 2004;99(8):1455–60.
73. Jang HW, Lee KJ, Jung MJ, Jung JW, Park JY, Park SW, et al. Endoscopic papillary large balloon dilatation alone is safe and effective for the treatment of difficult choledocholithiasis in cases of Billroth II gastrectomy: a single center experience. Dig Dis Sci. 2013;58(6):1737–43.
74. Lai K-H, Chan H-H, Tsai T-J, Cheng J-S, Hsu P-I. Reappraisal of endoscopic papillary balloon dilation for the management of common bile duct stones. World J Gastrointest Endosc. 2015;7(2):77–86.
75. Kim KH, Kim TN. Endoscopic papillary large balloon dilation in patients with periampullary diverticula. World J Gastroenterol. 2013;19(41):7168–76.

76. Poincloux L, Rouquette O, Privat J, Gorce D, Abergel A, Dapoigny M, et al. Large-balloon dilation of the sphincter of Oddi after sphincterotomy or infundibulotomy to extract large calculi or multiple common bile duct stones without using mechanical lithotripsy. Scand J Gastroenterol. 2013;48(2):246–51.
77. Sakai Y, Tsuyuguchi T, Sugiyama H, Nishikawa T, Kurosawa J, Saito M, et al. Endoscopic sphincterotomy combined with large balloon dilation for removal of large bile duct stones. Hepatogastroenterology. 2013;60(121):58–64.
78. Shirai N, Hanai H, Kajimura M, Kataoka H, Yoshida K, Nakagawara M, et al. Successful treatment of percutaneous transhepatic papillary dilation in patients with obstructive jaundice due to common bile duct stones after Billroth II gastrectomy: report of two emergent cases. J Clin Gastroenterol. 2000;30(1):91–3.
79. Ozcan N, Kahriman G, Mavili E. Percutaneous transhepatic removal of bile duct stones: results of 261 patients. Cardiovasc Intervent Radiol. 2012;35(4):890–7.
80. Kumar A, Martinez JM. Surgical treatment and outcomes. In: Hazey JW, Conwell DL, Guy GE, editors. Multidisciplinary management of common bile duct stones. Cham: Springer International Publishing; 2016. p. 93–100.
81. Masoni L, Mari FS, Pietropaolo V, Onorato M, Meucci M, Brescia A. Laparoscopic treatment for unsuspected common bile duct stones by transcystic sphincter of Oddi pneumatic balloon dilation and pressure-washing technique. World J Surg. 2013;37(6):1258–62.
82. Shen YH, Yang LQ, Yao YL, Wang L, Zhang YY, Cao J, He QB, Zou XP, Li YH. Dilation time in endoscopic papillary balloon dilation for common bile duct stones. Surg Laparosc Endosc Percutan Tech. 2017;27(5):351–5.
83. Seo YR, Moon JH, Choi HJ, Kim DC, Lee TH, Cha S-W, et al. Papillary balloon dilation is not itself a cause of post-endoscopic retrograde cholangiopancreatography pancreatitis; results of anterograde and retrograde papillary balloon dilation. J Gastroenterol Hepatol. 2013;28(8):1416–21.
84. Born P, Sandschin W, Rösch T. Percutaneous antegrade sphincterotomy under endoscopic retrograde control: report of two cases. Endoscopy. 2002;34(6):512–3.
85. DePaula AL, Hashiba K, Bafutto M, Zago R, Machado MM. Laparoscopic antegrade sphincterotomy. Surg Laparosc Endosc. 1993;3(3):157–60.
86. Hunter JG, Pham TH. Laparoscopic cholecystectomy, intraoperative cholangiography, and common bile duct exploration. In: Fischer JE, editor. Mastery of surgery. Philadelphia: Lippincott Williams and Wilkins; 2006. p. 1265–77.
87. Tekin A, Ogetman Z, Altunel E. Laparoendoscopic "rendezvous" versus laparoscopic antegrade sphincterotomy for choledocholithiasis. Surgery. 2008;144(3):442–7.

Chapter 10
Open Common Bile Duct Exploration

David W. Rattner

Open Common Bile Duct Exploration: Historical Perspective

The management of biliary disease has undergone a radical transformation over the past 30 years. The introduction of therapeutic biliary endoscopy in the 1980s followed by laparoscopic cholecystectomy at the end of that decade greatly benefited patients. In spite of ever-improving technology, there are still situations that require traditional surgical procedures including open common bile duct exploration (OCBDE). For surgeons now in their late 50s or older, OCBDE was a staple of their surgical training and early career. In contrast, few surgeons younger than 50 years old have ever performed OCBDE unless their practice is focused on hepatobiliary disease. This generational divide combined with the shrinking indications for OCBDE has implications for how best to manage patients with choledocholithiasis when endoscopic means are unsuccessful or not possible. In the hands of experienced surgeons, OCBDE is a safe procedure albeit one that historically has been plagued by retained common duct stones in 4–10% of patients [1–3]. Since OCBDE is now infrequently performed, there are no current reported series to draw conclusions from that would lead one to believe we are doing any better than our surgical forefathers.

D. W. Rattner, MD
Department of Surgery, Division of General and Gastrointestinal Surgery,
Massachusetts General Hospital, Harvard Medical School, Boston, MA, USA
e-mail: drattner@partners.org; drattner@mgh.harvard.edu

© Springer International Publishing AG, part of Springer Nature 2018

B. F. Santos, N. Soper (eds.), *Choledocholithiasis*,
https://doi.org/10.1007/978-3-319-74503-9_10

Indications for Open Common Bile Duct Exploration

Although there are circumstances where OCBDE is the only way to manage choledocholithiasis, the ever-expanding therapeutic armamentarium of interventional endoscopic and radiologic techniques often provides multiple options to consider. The optimal diagnostic and therapeutic strategy depends on both the clinical circumstances and the local expertise of multiple disciplines. Surgeons who completed their training more than two decades ago when interventional endoscopic techniques were not as widely utilized are more likely to be comfortable performing OCBDE than their younger colleagues. While textbooks and videos are instructive, there is unfortunately no substitute for the experience of performing OBCDE, as tactile feedback is especially important in this procedure. Deciding between performing OCBDE and pursuing an alternative that will require multiple interventional endoscopic and radiologic procedures should take into account the local surgical expertise. Another key factor to consider is the diameter of the common bile duct. If the common bile duct diameter is <6 mm, the risk of stricture following choledochotomy is significant. Trans-ampullary approaches, if feasible, eliminate this risk. On the other hand, a dilated common duct is the surgeon's friend, and a choledochotomy is safe and easy and in many instances can be closed without the use of a T-tube. Nonetheless, if there is no experience with OCBDE in an institution that also lacks hepatobiliary surgical expertise, consideration should be given to transferring the patient to a center with this capability. The risks of bile duct injury and subsequent stricture formation need to be considered in the decision-making process.

In spite of the need for a laparotomy incision, there are circumstances where OCBDE offers advantages over interventional endoscopic and radiologic techniques to treat choledocholithiasis. First and foremost, OCBDE can accomplish complete resolution of biliary pathology in one step. Although it is standard practice in many locations to rely on endoscopic removal of retained common duct stones following cholecystectomy, it bears noting that endoscopic sphincterotomy (ES) is not a benign procedure. Morbidity rates of 10% persist, half of these considered major complications, and mortality rates of 0.5% are well established [4–7]. Although there is no level I evidence comparing OCBDE with ES to treat choledocholithiasis, one needs to remember that even if ES is less invasive, it still carries substantial risk of complications, and hence invasiveness should not be the sole criteria upon which to base therapeutic decisions. Consider, for example, the situation of a difficult laparoscopic cholecystectomy requiring conversion to open cholecystectomy. Once a laparotomy is performed, it would be less morbid to deal with concurrent choledocholithiasis using OCBDE than completing the cholecystectomy and referring the patient for a post-op endoscopic retrograde cholangiopancreatography (ERCP) and ES.

Open common bile duct exploration is the preferred approach in patients with large common duct stones. If treated via ES, these patients often require multiple trans-ampullary interventions to break up the stone and should be offered the option

Table 10.1 Indications for open common bile duct exploration

Converted laparoscopic cholecystectomy with choledocholithiasis
Mirizzi's syndrome
Large common duct stone (>2 cm)
Need for concomitant biliary drainage procedure
Inability to access ampulla for ERCP/ES • Long Roux-en-Y limb • Peri-ampullary diverticulum • Prior gastroduodenal surgery

of undergoing one definitive procedure. In some of these patients, particularly if they have recurrent choledocholithiasis, a biliary drainage procedure, such as choledochoduodenostomy, is indicated and can easily be performed at the time of OCBDE. While many of these interventions can also be performed laparoscopically, more tools are available for use with OCBDE that come in handy with difficult situations. Likewise, patients with large peri-ampullary duodenal diverticula may have an increased risk of perforation with ES and should be considered as candidates for OCBDE.

There is a growing population of patients in whom endoscopic access to the common bile duct is difficult. Patients with prior gastrectomies and weight loss procedures such as Roux-en-Y gastric bypass (RYGBP) or biliary pancreatic diversion (BPD) often develop choledocholithiasis. In RYGBP patients it is possible to perform ERCP and ES through the gastric remnant, but consideration should be given to direct choledochotomy (either laparoscopic or open) when the bile duct is dilated. In patients who have undergone BPD or gastrectomy with Roux-en-Y reconstruction, OCBDE may be the only way to access and clear the common duct (Table 10.1).

Technique for Open Common Bile Duct Exploration

Exposure

Open common bile duct exploration can be performed through either a midline, paramedian, or right subcostal incision. As with any surgical procedure, adequate exposure is an essential first step. Fixed retraction is extremely helpful if not essential. If the gallbladder is present, a cholecystectomy should be performed prior to exploring the common duct. Aside from obtaining a cholangiogram, there is little utility to performing trans-cystic maneuvers in the open surgical setting. More commonly the gallbladder will have been removed, and the procedure will commence with adhesiolysis and dissection of the portal structures. In setting up the operative field for OCBDE, the fixed retraction to push the liver cephalad, the hepatic flexure caudad, and the gastric antrum medially should be established. Once this has been performed, the next step is to kocherize the duodenum. It is best for the surgeon to stand on the patient's left side and then hold the duodenum and head of the pancreas in his/her left hand. A generous Kocher maneuver allows the surgeon to straighten out and put tension on the common bile duct, palpate the distal bile duct, and guide instruments into and through the papilla during exploration.

Choledochotomy

With the common duct clearly identified, a choledochotomy is performed. This should be performed distal to the cystic duct insertion and as close to the superior border of the duodenum as is comfortable. Placing the choledochotomy in this location allows for creation of a side-to-side choledochoduodenostomy should this become necessary during the case. A vertical or slightly oblique incision is preferred. It is helpful to place two traction sutures in the anterior wall prior to incising the duct, to prevent lacerating the posterior wall when the choledochotomy is made. Since the arterial blood supply to the common bile duct runs in the 3 and 9 o'clock positions, a transverse incision can interrupt both arteries leading to ischemia and stricture formation. The choledochotomy should begin as a 2 cm incision unless it is known that stones larger than this are present. Sometimes stones will pop out of the duct immediately. However, even if they do, a full exploration should be performed as follows:

Exploration

The key elements of OCBDE are clearing the bile duct of calculi, establishing that there is no obstruction at the ampullary level, and safe closure of the choledochotomy. Once the bile duct has been opened, the first maneuver is to flush the duct vigorously with saline. A semi-firm 10 Fr rubber catheter attached to a 60 cc syringe is the ideal tool. The catheter should first be directed proximally to irrigate the intrahepatic ducts. Then the catheter is directed distally for further irrigation. This often will wash the stone(s) out through the choledochotomy. Additionally, it allows the surgeon to see if the catheter can be guided through the ampulla and into the duodenum. Passage into the duodenum signifies that there is no ampullary stenosis as a cause for choledocholithiasis. One can easily ascertain if the catheter has traversed the duodenum by flushing with saline and observing that all the saline is filling the duodenum while no saline is exiting via the choledochotomy. If the number of stones known to be present preoperatively is retrieved by this maneuver, it is appropriate to proceed to imaging and closure (see later) or to intraoperative choledochoscopy. However, in most cases it will be necessary to perform further maneuvers to clear the ducts of stones. There are a variety of tools that can be used to retrieve common duct stones, and their utility depends heavily on surgeon familiarity and preference (Fig. 10.1). Stone scoops come in different sizes and are made with soft

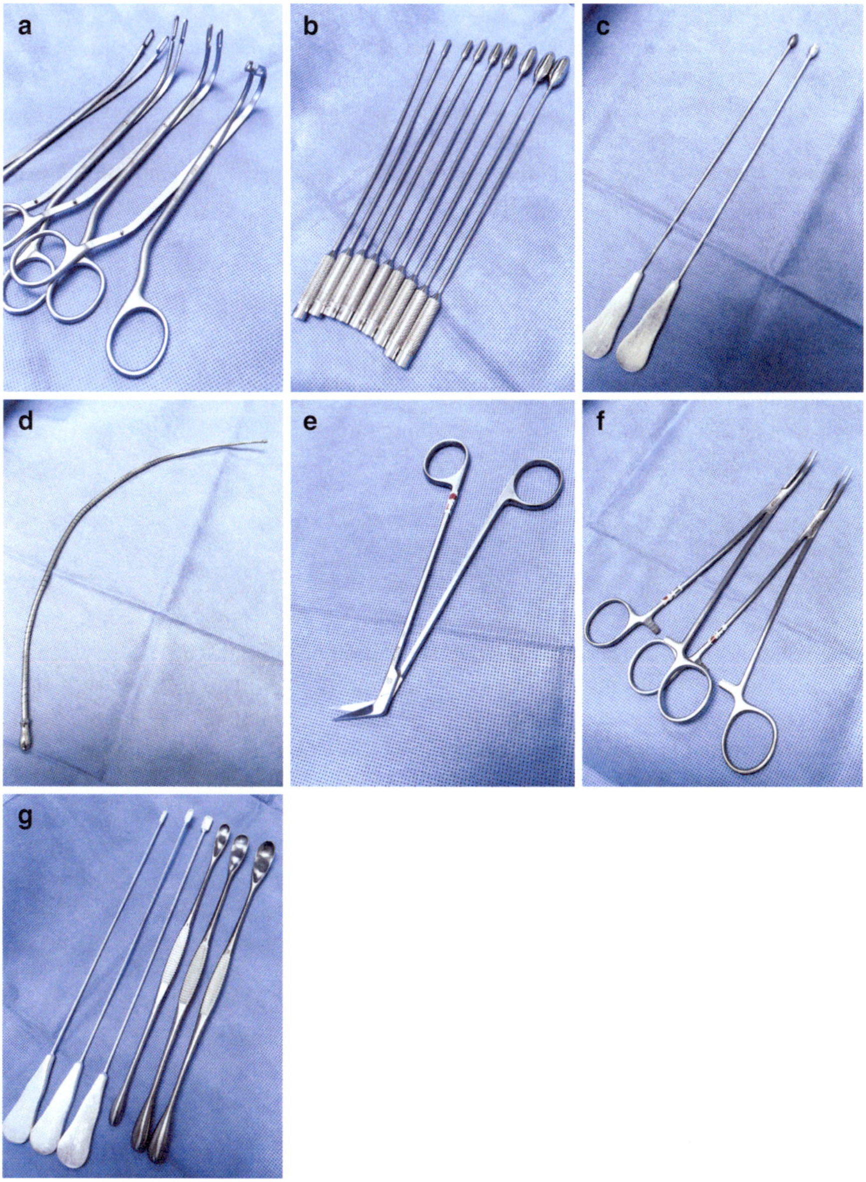

Fig. 10.1 Instruments for open common bile duct exploration. (**a**) Randall stone forceps. (**b**) Bakes dilators. (**c**) Mayo common duct probe. (**d**) Ochsner (Fenger) common duct probe. (**e**) Potts scissors. (**f**) Jake Schnidt. (**g**) Mayo and Ferguson common duct scoops. Photographs courtesy of B. Fernando Santos, MD

malleable shafts. This allows for bending into a C-shaped configuration in order to insert them into the common duct without restriction from the fixed retractors. Stone forceps are not malleable but can grasp and maneuver stones nicely. Irrespective of which tool is chosen, the surgeon's left hand should be holding the duodenum and guiding the distal bile duct onto the exploring instrument. Hence the exploratory process is bimanual, and tactile feedback is the key to success. An additional instrument commonly found in the OCBDE set is a Bakes dilator. Like the stone scoops, these come in a variety of sizes and are malleable. Their primary purpose is to provide a rigid object within the duct for palpation and to confirm patency of the ampulla. Although designed to dilate the ampulla, this practice should be considered outmoded in the current era, and one should not force these dilators into the duodenum if they do not go easily. Excessive force can create perforation of the distal bile duct or damage the ampulla leading to postoperative pancreatitis or worse. In general, one should not use anything larger than a 3–4 mm Bakes dilator.

Confirmation

Once all the stones have been retrieved and patency of the ampulla established, it is wise to confirm that a successful OCBDE has indeed been achieved. This can be confirmed either by choledochoscopy or cholangiography. Both techniques have been shown to reduce the incidence of retained stones. Since in the modern era, the use of OCBDE is generally restricted to situations in which it is difficult to access the common duct via endoscopic methods, it is very important to be as certain as possible that there are no remaining stones in the bile ducts. Choledochoscopy has several advantages over T-tube cholangiography. It can be performed prior to closing the choledochotomy and can also be combined with therapy. For example, if a completion choledochoscopy detected a stone in the proximal hepatic duct, basket retrieval under direct vision would be possible. Choledochoscopy can be performed with a variety of different instruments (flexible choledochoscopes, ureteroscopes, and even pediatric bronchoscopes as well as rigid nephroscopes), depending on institutional availability. If choledochoscopy is not available, a completion T-tube cholangiogram should be obtained.

Bile Duct Closure

It is traditional to leave a T-tube after performing OCBDE. The rationale for placing T-tubes is to allow fluoroscopic retrieval of retained stones, protect against bile leakage when ampullary edema develops following the trauma of exploration, and to stent the closure of small ducts. While there is a recent trend to omit this step, particularly when performing laparoscopic CBDE, one needs to carefully consider the indication for OCBDE before electing to close the choledochotomy primarily. If one is certain that there are no retained stones in the CBD, the ampulla is patent, and

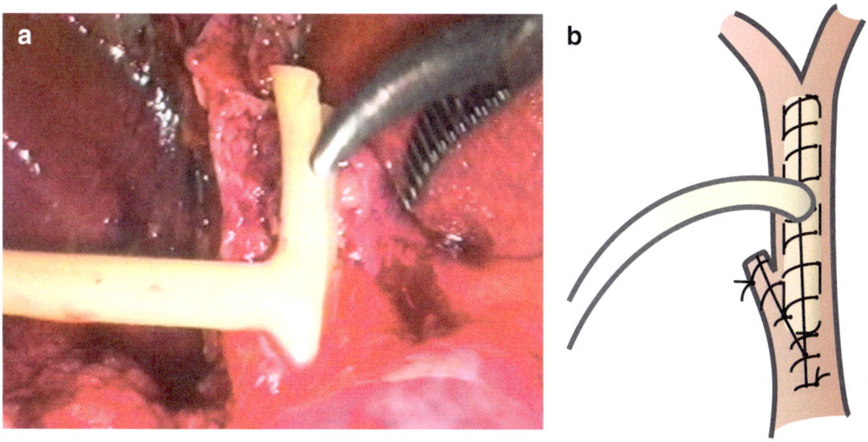

Fig. 10.2 T-tube placement. (**a**) Insertion of T-tube. Note that length of the “T” is longer than the choledochotomy. (**b**) Closure of choledochotomy with absorbable suture (suture locked around T-tube)

the duct is large, primary closure of the common bile duct is appropriate. However, absent perfect conditions, it is probably safer to leave a T-tube when closing. No matter how careful the exploration and how good the completion imaging seem to be, there is a persistent rate of retained common duct stones ranging from 3–10%. Since performing an OCBDE is necessitated by circumstances that precluded less-invasive approaches, a retained stone is likely to require re-laparotomy to address it, and hence a conservative approach seems prudent in this population. The size of the T-tube depends on the diameter of the bile duct but rarely needs to be larger than 16 Fr. Closure should be performed with an absorbable suture material (Fig. 10.2). It is common practice to place a closed suction drain in Morrison’s pouch to collect any bile that leaks from needle holes in the closure. T-tubes should remain in place at least 3 weeks post-op to ensure that a tract is formed, and a T-tube cholangiogram should be obtained just prior to removing the T-tube to ensure that the biliary tree is patent and that there are no retained stones (Table 10.2).

Table 10.2 Key components of open common bile duct exploration

Exposure • Fixed retraction • Kocher maneuver
Clearance of bile duct stones • Latex catheter, 14–18 Fr for flushing • Palpable stone? – Yes → stone forceps, etc. – No → choledochoscopy
Establish patency of ampulla
Confirm adequacy of stone clearance by choledochoscopy or completion cholangiogram
T-tube placement in most circumstances

Complications of Open Common Duct Exploration

Intraoperative Complications

As emphasized in the preceding sections, OCBDE is a two-handed operation that, performed in a careful manner, should have a very low incidence of intraoperative misadventures. Perforation of the bile duct or duodenum while instrumenting the common duct, although possible, should be avoidable. The more common intraoperative concerns are: (1) what to do when there is a stone impacted in the ampulla, or (2) there are so many stones present that the surgeon cannot be certain that complete clearance of the bile duct has been achieved. In the former circumstance, it is probably best to deal with the impacted stone in the operating room, since future endoscopic access is problematic. Overly aggressive attempts to crush the stone with a rigid instrument in the distal bile duct can lead to ampullary trauma. Therefore, if there is an inability to easily disrupt or dislodge the stone, the surgeon should perform a duodenotomy and sphincterotomy. Since the stone is impacted, this is quite easy to accomplish by cutting the mucosa of the ampulla directly onto the impacted stone. The incision should be made at the 11 o'clock position to avoid proximity to the pancreatic duct's entrance into the ampulla. A formal sphincteroplasty is not necessary. In the latter circumstance, the options are to leave a T-tube and plan on trying to clear any residual stones under fluoroscopic guidance via the T-tube tract 6 weeks post-op or proceeding to a biliary drainage procedure. In general this author prefers proceeding directly to performance of a side-to-side choledochoduodenostomy, as this will allow any retained stones to pass easily into the duodenum without consequence or need for further interventional procedures.

Early Postoperative Complications

T-tube dislodgement in the early post-op period can lead to bile peritonitis or a biliary fistula. Hence it is important to secure the tube to the skin carefully at the conclusion of the operative procedure. The presence of a closed suction drain near the choledochotomy mitigates this problem to a large extent. Postoperative jaundice needs to be promptly evaluated to determine if there is obstruction caused by the T-tube or if there has been ischemic injury to the liver. Retained stones seen on T-tube cholangiograms can often be retrieved under fluoroscopic guidance using a Dormia basket passed through the T-tube tract. It is essential to allow the tract to mature—usually a 6-week period—before manipulating it. Inability to remove the T-tube occurs when a suture has caught part of the tube in the closure. One simply waits for the absorbable suture to dissolve before attempting removal again.

Late Postoperative Complications

The main late postoperative complication of OCBDE is development of a benign biliary stricture. This is heralded by elevation of serum alkaline phosphatase and ultimately dilation of the biliary tree proximal to the stricture. Since the biliary system has been instrumented, cholangitis can occur, and strictures need to be treated. In the patient population discussed in this chapter, a transhepatic approach will usually be necessary. Should this circumstance arise, patients with bile duct strictures following OCBDE should uniformly be referred to tertiary care centers with established hepatobiliary expertise.

Conclusion

In the modern era, OCBDE is infrequently performed. Nonetheless there remains a role for this procedure in patients lacking endoscopic access to the ampulla and in those with complex biliary conditions. Strange as it may seem, what once was a common operation for general surgeons now is considered a challenging and exotic case. Many operating rooms no longer stock all of the instruments described in this chapter. When in doubt or operating in an emergency setting, placing a T-tube in the common bile duct will allow for decompression as well as providing transcutaneous access to deal with choledocholithiasis and biliary obstruction. In the current era, it is worth considering if patients needing this procedure electively should be referred to centers with more specialty experience and appropriate equipment.

References

1. Rattner DW, Warshaw AL. Impact of choledochoscopy on the management of choledocholithiasis. Experience with 499 common duct explorations at the Massachusetts General Hospital. Ann Surg. 1981;194:76–9.
2. Bartlett MK, Dreyfuss JR. Residual common duct stones. Surgery. 1960;47:202–5.
3. Glenn F. Retained calculi within the biliary ductal system. Ann Surg. 1974;179:528–39.
4. Himal HS. Common bile duct stones: the role of pre-operative, intraoperative and postoperative ERCP. Semin Laparosc Surg. 2000;7:237–45.
5. Binmoeller KF, Schafer TW. Endoscopic management of bile duct stones. J Clin Gastroenterol. 2001;32:106–18.
6. Vitale GC, Zavaleta CM. Endoscopic retrograde cholangio-pancreatography for surgeons. Semin Laparosc Surg. 2003;10:19–27.
7. Freeman ML, Nelson DB, Sherman SS, Haber GB, Herman ME, Dorsher PJ, et al. Complications of endoscopic biliary sphincterotomy. N Engl J Med. 1996;335:909–19.

Chapter 11
Role of Bilioenteric Bypass in the Management of Biliary Stone Disease

Lucio Lucas Pereira and Horacio J. Asbun

Introduction

According to the National Institutes of Health (NIH), more than 20 million Americans are estimated to have cholelithiasis. Approximately 500,000 patients per year are going to have symptoms or complications of gallstones and require a cholecystectomy; 10% of them are estimated to have stones within the common bile duct [1]. Primary stones, however, arise from the bile ducts themselves, and their management is more challenging because of the need for a more complex drainage procedure and in most cases surgery. There is a significant geographic variance in the incidence of primary stones, and these can originate from the intra- or extrahepatic biliary tree.

Primary stones are thought to result from the combination of biliary stasis and bacterial infections in the bile ducts that may include abnormalities of the sphincter of Oddi. The bacteria most capable of causing biliary sludge and stone formation produce enzymes that lead to deconjugation of bilirubin diglucuronide, resulting in the precipitation of calcium bilirubinate [2]. Older adults with large bile ducts and periampullary diverticula are at elevated risk for the formation of primary bile duct stones. In patients <60 years of age undergoing cholecystectomy, the prevalence of common bile duct (CBD) stones is 8–15%, but it increases to 15–60% in elderly patients. Of all patients with choledocholithiasis, 3–5% are asymptomatic [3].

Electronic supplementary material The online version of this chapter (doi: 10.1007/978-3-319-74503-9_11) contains supplementary material, which is available to authorized users.

L. L. Pereira, MD
Department of General Surgery, Mayo Clinic Florida, Jacksonville, FL, USA

H. J. Asbun, MD, FACS (✉)
Department of Surgery, Mayo Clinic Florida, Jacksonville, FL, USA
e-mail: Asbun.Horacio@mayo.edu

© Springer International Publishing AG, part of Springer Nature 2018

B. F. Santos, N. Soper (eds.), *Choledocholithiasis*,
https://doi.org/10.1007/978-3-319-74503-9_11

Patients with primary stones usually present with pancreatitis, biliary colic, cholangitis, and/or jaundice. Patients presenting with pancreatitis and jaundice were found to have common duct stones 20% and 45% of the time, respectively [4].

In an analysis of 1002 patients, the independent predictors of a CBD stone in patients undergoing cholecystectomy were found to be elevated gamma-glutamyl transpeptidase, alkaline phosphatase, and total bilirubin [5]. Patients suspected of having choledocholithiasis are diagnosed with a combination of laboratory tests and imaging studies; in most cases, the diagnosis is established by ultrasound.

The results of laboratory testing and transabdominal ultrasound can be used to stratify a patient at risk for having choledocholithiasis according to the American Society for Gastrointestinal Endoscopy (ASGE) [6]:

- *Very strong predictors*:
  - The presence of a common bile duct stone on transabdominal ultrasound
  - Clinical acute cholangitis
  - A serum bilirubin >4 mg/dL (68 μmol/L)
- *Strong predictors*:
  - A dilated common bile duct on ultrasound (more than 6 mm in a patient with a gallbladder in situ)
  - A serum bilirubin of 1.8–4 mg/dL (31–68 μmol/L)
- *Moderate predictors*:
  - Abnormal liver biochemical test other than bilirubin
  - Age older than 55 years
  - Clinical gallstone pancreatitis

Using the aforementioned predictors, patients are stratified as:

- *High risk*
  - At least one very strong predictor and/or
  - Both strong predictors
- *Intermediate risk*
  - One strong predictor and/or
  - At least one moderate predictor
- *Low risk*
  - No predictors

Localization of the calculi and assessment of the anatomy of the biliary tract are best obtained by magnetic resonance cholangiopancreatography (MRCP) and endoscopic retrograde cholangiopancreatography (ERCP).

Considering the need for a wide open drainage to avoid stasis within the biliary tree, which would cause recurrent "de novo" stones, surgery is commonly indicated for a definitive treatment of patients who have undergone multiple endoscopic procedures. In this chapter we describe the surgical technique for the management of primary stones of the extrahepatic biliary tree, commonly in a patient who has undergone a cholecystectomy and multiple ERCP procedures to evacuate recurrent common bile duct stones. Surgical procedures are preferable as a definitive treatment in these patients to allow for symptom resolution and avoid risk of recurrent pancreatitis and cholangitis as well as the need for repeated ERCP procedures.

Once the decision to proceed with a surgical intervention for primary CBD stones is made, there are two main options: (1) choledochoduodenostomy, anastomosing the duodenum to the common bile duct in a side-to-side manner, and (2) hepaticojejunostomy—using the jejunum for an end-to-side anastomosis. According to recent studies, both procedures are safe and have the same overall results on perioperative morbidity and mortality [7, 8]. However the technique of the author's choice is the side-to-side choledochoduodenostomy, since it provides a much wider anastomosis and results in a low-pressure biliary system.

The procedure can be done through an open or laparoscopic approach depending on the surgeon's experience. Other than the access, the technical aspects of the anastomosis are the same for both approaches. Besides the inherent laparoscopic advantages of shorter hospital stay and less pain, the magnification of the surgical field, different angles of visualization, and a precise anastomosis are beneficial in this procedure. Advanced laparoscopic skills are needed.

Choledochoduodenostomy

Choledochoduodenostomy was first performed by Bernhard Moritz Carl Ludwig Riedel (a German surgeon) in 1888, but the patient died as a result of leakage into the peritoneal cavity. Oskar Sprengel (another German surgeon) in 1891 reported the first recovery following choledochoduodenostomy. William J. Mayo, in 1905, reported the successful treatment of a strictured common duct following cholecystectomy and choledochotomy by suturing the end of the dilated portion of the duct to the duodenum [9].

Choledochoduodenostomy is the procedure of choice for patients who had previous gastric bypass with bile duct stones that originate in the main bile duct [10, 11]. The surgery can be performed by laparotomy, laparoscopy, or robotic-assisted [12–14].

Patient Position and Operating Room Setup

The patient is placed in a supine position with both arms out. All pressure points are padded, and the patient is well secured to the table. Generally, 3-inch silk tape and/or safety straps are placed across the patient's chest, pelvis, and legs to avoid slippage during the procedure. Tilting of the operative table into the different potential positions is performed on the undraped patient to visually confirm the security of the positioning prior to prepping or draping. Sequential compression stockings are used (Fig. 11.1).

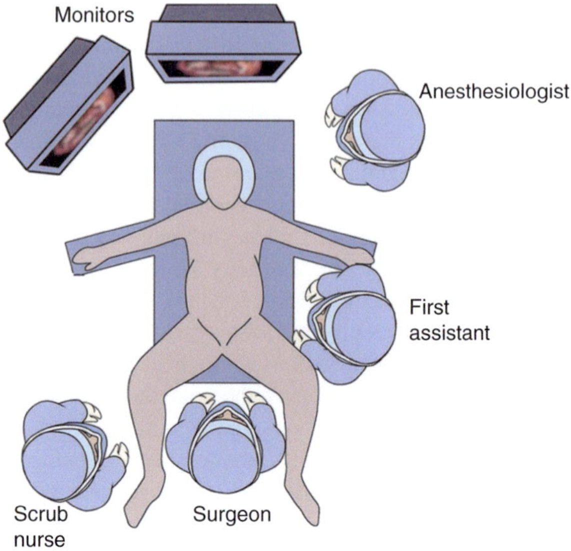

Fig. 11.1 Patient position for choledochoduodenostomy (Reprinted with permission from Asbun HJ, Stauffer J. Ch 11. Laparoscopic Bile Duct Resection and Hepaticojejunostomy for Type I Choledochal Cyst. In: Asbun HJ, Geller DA (eds). ACS Multimedia Atlas of Surgery: Liver Surgery Volume. Woodbury, CT: Ciné-Med. 2014)

Trocar Placement

The size and number of trocars can be varied according to the patient's body habitus and angle needed for exposure. The surgeon should have a general plan, but trocars can be added or changed to a larger size as needed. Similarly, the camera site and the side of the table on which the surgeon stands should be constantly assessed and changed as needed for better exposure or to facilitate a certain task. In general, the following is the most standard configuration: a 12 port in the midline, a high right lateral subcostal 5-mm trocar, a right hemiabdomen 12-mm port used for the camera, and a high left subcostal midaxillary 5-mm trocar. Additionally, a left hemiabdomen 5-mm trocar can be placed for an assistant (Fig. 11.2).

The procedure entails identification and dissection of the common bile duct, followed by a longitudinal choledochotomy with complete stone clearance of the biliary tree (Fig. 11.3). Reconstruction is performed by making a corresponding longitudinal incision on the anterior-superior wall of the duodenal bulb and performing an anastomosis (Fig. 11.4). The anastomosis between the two is then performed in a 4-quadrant, diamond-shaped fashion. Other techniques were used in the past [15]. For some surgeons, choledochoduodenostomy may be considered controversial because of the possibility of sump syndrome. However, if the choledochoduodenostomy is performed low on the common duct, thereby creating a wide, diamond-shaped anastomosis, the risk of sump syndrome is minimal with excellent long-term results [16, 17].

Laparoscopic choledochoduodenostomy can be also effective for biliary drainage in selected cases of benign or iatrogenic strictures of the distal common bile duct. Dilatation of the common bile duct (CBD) to >12–15 mm facilitates technical success of the operation. Steps of the operation include:

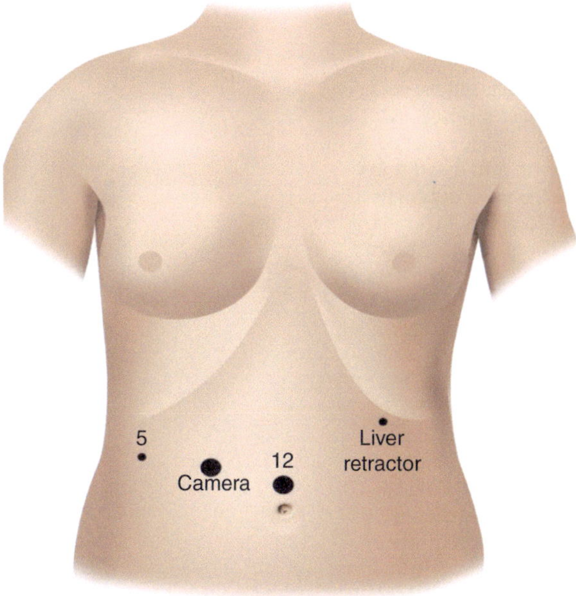

Fig. 11.2 Port placement. An extra port can be used if needed (Reprinted with permission from Asbun HJ, Stauffer J. Ch 11. Laparoscopic Bile Duct Resection and Hepaticojejunostomy for Type I Choledochal Cyst. In: Asbun HJ, Geller DA (eds). ACS Multimedia Atlas of Surgery: Liver Surgery Volume. Woodbury, CT: Ciné-Med. 2014)

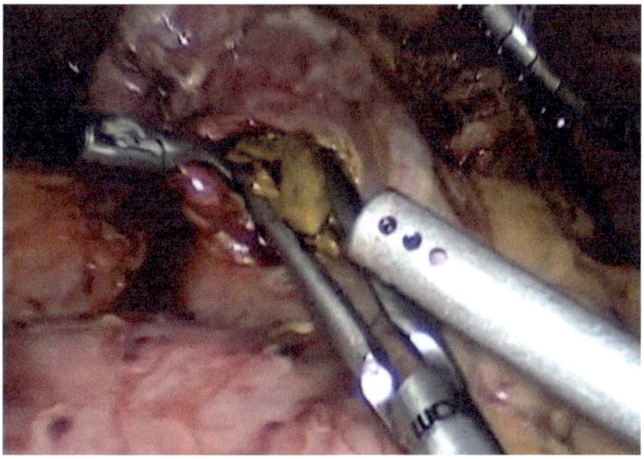

Fig. 11.3 A longitudinal choledochotomy has been performed. The stones are first retrieved with a grasper(Reprinted with permission from Asbun HJ, Stauffer J. Ch 11. Laparoscopic Bile Duct Resection and Hepaticojejunostomy for Type I Choledochal Cyst. In: Asbun HJ, Geller DA (eds). ACS Multimedia Atlas of Surgery: Liver Surgery Volume. Woodbury, CT: Ciné-Med. 2014)

- Identification and exposure of the CBD
- Wide Kocher maneuver of the duodenum
- Longitudinal choledochotomy >2 cm
- Clearance of all obstructing calculi from the biliary tree
- Longitudinal duodenotomy
- Choledochoduodenostomy anastomosis

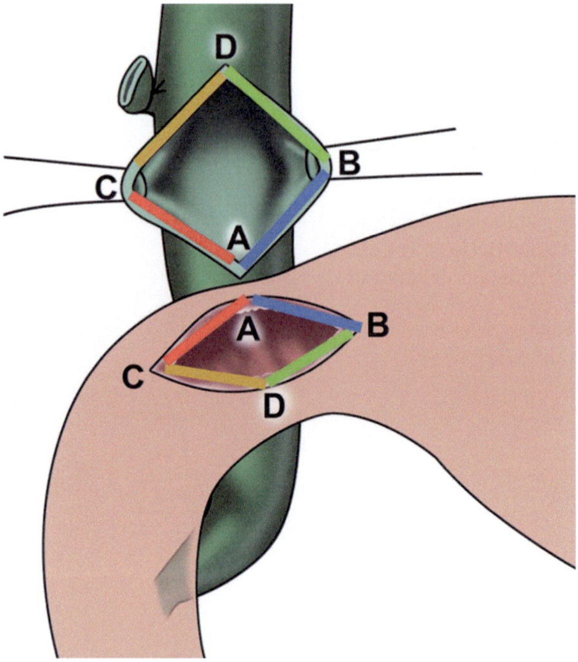

Fig. 11.4 A diamond-shaped, 4-quadrant anastomosis between the duodenum and the common bile duct is performed. The quadrants are matched as shown: A to B and A to C for the lower quadrants; C to D and B to D for the upper quadrants. The end result is a widely patent anastomosis (Reprinted with permission from Asbun HJ, Stauffer J. Ch 11. Laparoscopic Bile Duct Resection and Hepaticojejunostomy for Type I Choledochal Cyst. In: Asbun HJ, Geller DA (eds). ACS Multimedia Atlas of Surgery: Liver Surgery Volume. Woodbury, CT: Ciné-Med. 2014)

A full mobilization of the duodenum is carried out to allow a tension-free anastomosis. Care is taken to identify and dissect out the anterior wall of the common bile duct. A generous longitudinal choledochotomy is performed, and complete clearance of calculi from the CBD is performed. When necessary, choledochoscopy is used (Fig. 11.3, Video 11.1).

The anastomosis between the duodenum and the common bile duct is performed in a 4-quadrant method in a diamond shape (Fig. 11.4). A corresponding duodenotomy is made, and the inferior corner anchoring stitches are placed first. The two inferior quadrants are run proximally with a running 5-0 absorbable stitch (Fig. 11.5). Then, the medial and lateral stitches are placed and tied. These stitches are then run proximally to the superior corner, where they are tied, and the anastomosis is complete (Fig. 11.6, Video 11.2).

Hepaticojejunostomy

In 1908, Jacques-Ambroise Monprofit (France) described biliary-enteric anastomosis with a loop of small intestine Roux-en-Y as a way to reconstruct the biliary tract [18].

The hepaticojejunostomy differs from choledochoduodenostomy in many aspects. A complete transection of the main bile duct and closure of the distal duct

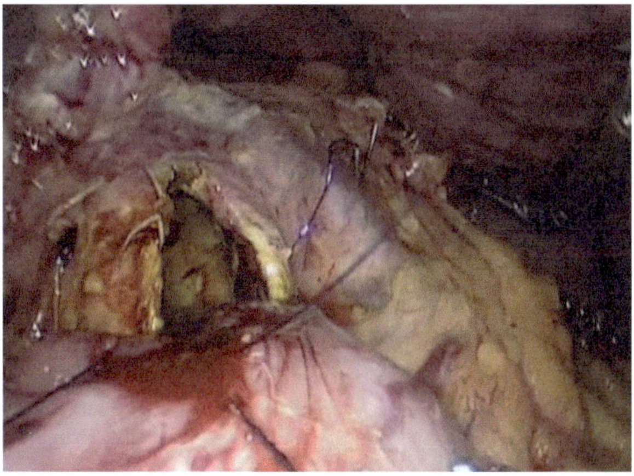

Fig. 11.5 Choledochoduodenostomy: the anastomosis of the lower two quadrants is completed, and the open upper half of the rhomboid is seen (Reprinted with permission from Asbun HJ, Stauffer J. Ch 11. Laparoscopic Bile Duct Resection and Hepaticojejunostomy for Type I Choledochal Cyst. In: Asbun HJ, Geller DA (eds). ACS Multimedia Atlas of Surgery: Liver Surgery Volume. Woodbury, CT: Ciné-Med. 2014)

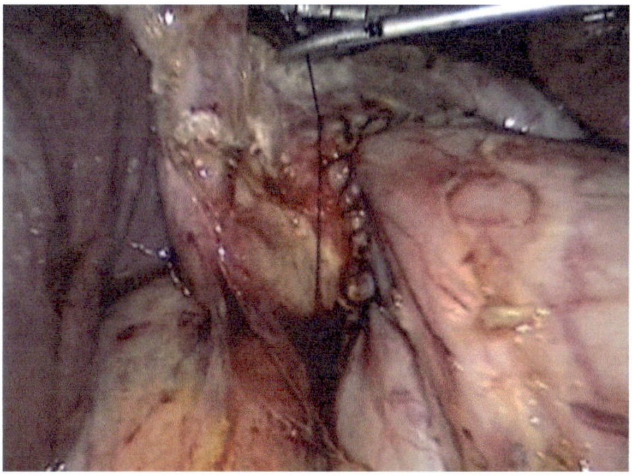

Fig. 11.6 Choledochoduodenostomy anastomosis is now completed (Reprinted with permission from Asbun HJ, Stauffer J. Ch 11. Laparoscopic Bile Duct Resection and Hepaticojejunostomy for Type I Choledochal Cyst. In: Asbun HJ, Geller DA (eds). ACS Multimedia Atlas of Surgery: Liver Surgery Volume. Woodbury, CT: Ciné-Med. 2014)

stump are performed (Fig. 11.7). Biliary-enteric flow is reestablished through a retrocolic duct to mucosa Roux-en-Y hepaticojejunostomy (Fig. 11.8). The procedure has very good results as reported in the literature and is an alternative to choledochoduodenostomy [19, 20].

Some authors suggest the use of a short limb for a Roux-en-Y hepaticojejunostomy to allow endoscope examination of the patient during follow-up [21]. The

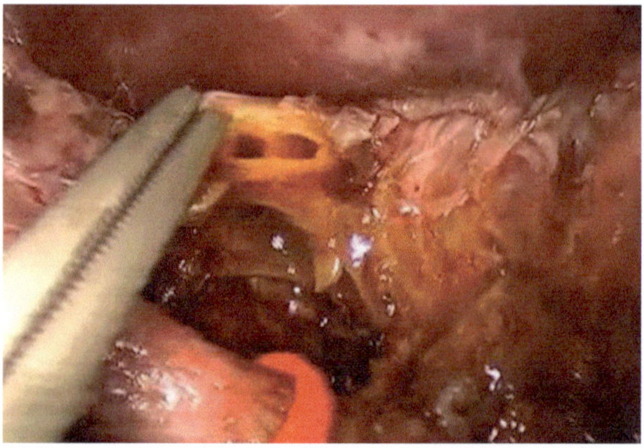

Fig. 11.7 Proximally, the division of the hepatic duct was performed near the bifurcation. The bifurcation into the right and left duct is shown (Reprinted with permission from Asbun HJ, Stauffer J. Ch 11. Laparoscopic Bile Duct Resection and Hepaticojejunostomy for Type I Choledochal Cyst. In: Asbun HJ, Geller DA (eds). ACS Multimedia Atlas of Surgery: Liver Surgery Volume. Woodbury, CT: Ciné-Med. 2014)

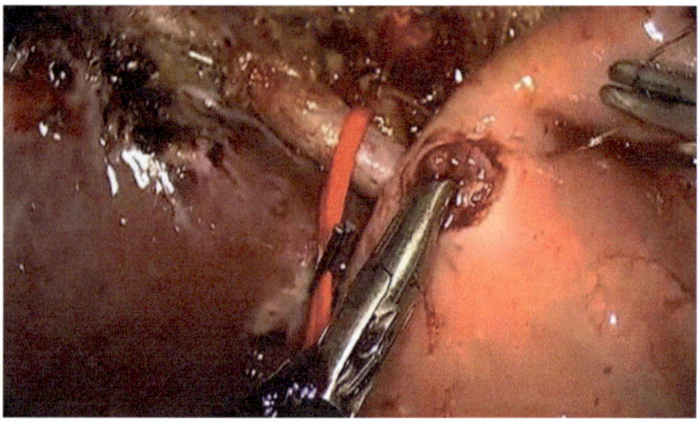

Fig. 11.8 The hepaticojejunostomy is begun. The red vessel loop is around the common hepatic artery (Reprinted with permission from Asbun HJ, Stauffer J. Ch 11. Laparoscopic Bile Duct Resection and Hepaticojejunostomy for Type I Choledochal Cyst. In: Asbun HJ, Geller DA (eds). ACS Multimedia Atlas of Surgery: Liver Surgery Volume. Woodbury, CT: Ciné-Med. 2014)

traditional operative technique was described via an open operation, but a minimal-access approach for this operation has been performed successfully with good outcomes [22]. Hepaticojejunostomy is used in a variety of procedures including pancreatoduodenectomy and is well described in the literature. A hepaticojejunostomy at the level of the bifurcation is illustrated in Figs. 11.7, 11.8, 11.9, and 11.10.

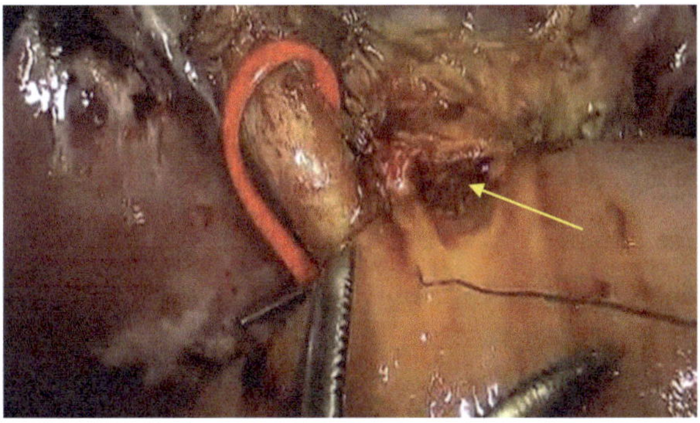

Fig. 11.9 The posterior running layer of the hepaticojejunostomy is completed (Reprinted with permission from Asbun HJ, Stauffer J. Ch 11. Laparoscopic Bile Duct Resection and Hepaticojejunostomy for Type I Choledochal Cyst. In: Asbun HJ, Geller DA (eds). ACS Multimedia Atlas of Surgery: Liver Surgery Volume. Woodbury, CT: Ciné-Med. 2014)

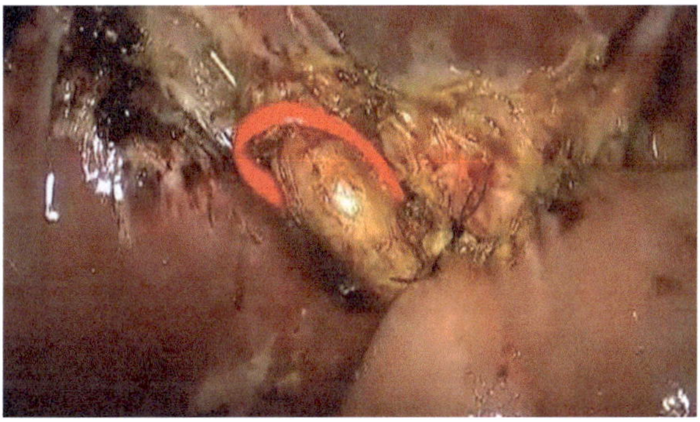

Fig. 11.10 The completed hepaticojejunostomy anastomosis is shown (Reprinted with permission from Asbun HJ, Stauffer J. Ch 11. Laparoscopic Bile Duct Resection and Hepaticojejunostomy for Type I Choledochal Cyst. In: Asbun HJ, Geller DA (eds). ACS Multimedia Atlas of Surgery: Liver Surgery Volume. Woodbury, CT: Ciné-Med. 2014)

References

1. Gallstones and laparoscopic cholecystectomy. NIH consensus statement. 1992;10(3):1–20.
2. Leung JW, Liu YL, Leung PS, Chan RC, Inciardi JF, Cheng AF. Expression of bacterial β-glucuronidase in human bile: an in vitro study. Gastrointest Endosc. 2001;54(3):346–50.
3. Scientific Committee of the European Association for Endoscopic Surgery (EAES). Diagnosis and treatment of common bile duct stones (CBDS). Results of a consensus development conference. Surg Endosc. 1998;12:856–64.
4. Hungness ES, Soper NJ. Management of common bile duct stones. J Gastrointest Surg. 2006;10:612–9.
5. Yang MH, Chen TH, Wang SE, Tsai YF, Su CH, Wu CW, et al. Biochemical predictors for absence of common bile duct stones in patients undergoing laparoscopic cholecystectomy. Surg Endosc. 2008;22:1620–4.

6. American Society for Gastrointestinal Endoscopy (A.S.G.E) Standards of Practice Committee. The role of endoscopy in the evaluation of suspected choledocholithiasis. Gastrointest Endosc. 2010;71:1–9.
7. Narayanan SK, Chen Y, Narasimhan KL, Cohen RC. Hepaticoduodenostomy versus hepaticojejunostomy after resection of choledochal cyst: a systematic review and meta-analysis. J Pediatr Surg. 2013;48(11):2336–42.
8. Luu C, Lee B, Stabile BE. Choledochoduodenostomy as the biliary-enteric bypass of choice for benign and malignant distal common bile duct strictures. Am Surg. 2013;79(10):1054–7.
9. Farrar T, Painter MW, Betz R. Choledochoduodenostomy. In the treatment of stenosis in the distal common duct. Arch Surg. 1969;98(4):442–6.
10. DuCoin C, Moon RC, Teixeira AF, Jawad MA. Laparoscopic choledochoduodenostomy as an alternate treatment for common bile duct stones after Roux-en-Y gastric bypass. Surg Obes Relat Dis. 2014;10(4):647–52.
11. Overby DW, Richardson W, Fanelli R. Choledocholithiasis after gastric bypass: a growing problem. Surg Obes Relat Dis. 2014;10(4):652–3.
12. Chander J, Mangla V, Vindal A, Lal P, Ramteke VK. Laparoscopic choledochoduodenostomy for biliary stone disease: a single-center 10-year experience. J Laparoendosc Adv Surg Tech A. 2012;22(1):81–4.
13. El Nakeeb A, Askr W, El Hanafy E, Atef E, Hamdy E, El Hemaly M, et al. Long term outcomes of choledochoduodenostomy for common bile duct stones in the era of laparoscopy and endoscopy. Hepato-Gastroenterology. 2015;62(137):6–10.
14. Priego P, Escrig J, Ángel V, Villegas C, Salvador JL. Laparoscopic choledochoduodenostomy: an option in cases of obstructive biliary tract. Am Surg. 2015;81(5):E195–7.
15. Lechaux J-P, Lechaux D. Anastomoses biliodigestives dans la lithiase biliaire. EMC - Techniques chirurgicales - Appareil digestif. 2007;2:1–9.
16. Malik AA, Rather SA, Bari SU, Wani KA. Long-term results of choledochoduodenostomy in benign biliary obstruction. World J Gastrointest Surg. 2012;4(2):36–40.
17. Matsushima K, Soybel DI. Operative management of recurrent choledocholithiasis. J Gastrointest Surg. 2012;16(12):2312–7.
18. Jabłońska B, Lampe P. Reconstructive biliary surgery in the treatment of iatrogenic bile duct injuries. J Gastrointest Surg. 2009;13(6):1084–93.
19. Kadaba RS, Bowers KA, Khorsandi S, Hutchins RR, Abraham AT, Sarker SJ, et al. Complications of biliary-enteric anastomoses. Ann R Coll Surg Engl. 2016;23:1–6.
20. Goessmann H, Lang SA, Fichtner-Feigl S, Scherer MN, Schlitt HJ, Stroszczynski C, et al. Biliodigestive anastomosis: indications, complications and interdisciplinary management. Chirurg. 2012;83(12):1097–108.
21. Felder SI, Menon VG, Nissen NN, Margulies DR, Lo S, Colquhoun SD. Hepaticojejunostomy using short-limb Roux-en-Y reconstruction. JAMA Surg. 2013;148(3):253–7. discussion 257–8.
22. Râmboiu S, Ghiţă F, Nicoli RE, Georgescu I. The role of biliodigestive derivations in the treatment of choledocholithiasis. Curr Health Sci J. 2011;37(4):181–4.

Chapter 12
Endoscopic Sphincterotomy for Choledocholithiasis

Varun Kapur, Victor Sandoval, and Jeffrey M. Marks

Introduction

Endoscopic retrograde cholangiopancreatography (ERCP), a procedure used to treat choledocholithiasis, came from humble beginnings more than 40 years ago. Numerous innovators in the field have advanced it into the procedure we know today. In the early 1960s, the first nonoperative pancreatography was described. A flexible catheter was inserted blindly into the duodenum; this was done several times until successful cannulation of the pancreatic duct was achieved. This idea eventually led to the first use of a fiber-optic duodenoscope to cannulate the ampulla of Vater by William McCune. But it was not until the 1970s that several famous endoscopists introduced the concept of endoscopic sphincterotomy. Now, this technology has moved from a diagnostic procedure to a viable therapeutic option for biliary decompression. Improvements in technology and technique in this field have led to what we know today as modern day interventional endoscopy.

Gallstone disease is one of the most common and costly digestive diseases in the United States, with estimated direct and indirect costs of 6.2 billion dollars annually

---

Electronic supplementary material The online version of this chapter (doi: 10.1007/978-3-319-74503-9_12) contains supplementary material, which is available to authorized users.

V. Kapur, MD
Department of General Surgery, University Hospitals Case Medical Center, Cleveland, OH, USA
e-mail: varunk.mamc@gmail.com

V. Sandoval, MD
Department of General Surgery, University Hospitals of Cleveland, Cleveland, OH, USA
e-mail: Victor.Sandoval@uhhospitals.org

J. M. Marks, MD, FACS, FASGE (✉)
Department of General Surgery, University Hospitals Cleveland Medical Center, Cleveland, OH, USA
e-mail: Jeffrey.marks@uhhospitals.org

© Springer International Publishing AG, part of Springer Nature 2018

B. F. Santos, N. Soper (eds.), *Choledocholithiasis*,
https://doi.org/10.1007/978-3-319-74503-9_12

[1]. The reported incidence of common bile duct (CBD) stones is also high, with stones present in up to 20% of patients with gallstone disease in Western countries [2]. Additionally, bile duct stones are incidentally found in up to 10% of patients during the evaluation of benign biliary disease. CBD stones can result in potential complications if untreated, and as such there is a clear need for effective methods of stone extraction.

Choledocholithiasis causes obstruction of the CBD as stones pass from the gallbladder via the cystic duct or from a stone that has formed within the CBD itself. Choledocholithiasis is the most frequent cause of extrahepatic biliary obstruction, and patients typically present with biliary colic, pancreatitis, jaundice, or cholangitis. Bile duct stones are classified into two groups: (1) primary (forming in the duct itself) and (2) secondary (forming elsewhere and having traveled into the duct). Approximately 85% of bile duct stones are secondary in nature, originating from the gallbladder. In contrast, primary stones are a consequence of bile stasis that can be associated with conditions such as biliary strictures, sclerosing cholangitis, choledochal cysts, or periampullary diverticula. These conditions share a common problematic outcome: their ability to slow the flow of bile, which subsequently promotes bacterial overgrowth. This, in turn, causes bilirubin deconjugation and the breakdown of biliary lipids—resulting in the formation of pigment stones.

Presentation, Diagnosis, and Indications

Presentation

Choledocholithiasis is usually found concomitantly in patients who present with symptomatic cholelithiasis or pancreatitis. Choledocholithiasis can be complicated by pancreatitis and acute cholangitis. These patients can present in extremis from severe cholangitis and may require emergent biliary decompression. Acute cholangitis is caused primarily by a bacterial infection. Bacterial organisms ascend from the duodenum, eventually travel into the portal venous system, and ultimately enter the systemic circulation. When the normal barrier mechanisms become dysfunctional or disrupted, bacteria are able to thrive in the biliary tree due to the bile stasis from the obstruction. The biliary obstruction causes an increase in the intrabiliary pressure (normal biliary pressures range from 5 to 15 cm H_2O) that results in an increase in permeability of the bile ductules, permitting the translocation of bacteria and/or toxins into the systemic circulation. The systemic symptoms of fever and chills are due to bacteremia from the translocation of bacteria into the venous and lymphatic systems that parallel the bile duct system.

Choledocholithiasis can present in several ways, but many patients are asymptomatic. The presence of symptoms is primarily contingent upon the size of the stones. Small stones usually pass into the duodenum without producing a primary blockage of the main ductal system. When a patient presents with choledocholithiasis, their most frequent complaint is acute onset pain located in the right upper quadrant or epigastric region. The pain is caused by the dilation of the CBD. This distension can be from partial or complete obstruction of the duct. Pain is typically epigastric or right upper quadrant, but the pain can be located anywhere in the abdomen and it can range from mild to severe. The pain is usually accompanied by nausea and/or vomiting.

Diagnosis

Laboratory abnormalities aid in the diagnosis of choledocholithiasis. Patients will typically have elevated alkaline phosphatase, conjugated bilirubinemia, and may have transaminitis. When a patient presents with acute abdominal pain, laboratory testing should be obtained along with an imaging study. Typical first-line testing for right upper quadrant pain that is biliary colic in nature is ultrasound. The advantages of ultrasound are numerous: it is widely available, is noninvasive, and is an inexpensive test. One limitation to ultrasound is that its efficacy is contingent upon the experience and technique of the operator, and it is unable to effectively image the distal common bile duct to look for stones. Sensitivity of ultrasound for the detection of biliary duct dilatation, an indirect sign indicating potential CBD stones, is reported as 55–91% [3]. A negative ultrasound, however, cannot eliminate the diagnosis of CBD stones. For computed tomography (CT) scans, the ability to identify CBD dilation has been reported to have a sensitivity of 87% [4]. Endoscopic ultrasound (EUS) and magnetic resonance cholangiopancreatography (MRCP) can detect stones 5 mm and greater in size. The sensitivity and specificity for both studies is approximately 95% [5].

Indications

The general indications for ERCP and sphincterotomy are symptomatic choledocholithiasis, patients undergoing elective cholecystectomy that preoperatively are found to have CBD stones, or patients who have undergone cholecystectomy but are suspected to have retained CBD stones (Table 12.1). For patients with normal anatomy and who are in post-cholecystectomy state, ERCP is the primary modality for clearance of common duct stones. For patients with gallbladder in situ, the role of

Table 12.1 Preoperative and postoperative indications for ERCP

Preoperative indications for ERCP	Postoperative indications for ERCP
Jaundice	Retained CBD stone
Elevated total bilirubin	Postoperative jaundice
Dilated CBD on US	Unsuccessful stone retrieval during laparoscopic CBD exploration
CBD stones on imaging	
Acute cholangitis	

ERCP endoscopic retrograde cholangiopancreatography, *CBD* common bile duct, *US* ultrasound

ERCP depends on the patient's condition and whether common bile duct exploration (CBDE) is available (see Chap. 3 for the recommended algorithm when intraoperative imaging and CBDE is an option). The care of patients with gallbladder in situ at centers where only ERCP is available or where it is preferentially utilized will be discussed. Patients who have undergone ultrasound and are found to have gallbladder stones, but have normal liver function tests (LFTs) and no evidence of CBD dilation or stones, should undergo cholecystectomy, as they will have a low likelihood of needing ERCP. Patients who are found to have gallbladder stones and CBD stones should undergo preoperative or intraoperative ERCP before cholecystectomy. Patients who fall into the category of ultrasound-proven gallbladder stones, CBD dilation, or abnormal LFTs may benefit from additional testing, especially if their pain is controlled and they do not have obvious signs of cholangitis. For example, some institutions obtain a non-contrast CT scan and if a CBD stone is found, they proceed for preoperative or intraoperative ERCP. Patients who are found to have ultrasound-proven gallbladder stones and CBD dilation and/or abnormal LFTs get an MRCP, with that procedure now becoming more widely available. If the findings of the MRCP support CBD stones, the patient then undergoes preoperative or intraoperative ERCP. Classical indications for preoperative ERCP included image-proven gallbladder stones plus any of the following: elevated liver enzymes (primarily elevated direct bilirubin and alkaline phosphatase), a dilated CBD or visible stones in the CBD, or acute gallstone pancreatitis. There is now evidence that most patients with gallstone pancreatitis do not benefit from preoperative ERCP, with a recommendation that ERCP be reserved for patients with evidence of concurrent cholangitis. Post-cholecystectomy indications for ERCP are primarily for retained common bile duct stones identified on intraoperative imaging or when the diagnosis is suspected due to postoperative problems. Retained common bile duct stones can cause significant morbidity and mortality. Retained stones should be suspected in patients who have continued postoperative pain that is more significant than typical postsurgical pain, continued jaundice, poor oral intake, or failure for LFTs to normalize. There is mounting evidence that asymptomatic CBD stones are not as benign as previously thought. There is a push to address and remove all CBD stones when found during cholecystectomy [6]. For this reason, it is incumbent upon the surgeon to risk-stratify all patients undergoing cholecystectomy for possible CBD stones and develop an evaluation and management plan to deal with this potential issue.

Indications for Emergent Endoscopic Retrograde Cholangiopancreatography

Emergent ERCP and biliary decompression are necessary in the setting of acute cholangitis and systemic signs of infection that have failed to resolve with medical management. Cholangitis can be caused not only by bile duct calculi (comprising >70% of all causes) but also by benign and malignant strictures or external compression from extrahepatic masses or Mirizzi's syndrome. The first line of treatment is intravenous (IV) hydration and antibiotics followed by biliary decompression. When acute cholangitis is left untreated, this disease process eventually leads to sepsis and septic shock. The type of decompression is typically based on the level at which the obstruction occurs. ERCP and sphincterotomy with stent placement are commonly used to alleviate the obstruction when it is localized to the extrahepatic ductal system and at the level of the ampulla of Vater.

Anatomic Anomalies of the Cystic and Common Bile Duct

The cystic duct drains the gallbladder and joins the CBD. Superior to this junction is the common hepatic duct and just below is the CBD. The cystic duct is approximately 5 cm in length but can be as short a few centimeters long and is typically 1–5 mm in diameter. There are several anatomic anomalies of cystic duct insertion (Table 12.2). These include takeoff directly from the right hepatic duct, parallel course with the common hepatic duct in which the cystic duct is enclosed in a fibrous sheath with a low takeoff, short cystic duct <5 mm, double cystic duct, very low medial insertion, and spiral course around the common hepatic duct in an anterior or posterior path inserting medially. The CBD is formed by the common hepatic and cystic duct. Its length ranges from 8 to 10 cm in length. Its diameter is typically between 5 and 9 mm and generally increases with age. When the duct reaches a size greater than 10 mm, it is considered enlarged. The CBD is commonly separated into thirds: the upper third is the supraduodenal, which courses cephalad from the superior edge of the duodenum, anterior to the portal vein, and lateral to the hepatic artery; the middle third is the retroduodenal that lies posterior to the duodenum, lateral to the portal vein, and in front of the inferior vena cava; and the lower third is the intrapancreatic segment, which runs posteriorly along the pancreas, enters the duodenum, and then joins the pancreatic duct becoming intraduodenal. Once intraduodenal, the CBD passes at an angle through the papilla of Vater. The blood supply of the CBD runs in the 3 and 9 o'clock positions when seen in cross section. Knowledge of the common relationship between the CBD and the pancreatic duct is important due to its variability (Table 12.3). Typically, the two ducts run parallel and then join with the wall of the duodenum to form a common channel. But, they

Table 12.2 Anatomical variations of the cystic duct

Anatomical variations of the cystic duct
1. Takeoff directly from the right hepatic duct
2. Parallel course with the common hepatic duct with the cystic duct enclosed in a fibrous sheath with a low takeoff
3. Short cystic duct
4. Double cystic duct
5. Low medial insertion with spiraling course around the common hepatic duct

Table 12.3 Variations in the common bile duct normal anatomical position

Variations in the common bile duct normal anatomical position
1. Various bifurcating ducts entering the stomach or duodenum
2. A separate CBD and separate pancreatic duct entering the duodenum
3. One common duct that enters at the level of the fundus
4. One common duct entering at the level of the pylorus

CBD common bile duct

can also join just before entering the duodenal wall, and, very rarely, they form two separate entry ports into the duodenum. As they enter the duodenal wall, the specialized muscle of the sphincter of Oddi encases the terminal portion of these ducts.

Endoscopic Retrograde Cholangiopancreatography Procedure

General Anesthesia Versus Moderate Sedation

Sedation and pain control are important to successful endoscopic procedures. The majority of endoscopic procedures (colonoscopies and upper endoscopies) are done under moderate sedation. The overall use of moderate sedation with ERCP is higher than the use of general anesthesia. It usually does not involve an anesthesiologist but requires a pre-procedure and physical history, American Society of Anesthesiologists (ASA) classification, IV access, supplemental oxygen, real-time vital sign monitoring (electrocardiogram, blood pressure, and pulse oximetry), personnel certified in basic life support (BLS)/advanced cardiac life support (ACLS), and familiarity with reversal agents for the sedatives being used. The most common complications related to sedation are cardiovascular compromise due to aspiration, hypoventilation, hypotension, arrhythmias, or hypoxia from airway obstruction. Commonly used sedation/analgesic regimens include a combination of opioid analgesics, short-acting benzodiazepine, or antihistamines. Studies have shown that between one-third to one-half of patients who undergo ERCP under moderate sedation experience pain and discomfort during the procedure [7]. This is likely due to the fact that ERCP is more complex and is typically of longer duration than an upper endoscopy or colonoscopy. A large retrospective review did not show a difference in morbidity or mortality for ERCP when comparing moderate sedation versus general anesthesia [8]. The typical reasons for the use of general anesthesia with ERCP are patients who have previously failed a prior ERCP attempt under moderate sedation; patients who demonstrate a high risk for aspiration, a concern for airway patency, and a lack of appropriate ancillary personnel in the general endoscopy procedure suites; or patients who may require prolonged sedation due to the complexity of the procedure and associated interventions. The drawbacks of general anesthesia are threefold: it adds time and extra personnel, adds additional risks specific to general anesthesia, and increases the overall cost of the procedure. All of these factors need to be taken into account when selecting the proper use of moderate sedation versus general anesthesia for a successful ERCP.

Room Setup

ERCP is generally performed in the hospital endoscopy suite, which in some hospitals may be shared with interventional radiology in order to conserve space. Depending upon acuity and comorbidities of the patient, it may also be performed in the operating room. In addition to the endoscopist, sedation/anesthesia staff, an endoscopy nurse/assistant, and a fluoroscopy technician should be in the room to assist.

Equipment

Duodenoscopes are specialized side-viewing endoscopes with controls for the manipulation of accessory devices. These scopes are equipped with an elevator control that is used to facilitate cannulation of the papilla by changing the angle from which the accessory exits the scope (Fig. 12.1). The therapeutic scopes are typically large channel scopes that are 125 cm in length. The working channels of the scope come in varying sizes of 2.8, 3.2, 4.2, and a larger 4.8 mm channel. The larger channel scope allows the operator to pass 10–11.5 Fr diameter catheters for therapeutic interventions and for the aspiration of duodenal contents while an accessory is being used. It also permits the simultaneous use of two guidewires or accessories. The larger endoscope with a 4.2 mm channel may be preferred in adults, while the

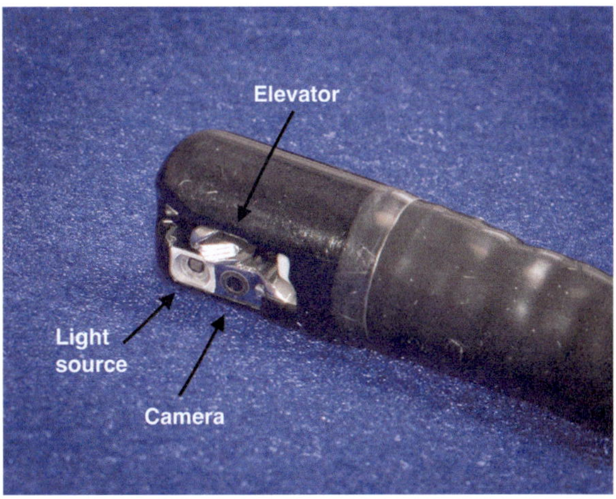

Fig. 12.1 Close-up view of duodenoscope tip showing the 90-degree side-viewing camera, light source, and instrument channel elevator. Photo credit: Kelsey Angell, PGY-3 General Surgery

smaller endoscope with a 3.2 mm working channel may be used when there is suspected narrowing of the lumen, and in children above the age of 2. Smaller pediatric duodenoscopes with a 2.0 mm channel may be used in neonates. In patients with altered anatomy such as post-Billroth II reconstruction or Roux-en-Y hepaticojejunostomy, it may be best to use a forward-viewing scope such as the pediatric colonoscope. An upper endoscope can sometimes be used to traverse a prior choledochoduodenostomy to access the intrahepatic ducts. Laparoscopic assistance may be needed to access the remnant stomach in post-gastric bypass patients.

Contrast

There are several available options on the market. The contrast used is iodine-based and water soluble. Currently, there is limited data on the adverse effects of contrast that is used with ERCP. Previously, high osmolality agents were primarily used. Now, low-osmolality forms are available but with an approximately tenfold higher cost. It is thought that these newer low-osmolality forms are safer, but this is based on extrapolation of data from radiologic literature on IV contrast, which may not apply to ERCP. The danger of contrast-related reactions is thought to be mainly related to the ability of a contrast agent to be absorbed systemically. Similar to the iodine-based oral contrast media used with CT scans, contrast within the hepatobiliary system has only a fraction of the systemic absorption seen with administration of IV contrast. The quality of the imaging from contrast media is a direct result of its overall viscosity, density, and osmolality and does not seem to vary significantly when using high- versus low-osmolality contrast. There are documented reports of adverse reactions from the contrast media use, but the overall incidence is unknown [9]. For patients deemed high risk or who have had a previously documented contrast-related reaction, standard prophylactic and pretreatment may be considered; however, there is no evidence-based, standard practice in this regard for ERCP. Most institutions have established protocols that are largely based on IV-mediated contrast reactions. These protocols typically involve pre- and posttreatment with a systemic corticosteroid and a combination of antihistamines.

Accessories

Guidewires

As with most interventional radiology procedures, guidewires are a key component of ERCP [10]. Using Seldinger technique with fluoroscopy, guidewires are used for accessing the papilla, maintaining bile duct and pancreatic duct access, and for placing different diagnostic devices (manometry devices, tissue sampling, and injections of contrast media) or therapeutic accessories (balloons, baskets, stents, sphincterotomes, etc.). Specific wire characteristics assist in the guided cannulation of the papilla and ductal system. It is recommended that a short, straight wire that is soft and flexible but not overly floppy be selected initially, but an angle tip wire may be useful in some situations. A 0.89 mm (0.35 in) wire is generally preferred for pushability and stability. Wire length is variable from 260 to 400 cm. The longer wires are used for exchanging devices, and specially coated wires are used for electrosurgery devices. Wires come in a variety of lengths and flexibility strengths and can be coated with hydrophilic resin to pass easily through the papilla. Typically, the more flexible, slick wires are used for initial access into the ductal system, whereas the stiffer wires are used for the passage of dilators and/or stents. As the stiffness of a wire increases, the endoscopist is able to minimize the lateral deviation while maintaining a stronger forward movement of the wire. Wires used for therapeutic device deployment have distance markers that are easily viewed with fluoroscopy.

Sphincterotomes/Papillotome

Sphincterotomes can be broadly classified as "push," "pull," or "needle knife." Standard sphincterotomes are the "pull-type" plastic catheters with an exposed 2–3 cm wire loop partially enclosed in the catheter for coagulation and cutting (Fig. 12.2). With the "pull type," the papilla is identified and cannulated with the sphincterotome, which is then inserted and slowly withdrawn until a portion of the wire is exposed. Once exposed, the sphincterotome is bowed. The cutting portion of the wire is in contact with the superior portion of the papilla. Using the elevators of the duodenoscope and using short bursts of thermal energy, a papillotomy is completed. They also have one or two channels for injection and guidewires. The

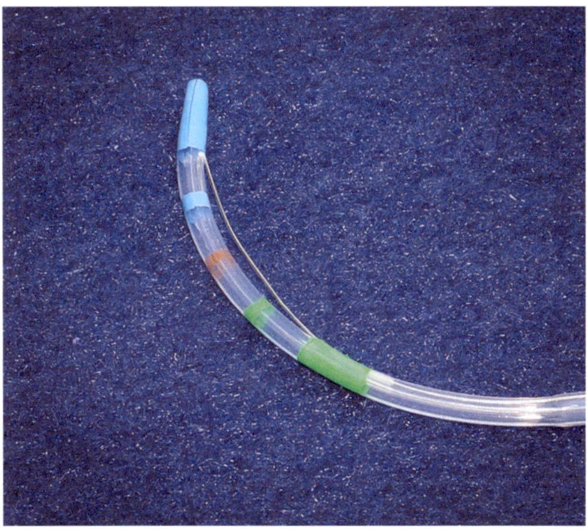

Fig. 12.2 "Pull-type" sphincterotome tip is seen. The cutting wire is visible along the side of the sphincterotome. Photo credit: Kelsey Angell, PGY-3 General Surgery

"needle knife" sphincterotome is a simple catheter with a central short, extendable cutting wire that projects approximately 5 mm past the tip of the catheter. It can be used to obtain access to the bile duct when standard approaches fail (with or without an indwelling stent). There are also sphincterotomes available that can rotate and may facilitate better sphincterotome and cutting wire orientation [11].

Catheters

Catheters are long plastic tubes used for injection of contrast and for insertion of guidewires. Multichannel catheters are more efficient and are preferred. The main difference between a standard catheter and a sphincterotome is that a sphincterotome has an electrosurgical cutting wire at the distal end of the catheter. When choosing a sphincterotome for cannulation, the short cutting wire is used to allow the scope to remain close to the papilla and maintain device stability while changing the angulation of the sphincterotome [12].

Stone Extraction Balloons and Baskets

Balloons and baskets are used for removing stones from the bile duct or pancreatic duct depending on the size and location of the stones and the exit passage. Balloons can be double lumen or triple lumen (allowing passage of a guidewire and/or contrast injection) and are advanced in a closed fashion above the stones, inflated so they are flush with the bile duct wall, and then withdrawn through the sphincterotomy to sweep out stones (Fig. 12.3). The extraction balloon is also used to perform an occlusion cholangiogram, in which the balloon is inflated to create a seal against

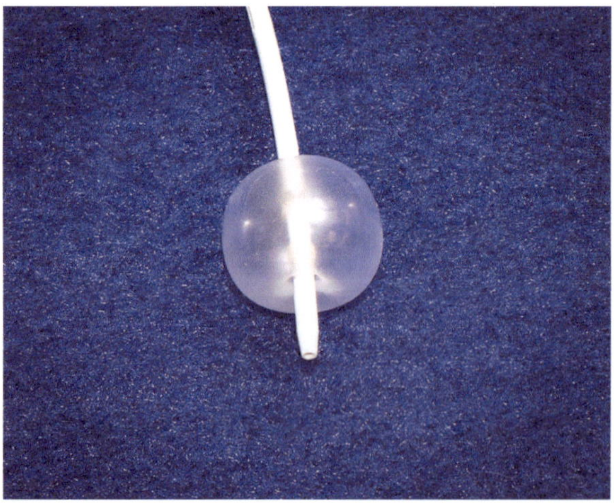

Fig. 12.3 Close-up view of a stone extraction balloon. A lumen is visible allowing passage of the balloon over a guidewire as well as injection of contrast. Photo credit: Kelsey Angell, PGY-3 General Surgery

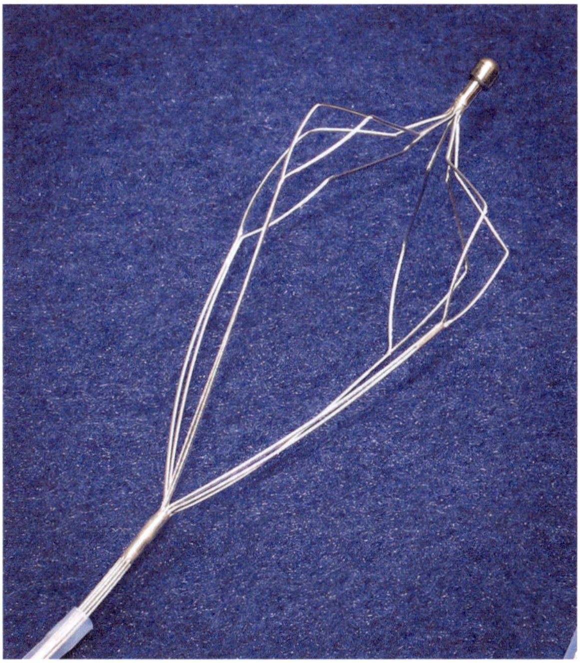

Fig. 12.4 Close-up view of a stone retrieval basket. Photo credit: Kelsey Angell, PGY-3 General Surgery

the bile duct while injecting contrast to distend the bile duct. The balloons may also be used for testing the adequacy of a sphincterotomy by pulling an inflated 10 mm balloon through the sphincterotomy and observing whether it deforms (an adequate sphincterotomy should not deform the balloon). The balloon extractor can also be used to check whether the dilation of a bile duct stricture is adequate in a similar fashion. Retrieval baskets (Fig. 12.4) typically have four wires in a hexagonal configuration and are used to capture larger stones, with some being designed for lithotripsy (see section on lithotripsy for stone fragmentation).

Stents

Stents are broadly divided into plastic and self-expandable metal stents. These are used for temporary drainage of the biliary system in patients with obstructing stones and/or cholangitis. In patients with cholangitis who require emergent drainage but who otherwise have contraindications to sphincterotomy (due to bleeding risk, dual-antiplatelet therapy, thrombocytopenia, etc.), stents are placed beyond the obstructing stone. Commonly used biliary stents are 7 and 10 Fr in size. They can be straight with flaps at both ends for retention or with a pigtail component at the end to prevent migration.

Basic Endoscopic Retrograde Cholangiopancreatography Technique

1. The side-viewing duodenoscope should be gently inserted past the upper esophageal sphincter. Once the esophagus is identified, the scope is gradually advanced to the duodenum where the ampulla of Vater is identified.
2. Cannulation of the CBD is commonly performed using a catheter or sphincterotome; a guidewire may be used to facilitate access. The risk of post-ERCP pancreatitis can be reduced by avoiding trauma to or injection of contrast into the pancreatic duct [13]. Other commonly used techniques used for a difficult biliary cannulation are listed in Table 12.4 [12]. The path of the guidewire can be observed under fluoroscopy to infer which duct has been cannulated. A relatively horizontal path that crosses the midline is consistent with pancreatic duct cannulation. A rounded cephalad path is consistent with common duct cannulation. A cholangiogram is then obtained by injecting contrast into the biliary tree, to identify anatomy and confirm cannulation of the correct duct.
3. Sphincterotomy: The goal of sphincterotomy is to open the terminal orifice of the CBD or pancreatic duct. This is achieved by disrupting the papilla and associated sphincter muscles. With this completed, access for a therapeutic intervention of the ducts is possible. A straightforward sphincterotomy is performed by positioning the sphincterotome across the papilla. With approximately one-third of the length of the sphincterotome cutting wire inside the papilla, the sphincterotome is flexed by tensioning the wire so that it comes into apposition with the wall of the papilla toward the 11 o'clock position. Electrosurgical energy is delivered through the cutting wire to incise the papilla to approximately 10 mm (up to but not beyond the first transverse mucosal fold) (Video 12.1). A "precut" sphincterotomy is used when a duct is blocked with an impacted stone or is a difficult cannulation. This technique is used for initial access and then is followed by conventional sphincterotomy. The papilla is first incised prior to deep cannulation. The most widely used technique for sphincterotomy is the freehand "needle knife" technique. This technique uses an endoscopic cutting needle knife rather than the standard sphincterotome, with the endoscopist making an incision at the papilla traveling cephalad. The discussion of techniques for difficult ERCP (e.g., due to aberrant anatomy or surgically altered anatomy due to Roux-en-Y gastric bypass surgery) is beyond the scope of this chapter.

Table 12.4 Biliary cannulation techniques

Biliary cannulation techniques
1. Pancreatic access (guidewire or stent) placement to assist biliary cannulation
2. Precut access sphincterotomy
3. Endoscopic scissors, endoscopic dissection techniques
4. Sphincterectomy

Lithotripsy for Stone Fragmentation

Lithotripsy has fallen out of favor over the years and now is employed only when other methods have failed. There are two primary setup types: through-the-scope devices and over-the-scope devices. Currently available types of lithotripsy are mechanical, extracorporeal shock wave (ESWL), electrohydraulic, chemical dissolution, and laser. These devices function by fragmenting large stones into smaller, more manageable pieces, which are then removed with a basket. Mechanical lithotripsy devices are used for the removal of stones >15 mm and work by crushing an entrapped stone between basket wires that are tightened against a metal catheter sheath using a locking crank handle. Several studies have shown that success rates for mechanical lithotripsy are >75% and that a major predictor for success is whether or not the stone is impacted in the bile duct [14]. Similar success rates have been demonstrated for ESWL and laser fragmentation [15]. Laser lithotripsy functions by using amplified light energy at a certain wavelength focused into a single unit of light and projected onto a CBD stone to break up the stone. There are studies that have shown successful fragmentation in 70–95% of cases [16]. ESWL (first used in urology for the fragmentation of renal calculi) was first applied to the treatment of gallstones in the 1980s. It works by fluoroscopy or ultrasound-guided percutaneous administration of sound waves focused on the gallstones and CBD stones. Since most stones are primarily cholesterol stones, they are not radiopaque. A nasobiliary tube is placed to prevent occlusion of the common duct, and contrast is used to visualize the stones and monitor progress. There has been a reported 90% successful fragmentation rate with this technique for common bile duct stones [17]. Once the treatment is completed, the patient undergoes ERCP for retrieval of the smaller stones. Overall, this treatment is well tolerated but it can require several sessions to achieve the desired fragmentation. Electrohydraulic lithotripsy (EHL) uses a bipolar probe that discharges sparks underwater. This creates high frequency pressure waves that disperse the energy equally through nearby biliary duct stones. This energy is very effective at fragmenting stones. This technique can be done under fluoroscopic guidance or directly under cholangioscopic guidance and visualization. Despite the various forms of fragmentation and newer technologies, the most common form is mechanical fragmentation. This is primarily due to cost, availability, safety, and training patterns.

Endoscopic Retrograde Cholangiopancreatography in Pediatric Patients

There is a relatively lower incidence of patients requiring ERCP for choledocholithiasis in the pediatric population. Common duct stones are most commonly seen in the setting of hemolytic disorders, which lead to increased formation of calcium bilirubinate and primary CBD stones. Other indications for ERCP in pediatrics include evaluations for choledochal cysts, post-cholecystectomy bile duct injury, and trauma. Recent studies have suggested that ERCP in the pediatric population can be safely and reliably performed by well-trained adult endoscopists [18].

Endoscopic Retrograde Cholangiopancreatography in Pregnant Patients

ERCP has not been well studied during pregnancy, with most data coming from observational studies. Invasive procedures during pregnancy should be undertaken when failure to intervene would pose harm to the mother or fetus [19]. In situations where therapeutic intervention is necessary, endoscopy does provide a safer alternative to surgical or radiologic procedures. Biliary pancreatitis, cholangitis, and symptomatic choledocholithiasis all require prompt intervention due to the potential for fetal loss if left untreated.

Intervention should be undertaken during the second trimester, if possible, and an obstetrician should always be consulted. Radiation should be minimized or strategies used to confirm deep cannulation without fluoroscopy, such as cannulation over a wire with aspirating of bile to confirm position in the common bile duct. Bipolar electrosurgery devices are preferred, but monopolar devices for sphincterotomy can still be used safely with proper positioning of the return electrode so that the uterus is not between the monopolar device and the return electrode [19]. The risk of post-ERCP pancreatitis is significantly higher in this population and also when done in a community hospital. Transfer to a tertiary referral center should be considered in these cases.

Complications and Management

Pancreatitis

Pancreatitis is the most common, severe adverse event associated with ERCP [20, 21]. In systematic reviews and meta-analysis, the incidence of pancreatitis is 3–10% [20, 21]. Post-ERCP pancreatitis (PEP) constitutes a syndrome of abdominal pain associated with hyperamylasemia requiring hospitalization (Table 12.5). A finding of elevated pancreatic enzymes alone does not constitute pancreatitis, as they may

Table 12.5 Risk factors associated with PEP

Risk factors associated with PEP include	
Patient factors	Sphincter of Oddi dysfunction, pregnancy, recurrent pancreatitis, prior history of PEP
Procedure-related factors	Difficult cannulation, endoscopic large balloon dilation
Operator factors	Inadequate experience

PEP post-endoscopic retrograde cholangiopancreatography pancreatitis be elevated in more than 75% of patients. Two important factors implicated in pancreatitis are mechanical trauma from duct instrumentation and hydrostatic injury from contrast injection.

Management IV hydration in the periprocedural period can decrease the rate of hypoperfusion and subsequent development of pancreatitis. Methods to reduce PEP include appropriate patient selection and guidewire cannulation. Early precut sphincterotomy can reduce the risk of mechanical trauma with repeated cannulation attempts in a difficult case and can decrease the risk of pancreatitis [13]. Also, pancreatic duct stent placement in patients at high risk of developing PEP should be considered. Pharmacological prophylaxis with indomethacin, by interrupting the inflammatory cascade, has also been shown to significantly reduce the rate of PEP [21].

Bleeding

Bleeding is most commonly seen after biliary or pancreatic sphincterotomy. It may occur immediately post-procedure or may be delayed in presentation from several hours to even weeks. Bleeding is classified as mild, moderate, or severe, based on number of blood transfusions and whether there is a need for surgical or angiographic intervention (Table 12.6) [22].

Prevention Steps to minimize bleeding include avoiding unnecessary sphincterotomy (in cases of cholangitis, endoscopic papillary large balloon dilation and stent placement alone without sphincterotomy are alternatives when there is a high risk of post-sphincterotomy bleeding), using a blended mode of electrosurgery rather than a pure-cut waveform, and prophylactic injection of hypertonic saline and epinephrine.

Infection

While ERCP is the endoscopic modality of choice for treatment of cholangitis, it may also contribute to causing this complication [21]. In 0.5–3% of individuals, infection may occur when ERCP is performed for choledocholithiasis, and incomplete biliary drainage is achieved. The most frequent microbes associated with post-ERCP infection are enteric bacteria. In recent years, however, there has been a rise in scope-related transmission of infection. In 2013, an outbreak of carbapenem-resistant Enterobacteriaceae (CRE) infections associated with duodenoscopes was identified

Table 12.6 Risk factors associated with bleeding

Risk factors associated with bleeding include	
Patient factors	Coagulopathy, active cholangitis, anticoagulation within 3 days of ERCP
Technical	Type of current used. Pure cut is associated with a higher risk of bleeding compared to blended current
Operator	Endoscopist case volume (<1/week)

ERCP endoscopic retrograde cholangiopancreatography

and investigated by the US Food and Drug Administration (FDA). Given the unique design of the duodenoscope elevator, it was concluded that this part of the instrument was difficult to effectively clean and disinfect in duodenoscopes and likely led to the transmission of infections between patients. The FDA subsequently released guidelines in 2015 for the reprocessing of scopes to reduce the risk of infection transmission [23]. Per the Centers for Disease Control and Prevention (CDC), currently, there is limited data to support the practice of routine performance of surveillance cultures to assess endoscope reprocessing outside of recognized outbreak settings. Given the potential for infection transmission, it is important that endoscopists adhere to appropriate indications for ERCP to minimize the occurrence of this complication [24].

Perforation

The incidence of perforation from ERCP has been reported as 0.05–1.0% [25, 26]. Perforations are commonly associated with sphincterotomy but can also be associated with endoscope insertion into the duodenum or from the placement of the guidewire. They are classified into different types as: (1) free bowel wall perforation, (2) retroperitoneal perforation secondary to periampullary injury, (3) perforation of the bile duct or pancreatic duct, and (4) isolated retroperitoneal air [26]. The most common perforation is a class 1 located in the retroperitoneal duodenum. This is caused by the endoscope perforating the lateral wall of the duodenum. Class 3 injuries typically occur from the sphincterotomy; for example, if the cut is carried too far along the bile duct, causing a full-thickness duodenal wall injury resulting in a perforation. Perforations can also be caused by cannulation, dilation, or from the guidewire itself. Extraction of large, difficult stones may also lead to perforations within the ductal system. The clinical presentation of patients who have ERCP-related perforation ranges from asymptomatic pneumoperitoneum and retroperitoneal air to generalized peritonitis. Most symptoms start as mild epigastric pain and worsen over the course of hours depending on the type and severity of the injury. The management of the perforation starts with identification. The majority of these injuries can be seen or suspected during the procedure. The remaining patients are identified due to ongoing pain or abnormal findings on imaging. Management begins with bowel rest, IV hydration, and broad-spectrum antibiotics covering typical organisms found in the proximal gastrointestinal (GI) tract and should include antifungal coverage. A contrast upper gastrointestinal study (UGI) is done to help identify the approximate location of the perforation and, to some extent, the degree of perforation. This is important because small leaks can be managed with close observation and antibiotics. Surgery is indicated for patients with failed nonoperative management (persistent leukocytosis, fevers, and pain), retained hardware, large contrast extravasation on UGI, large fluid collections on imaging studies, or who show signs of sepsis. Isolated retroperitoneal air found on imaging after an ERCP is not infrequent, and without associated clinical symptoms, is not an indication by itself for surgical intervention [26, 27].

Endoscopic Retrograde Cholangiopancreatography: Training, Competency Assessment

ERCP is currently the most common complex endoscopic procedure and carries with it a significant risk of failure, adverse events, and possible medicolegal jeopardy. Thus it is necessary that credentialing to perform ERCP is granted conscientiously. For the purposes of training and credentialing, successful performance of ERCP is defined as the deep cannulation of the bile duct. Historically, a bench mark of 180 procedures with a minimum cannulation rate of 80% was considered necessary for a trainee to acquire a level of competence in diagnostic and therapeutic ERCP; recently a minimum of 200 procedures has been proposed [28]. Despite these minimum case number recommendations, however, it is increasingly being recognized that case volume does not always equal technical competence, and that use of validated assessment tools and direct observation of cases by a qualified, unbiased endoscopist may be better ways of assessing competence [29]. Also, cannulation is only one diagnostic component of an ERCP, and other aspects of the procedure—including sphincterotomy, stone extraction, stricture dilation, stent placement, and tissue sampling techniques—must also be assessed. An adequate volume of activity is also needed to maintain proficiency. It has been shown that individual endoscopists who perform more than 40 endoscopic sphincterotomies per year or at least 1 per week have a lower complication rate than those who perform fewer procedures.

Training

ERCP training is usually a part of an interventional gastroenterology fellowship or an advanced endoscopic surgery fellowship. In many countries, and especially in the United States, there is no limitation to the training positions, resulting in significant variability in the training experience and procedure numbers among trainees. Also, there is considerable variation in the extent of hands-on involvement in different fellowships, with the result that many fellowship graduates may feel inadequate in performing the procedure with the need to do an additional fellowship to gain confidence. It is incumbent upon training programs to ensure that trainees are able to reach an acceptable level of competence for safe independent practice. Increasingly, programs are supplementing clinical hands-on work experience with simulation and animal lab experience. These training models may improve the trainee's understanding of the anatomy, endoscopic accessories, and basic techniques of scope handling, manipulation of accessories, and coordination with the assistant without involving a patient and augment the clinical experience.

References

1. Stinton LM, Shaffer EA. Epidemiology of gallbladder disease: cholelithiasis and cancer. Gut Liver. 2012;6(2):172–87.
2. Cai J-S, Qiang S, Bao-Bing Y. Advances of recurrent risk factors and management of choledocholithiasis. Scand J Gastroenterol. 2016;52(1):1–10.
3. Liu TH, Consorti ET, Kawashima A, Tamm EP, Kwong KL, Gill BS, et al. Patient evaluation and management with selective use of magnetic resonance cholangiography and endoscopic retrograde cholangiopancreatography before laparoscopic cholecystectomy. Ann Surg. 2001;234(1):33–40.
4. Mitchell SE, Clark RA. A comparison of computed tomography and sonography in choledocholithiasis. AJR Am J Roentgenol. 1984;142(4):729–33.
5. Giljaca V, Gurusamy KS, Takwoingi Y, Higgie D, Poropat G, Štimac D, et al. Endoscopic ultrasound versus magnetic resonance cholangiopancreatography for common bile duct stones. Cochrane Database Syst Rev. 2015;2:CD011549.
6. Möller M, Gustafsson U, Rasmussen F, Persson G, Thorell A. Natural course vs interventions to clear common bile duct stones. JAMA Surg. 2014;149(10):1008–13.
7. Jeurnink SM, Steyerberg EW, Kuipers EJ, Siersema PD. The burden of endoscopic retrograde cholangiopancreatography (ERCP) performed with the patient under conscious sedation. Surg Endosc. 2012;26(8):2213–9.
8. Garewal D, Powell S, Milan SJ, Nordmeyer J, Waikar P. Sedative techniques for endoscopic retrograde cholangiopancreatography. Cochrane Database Syst Rev. 2012;6:CD007274.
9. Mishkin D, Carpenter S, Croffie J, Chuttani R, DiSario J, Hussain N, Technology Assessment Committee, American Society for Gastrointestinal Endoscopy, et al. ASGE technology status evaluation report: radiographic contrast media used in ERCP. Gastrointest Endosc. 2005;62(4):480–4.
10. Singhvi G, Dea SK. Guidewires in ERCP. Gastrointest Endosc. 2013;77(6):938–40.
11. Cotton PB, Leung J. ERCP: the fundamentals. 2nd ed. West Sussex: Wiley; 2015.
12. Kethu SR, Adler DG, Conway JD, Diehl DL, Farraye FA, Kantsevoy SV, Kaul V, Kwon RS, Mamula P, Pedrosa MC, Rodriguez SA, The ASGE Technology Committee. ERCP cannulation and sphincterotomy devices. Gastrointest Endosc. 2010;71(3):435–45.
13. Zagalsky D, Guidi M, Curvale C, Lasa J, de Maria J, Ianniccillo H, et al. Early precut is as efficient as pancreatic stent in preventing post-ERCP pancreatitis in high-risk subjects–a randomized study. Rev Esp Enferm Dig. 2016;108(9):558–62.
14. Garg PK, Tandon RK, Ahuja V, Makharia GK, Batra Y. Predictors of unsuccessful mechanical lithotripsy and endoscopic clearance of large bile duct stones. Gastrointest Endosc. 2004;59(6):601–5.
15. Amplatz S, Piazzi L, Felder M, Comberlato M, Benvenuti S, Zancanella L, et al. Extracorporeal shock wave lithotripsy for clearance of refractory bile duct stones. Dig Liver Dis. 2007;39:267–72.
16. Prat F, Fritsch J, Choury AD, Frouge C, Marteau V, Etienne JP. Laser lithotripsy of difficult biliary stones. Gastrointest Endosc. 1994;40(3):290–5.
17. Sauerbruch T, Stern M. Fragmentation of bile duct stones by extracorporeal shock waves. A new approach to biliary calculi after failure of routine endoscopic measures. Gastroenterology. 1989;96(1):146–52.
18. Yıldırım A, Altun R, Ocal S, Kormaz M, Ozcay F, Selcuk H. The safety and efficacy of ERCP in the pediatric population with standard scopes: does size really matter? Spring. 2016;5:128.
19. ASGE Standard of Practice Committee, Shergill AK, Ben-Menachem T, Chandrasekhara V, Chathadi K, Decker GA, Evans JA, et al. Guidelines for endoscopy in pregnant and lactating women. Gastrointest Endosc. 2012;76(1):18–24.
20. ASGE Standards of Practice Committee, Chandrasekhara V, Khashab MA, Muthusamy VR, Acosta RD, Agrawal D, Bruining DH, et al. Adverse events associated with ERCP. Gastrointest Endosc. 2017;85(1):32–47.

21. Freeman ML. Adverse outcomes of ERCP. Gastrointest Endosc. 2002;56(6B):a129028.
22. Cotton PB, Lehman G, Vennes J, Geenen JE, Russell RC, Meyers WC, et al. Endoscopic sphincterotomy complications and their management: an attempt at consensus. Gastrointest Endosc. 1991;37(3):383–93.
23. FDA Executive Summary. Effective reprocessing of endoscopes used in endoscopic retrograde cholangiopancreatography (ERCP) procedures. May 2015. https://www.fda.gov/downloads/AdvisoryCommittees/CommitteesMeetingMaterials/MedicalDevices/MedicalDevicesAdvisoryCommittee/Gastroenterology-UrologyDevicesPanel/UCM445592.pdf. Accessed 08 Aug 2017.
24. Keswani RN, Soper NJ. Endoscopes and the "Superbug" outbreak. JAMA Surg. 2015;150(9):831–2.
25. Masci E, Toti G, Mariani A, Curioni S, Lomazzi A, Dinelli M, et al. Complications of diagnostic and therapeutic ERCP: a prospective multicenter study. Am J Gastroenterol. 2001;96(2):417–23.
26. Stapfer M, Selby RR, Stain SC, Katkhouda N, Parekh D, Jabbour N, et al. Management of duodenal perforation after endoscopic retrograde cholangiopancreatography and sphincterotomy. Ann Surg. 2000;232(2):191–8.
27. Genzlinger JL, McPhee MS, Fisher JK, Jacob KM, Helzberg JH. Significance of retroperitoneal air after endoscopic retrograde cholangiopancreatography with sphincterotomy. Am J Gastroenterol. 1999;94(5):1267–70.
28. ASGE Standards of Practice Committee, Faulx AL, Lightdale JR, Acosta RD, Agrawal D, Bruining DH, Chandrasekhara V, et al. Guidelines for privileging, credentialing, and proctoring to perform GI endoscopy. Gastrointest Endosc. 2017;85(2):273–81.
29. Pearl J, Fellinger E, Dunkin B, Pauli E, Trus T, Marks J, Fanelli R, Meara M, Stefanidis D, Richardson W. Guidelines for privileging and credentialing physicians in gastrointestinal endoscopy. Surg Endosc. 2016;30(8):3184–90.

Chapter 13
Endoscopic Ultrasound in the Management of Biliary Stone Disease

Robert D. Fanelli and Todd H. Baron

Introduction

Choledocholithiasis is identified frequently in patients with gallstone disease, occurring in 5–15% of patients undergoing cholecystectomy. The incidence of choledocholithiasis increases with age, and common bile duct stones (CBDS) are identified in up to 30–60% of patients over age 70 years who present for cholecystectomy. CBDS can be occult and asymptomatic and may not be associated with biochemical abnormalities [1–4]. Although it is commonly accepted that up to 30% of CBDS will pass spontaneously, it is not possible to predict reliably which patients will pass CBDS or if all stones will be cleared without the need for intervention. CBDS are clinically significant because they may cause jaundice, biliary pancreatitis, and cholangitis, each of which may be associated with morbidity or even mortality.

CBDS are classified as primary stones and secondary stones. Primary stones form in the intrahepatic or extrahepatic bile ducts and typically are comprised of calcium bilirubinate, cholesterol, and calcium salts. Primary stones also are referred to as pigment stones. Secondary CBDS, those that form in the gallbladder and then advance into the common bile duct through the cystic duct, typically are comprised of cholesterol, bile salts, and phospholipids. Secondary CBDS tend to be much more common than primary CBDS in the United States and other developed nations.

CBDS can be managed preoperatively, intraoperatively, or postoperatively, depending on the clinical scenario, individual patient needs, and available expertise.

R. D. Fanelli, MD, MHA, FACS, FASGE (✉)
Department of Surgery, The Guthrie Clinic, Sayre, PA, USA
e-mail: surgical.presentations@gmail.com

T. H. Baron, MD, FASGE
Department of Medicine, Division of Gastroenterology and Hepatology, University of North Carolina, Chapel Hill, NC, USA
e-mail: todd_baron@med.unc.edu

© Springer International Publishing AG, part of Springer Nature 2018
B. F. Santos, N. Soper (eds.), *Choledocholithiasis*,
https://doi.org/10.1007/978-3-319-74503-9_13

Evaluation for CBDS begins with a high degree of suspicion when treating patients with gallstone disease, especially those at a higher than average risk for CBDS. The primary goal in treating patients with gallstone disease is reducing the likelihood of recurrent symptoms and limiting occurrence of associated complications such as sepsis and pancreatitis.

Endoscopic ultrasound (EUS) is an effective and efficient technique for identification of CBDS and in patients with altered anatomy is effective in providing alternate access to the common bile duct for stone removal. In order to select patients appropriately for EUS, individual patient risks for CBDS must be stratified and an algorithmic approach used to guide clinical management.

Endoscopic Ultrasound as a Diagnostic Modality

Because of the proximity of the ultrasound transducer to the biliary tree when the echoendoscope is passed into the duodenum, the loss of echo due to distance is eliminated. Thus, high frequency can be used (up to 10 mhz), making the resolution markedly superior to transabdominal ultrasound (TUS). It has been demonstrated that EUS provides excellent accuracy in the diagnoses of CBDS. Given a sensitivity of 89–98% and a specificity of 94–100% [1, 5, 6], EUS is comparable to endoscopic retrograde cholangiopancreatography (ERCP), but EUS has a lower risk of adverse events (AEs) than ERCP. Diagnostic EUS serves as an effective tool that can prevent unnecessary ERCP in patients who do not have CBDS, eliminating ERCP-related AEs in those shown not to have CBDS by EUS. Using this staged approach based on EUS-directed ERCP, unnecessary ERCP can be avoided in 30–75% of patients initially suspected of having CBDS, resulting in fewer complications and less cost than when direct ERCP is utilized [7–9]. For patients in whom CBDS have already been demonstrated or for those in need of bile duct decompression for biliary sepsis, direct ERCP remains more cost-effective [7, 8].

EUS has emerged as a superb diagnostic modality for the identification of CBDS and improves the safety of endoscopic management of biliary stone disease by eliminating ERCP in all but those circumstances where it is necessary for therapeutic intervention. The value of EUS is better appreciated when it is compared with other diagnostic modalities commonly used in the clinical evaluation of patients with suspected CBDS.

Competing Diagnostic Modalities

Clinical Presentation

CBDS may be asymptomatic and clinically silent or might be manifested as biliary colic, jaundice, biliary stricture, pancreatitis, cholangitis, and sepsis or present synchronously with biliopancreatic malignancy. Certain clinical disorders, such as biliary pancreatitis and acute cholangitis, traditionally have been accepted as evidence supporting the diagnosis of CBDS by mere virtue of their presence. Counterintuitively, however, biliary pancreatitis may not be a good indicator for the presence of CBDS. The risk of persistent CBDS has been shown to decline both after the onset of, and recovery from, biliary pancreatitis, likely because CBDS have already passed through the ampulla spontaneously [10]. A prospective population-based cohort study of 1171 patients revealed that CBDS were not significantly predicted by biliary pancreatitis or cholecystitis and that the highest predictability of CBDS was seen in electively treated patients with elevated liver chemistries without pancreatitis or cholecystitis [11]. These data suggest that patients presenting with biliary pancreatitis undergo invasive biliary intervention more often than necessary, given the infrequent presence of CBDS in this clinical setting [10]. EUS represents a safe and effective alternative approach for the evaluation of patients with biliary pancreatitis, and those considered at high risk for CBDS, which avoids the associated risks and complications of direct ERCP often utilized in these clinical scenarios.

Cholangitis, unlike biliary pancreatitis, is associated with a very high risk of persistent CBDS. Patients presenting with biliary sepsis should undergo ERCP without much further investigation, as the emphasis is less on diagnosis and more on therapy for sepsis [1, 12].

The combined findings of jaundice and right upper quadrant abdominal pain suggest the presence of CBDS. A prospective study showed that jaundice is significant as a predictor of CBDS on univariate analysis but fails to reach significance when multiple logistic regression analysis is applied [12]. Therefore, patients with jaundice unaccompanied by other signs of biliary obstruction should undergo evaluation for non-biliary causes of jaundice before invasive evaluation of the biliary tree is considered. Table 13.1 presents the American Society for Gastrointestinal Endoscopy (ASGE) risk stratification criteria, widely used for categorizing patients according to their risk of CBDS [1]. The sensitivity and specificity of these criteria have been questioned; however, with one study showing that of patients meeting high-probability criteria, only 54.9% were ultimately found to have CBDS, while patients meeting low or intermediate probability were found to have CBDS 31.4% of the time, resulting in an overall sensitivity and specificity of 54.9% and 68%, respectively [13].

Biochemical Testing

Obstruction from CBDS may not represent a static process. Obstruction from CBDS may be intermittent and may be related to stone migration through the common bile duct (CBD). CBDS may become trapped within the CBD in a completely obstructing, partially obstructing, or non-obstructing manner. For these reasons, liver chemistry measurements may be variable and may alone be unreliable indicators of the presence of CBDS. The diagnostic utility of liver chemistries is further limited by the lag time that exists between actual mechanical obstruction and rising and falling

Table 13.1 Predictors of common bile duct stones (CBDS)

Moderate risk predictors for CBDS	
• Liver function test other than bilirubin abnormal	
• Age >55 years	
• Gallstone pancreatitis on presentation	
Strong risk predictors for CBDS	
• Bilirubin greater than 1.8 but less than 4.0 mg/dL	
• Dilated bile duct on transabdominal ultrasound >8 mm	
Very strong risk predictors for CBDS	
• Bilirubin >4 mg/dL	
• CBDS identified on transabdominal ultrasound	
• Cholangitis on presentation	
Predictors present	*Risk for CBDS*
None	Low
One, two, or three moderate	Intermediate
One strong with/without moderate	Intermediate
Two strong	High
One or more very strong	High

Adapted from [1, 4]

chemistry levels [14]. Partially obstructing and non-obstructing CBDS may be associated with normal liver chemistries, especially early in the course of obstruction where biochemical lag is common [11].

However, false-negative liver chemistry results occur infrequently. In a study involving routine magnetic resonance cholangiopancreatography (MRCP) performed for patients with gallstone disease, only 4% of patients with normal liver chemistries had CBDS, yielding a negative predictive value of 96% [2]. Improved liver chemistries that accompany improved clinical symptoms are generally thought to suggest spontaneous clearance of CBDS, with increasing chemistry levels suggesting retained CBDS [15, 16]. However, incorporating a second set of liver enzymes into the ASGE risk stratification criteria does not improve its accuracy, and declining liver function tests do not reliably predict spontaneous stone passage [13]. Liver chemistries alone cannot be relied upon to accurately direct the patient to ERCP or other invasive therapy for clearance of suspected CBDS.

Despite limitations, liver chemistries play a significant role in selecting patients for further study aimed at identifying and treating CBDS. Individual liver chemistry values have greater utility in excluding CBDS than in predicting their presence. Bilirubin, alkaline phosphatase, γ(gamma)-glutamyl transpeptidase (GGT), aspartate aminotransferase (AST), and alanine aminotransferase (ALT) each have a positive predictive value between 25% and 50%, and each has a negative predictive value between 94% and 99% [1–3, 11, 12, 17, 18]. In aggregate, however, liver chemistries have an increased predictive utility, and as more individual studies become abnormal, this implies an increased risk of CBDS. Table 13.2 presents sensitivity and specificity ranges for laboratory and imaging tests commonly used in the evaluation of patients in whom CBDS are suspected [4].

Table 13.2 Sensitivity and specificity ranges for studies commonly used when evaluating patients for common bile duct stones (CBDS)

	Sensitivity (%)	Specificity (%)
Laboratory studies for detecting CBDS		
Total bilirubin (TB)	34–49	60–88
Alkaline phosphatase (AP)	41–80	88–73
Gamma-glutamyl transpeptidase (GGT)	63–84	72–73
Aspartate transaminase (AST)	44–64	79–86
Alanine transaminase (ALT)	50–72	68–81
At least one component elevated from the panel		
TB—AP—GGT—AST—ALT	52–88	53–91
Imaging studies for detecting CBDS		
Transabdominal ultrasound (US)	20–58	68–91
Computed tomography (CT)	50–88	84–98
Magnetic resonance cholangiopancreatography (MRCP)	85–95	91–100
Endoscopic retrograde cholangiopancreatography (ERCP)	89–93	98–100
Endoscopic ultrasound (EUS)	89–98	94–100

Modified with permission from Fanelli RD, Andrew BD. Making the Diagnosis: Surgery, a Rational Approach to the Patient with Suspected CBD Stones. In: Hazey JW, Conwell DL, Guy GE (eds). Multidisciplinary Management of Common Bile Duct Stones: An Interdisciplinary Textbook. New York, NY: Springer International Publishing Company; 2016:37–48.

Transabdominal Ultrasound

Limited transabdominal ultrasound frequently is used in the evaluation of abdominal pain suspected to be of biliary origin. However, TUS is not well suited for direct identification of CBDS. Sensitivity and specificity for TUS in detecting CBDS range from 20% to 58% and 68% to 91%, respectively [3, 14].

Poor sensitivity and specificity are attributable to the many physical limitations plaguing TUS. In general, a refractive border between the CBD wall and common duct stones themselves is absent, making delineation of CBDS difficult using TUS. Body fat and intestinal gas interfere with TUS transduction, and CBDS located in the intraduodenal and intrapancreatic CBD are particularly difficult to identify on TUS because of these same interfering factors. TUS is extremely dependent on technician experience. For example, Rickes et al. demonstrated that experienced sonographers are more accurate in diagnosing CBDS (83% vs. 64%) compared to their less experienced colleagues [19]. As part of an algorithmic diagnostic approach to CBDS, TUS is useful in detecting signs that are suggestive of CBDS. For example, a normal CBD on TUS in the setting of normal liver chemistries has a negative predictive value for CBDS of 95%. A dilated CBD on TUS in the same clinical and laboratory value setting raises the risk of CBDS to intermediate [1, 15, 20, 21]. TUS remains an important screening tool for patients with biliary stone disease, but its limitations and inferiority to EUS must be considered in patients at risk for CBDS.

Computed Tomography

Although computed tomography (CT) provides excellent diagnostic utility for general abdominal pathology, it has not proven to be particularly effective in diagnosing CBDS. Continuing advancements in CT technology have led to improved utility in vascular, oncologic, and general abdominal radiology, but sensitivity and specificity for detecting CBDS remain limited, ranging from 50% to 88% and 84% and 98%, respectively [22, 23]. Sensitivity is further diminished when CBDS are comprised primarily of cholesterol—the most common composition of secondary stones in Western countries. The size of CBDS affects the diagnostic capabilities of CT, as stones smaller than 5 mm are less commonly diagnosed compared with stones larger than 5 mm (57% vs. 81%) [22]. CT often is performed early in the evaluation of patients with abdominal pain, but in patients suspected to be at risk for CBDS, a negative CT does not exclude CBDS. In situations where suspicion for CBDS remains high, a negative CT should not preclude EUS.

Computed Tomographic Cholangiography

CT cholangiography (CTC)—abdominal CT performed after administration of contrast designed specifically for biliary excretion—is rarely used clinically. Because of the unnecessary radiation exposure associated with CTC, the potential for contrast toxicity specific to intravenous (IV) biliary contrast, and the fact that contrast excretion is hampered in the setting of biliary obstruction, most clinicians prefer magnetic resonance imaging (MRI) and magnetic resonance cholangiopancreatography rather than CTC when advanced imaging is needed in the evaluation of CBDS [1, 24].

Magnetic Resonance Cholangiopancreatography

MRCP most often is utilized to evaluate patients at intermediate risk for CBDS. Low-risk patients will not benefit from MRCP, and high-risk patients typically benefit most from EUS-directed ERCP, direct ERCP, or common bile duct exploration. The sensitivity of MRCP in detecting CBDS is 85–95%, and its specificity is 91–100% [1, 3, 5, 25–29]. As seen with CT, sensitivity is lower when smaller stones are present but is dependent on slice thickness used for image acquisition. When MRCP slice thickness is set to 5 mm, sensitivity for detecting CBDS smaller than 6 mm is 33–71% [3, 27]; a slice thickness of 3 mm is associated with 100% sensitivity for CBDS as small as 3 mm [30]. Evidence suggests that clinical improvement, normalization of previously abnormal laboratory tests, and a negative MRCP indicate spontaneous clearance of CBDS [16].

Diagnostic algorithms favor MRCP over ERCP when CBDS are suspected and EUS is not available. MRCP is noninvasive and has virtually no associated complications; it is superior to ERCP, which has a serious adverse event rate of 1–7% [10]. Using MRCP to evaluate patients suspected of having CBDS with moderate risk factors helps avoid unnecessary ERCP in 43–80% of patients who have a negative MRCP in this setting [21, 26, 27, 31]. Liberal use of MRCP in intermediate-risk scenarios for CBDS may limit the need for EUS in some patients, but cost, available expertise, and the ability to follow diagnostic EUS with therapeutic ERCP when needed may influence MRCP utilization.

Endoscopic Retrograde Cholangiopancreatography

ERCP is both diagnostic and therapeutic in the treatment of CBDS and holds advantages over almost all other modalities used in this setting. As a diagnostic modality, ERCP has a sensitivity for CBDS of 89–93% and a specificity of 98–100% [1, 3, 27]. ERCP may miss smaller CBDS, but the clinical significance of these small stones remains unclear [1, 32], especially when most endoscopists perform empiric biliary sphincterotomy and duct sweeping even if no stones are identified. Although ERCP is of great utility in the management of CBDS, its application as a diagnostic modality is associated with morbidity ranging from 2% to 7%; AEs include pancreatitis, hemorrhage, and duodenal perforation, among others. Mortality from diagnostic ERCP is approximately 1%. ERCP adds cost to the management of patients at low and moderate risk for CBDS, whether performed preoperatively or postoperatively, but when utilized in patients whose risk for CBDS exceeds 80%, ERCP becomes a cost-effective choice [33]. AEs related to ERCP can be limited with the use of rectally administered nonsteroidal agents and placement of prophylactic pancreatic stents. Utilizing less invasive confirmatory studies or approaches such as EUS-directed ERCP decreases utilization of ERCP by 30–80%, largely by eliminating the need for diagnostic ERCP in patients in whom no CBDS are found during EUS [7, 21, 26, 27, 31].

ERCP will have a place in the management of CBDS for the foreseeable future, but its role has nearly evolved to entirely therapeutic, as the superior performance and safety parameters of EUS for diagnosis and for selecting patients who require therapeutic ERCP are difficult to ignore.

Summary

EUS has superior sensitivity and specificity (89–98% and 84–100%, respectively) for the diagnosis of CBDS compared with clinical presentation, biochemical testing, transabdominal ultrasound, CT, CT cholangiography, and MRI/MRCP. It is marginally superior to ERCP for the diagnosis of CBDS but affords patients suspected of having CBDS a significant margin of safety over diagnostic ERCP. ERCP, like surgical common bile duct exploration, should be reserved for the definitive treatment of patients confirmed to have CBDS. When expertise is available, EUS is the diagnostic procedure of choice in patients suspected of having CBDS who may require ERCP.

Endoscopic Ultrasound as a Therapeutic Modality

EUS is an endoscopic tool that has wide applications in the evaluation and treatment of abnormalities of the gastrointestinal tract. Target lesions are those that occur within the luminal organs of the foregut and rectum and those solid organs within reasonable proximity to these points of entry. Sonographic evaluation, and sampling of fluid or tissue for analysis through adjunctive procedures such as fine needle aspiration (FNA), lends diagnostic accuracy to the evaluation of mucosal lesions, submucosal nodules, solid tumors of the pancreas, liver, lymph nodes, and other structures. It also promotes the accurate staging of thoracic and abdominal malignancy to better tailor systemic chemotherapy, radiation therapy, and oncologic surgery.

EUS also is useful for evaluating inflammatory conditions such as pancreatitis and for draining inflammatory collections, such as pancreatic pseudocysts and even gallbladders distended as the result of acute cholecystitis in some cases. Newer techniques, such as the placement of EUS-guided lumen-apposing stents, allow the creation of pathways not native to the gastrointestinal tract [34–36]. For the remainder of this chapter, we will focus on the role that EUS plays in the diagnosis and management of biliary stone disease, in patients with normal and surgically altered anatomy.

Normal Anatomy

With respect to CBDS, the primary role for EUS is to identify patients with common duct stones that were not identified using another modality, so that they then can be treated by CBDS clearance using ERCP (Figs. 13.1 and 13.2).

Figures 13.1 and 13.2 demonstrate CBDS identified in different patients during EUS. EUS-directed ERCP has become a standard approach for the treatment of CBDS, with ERCP following EUS immediately in many centers [1].

It is not uncommon for patients with biliary pancreatitis to be referred for inpatient ERCP, both for confirmation of the suspected etiology and in preparation for cholecystectomy. Studies suggest that EUS provides the advantage of confirming a biliary origin in patients in whom traditional radiographic analysis failed to localize the source of pancreatitis and that EUS done early in the course of illness may be useful in predicting the severity of pancreatitis, length of hospital stay, and illness severity and mortality [37–39].

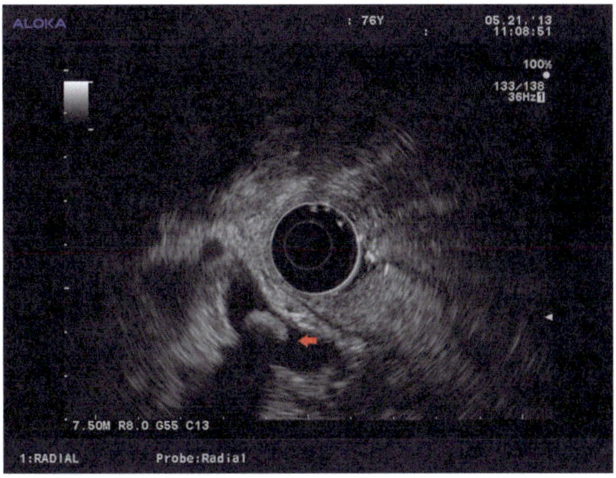

Fig. 13.1 Shadowing CBD stone (red arrow) identified in a dilated bile duct during radial EUS examination

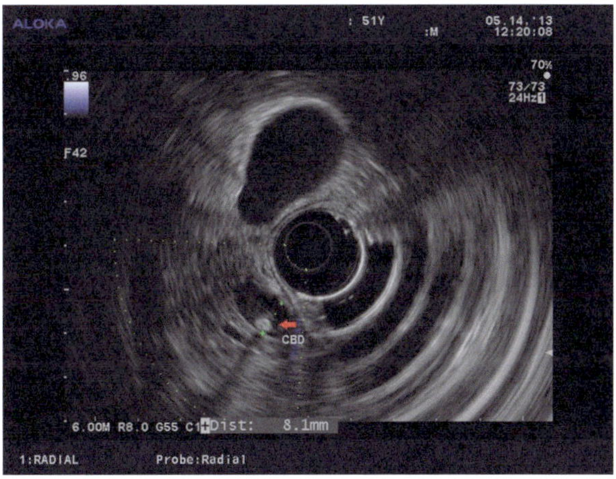

Fig. 13.2 Small CBD stone (red arrow) identified in a mildly dilated bile duct during radial EUS examination

Therapeutic Applications of Endoscopic Ultrasound in Patients with Common Bile Duct Stones

Failed Endoscopic Retrograde Cholangiopancreatography in Patients with Native Gastrointestinal Anatomy

In patients with established CBDS, successful ERCP cannulation is over 95%. However, in patients with acute pancreatitis, severe duodenal edema may preclude identification of the papilla due to edema in the duodenal wall. In addition, periampullary diverticula are often present in elderly patients with CBDS, also making cannulation difficult, if not impossible. In these situations, EUS can be utilized for rendezvous to facilitate ERCP (Fig. 13.3a, b) [40, 41].

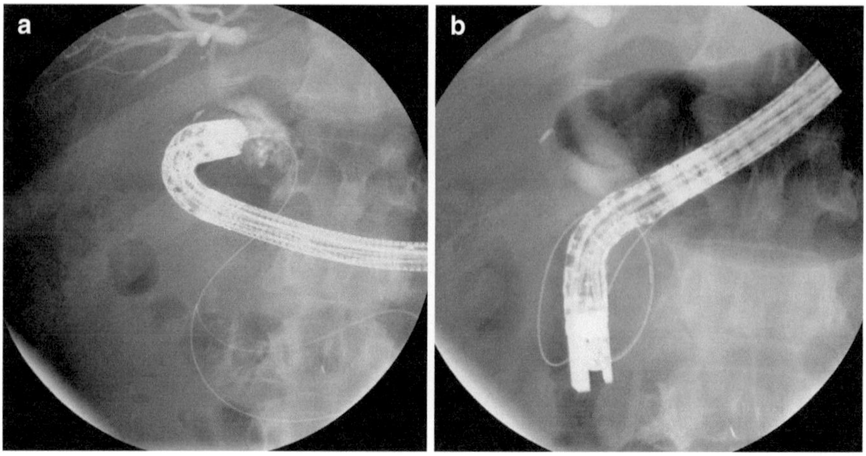

Fig. 13.3 EUS-guided rendezvous after failed ERCP cannulation in a patient with native anatomy. (**a**) Fluoroscopic image with forward-viewing linear echoendoscope positioned in the duodenum with a guidewire passed antegrade and looped in the duodenum. (**b**) Fluoroscopic image with duodenoscope positioned in the second duodenum with a sphincterotome passed retrograde. The indwelling stone was subsequently removed

This is performed using a linear echoendoscope, which allows real-time visualization of needle passage. With the echoendoscope positioned in the stomach or duodenum, the biliary system is punctured with a 22G or 19G needle transhepatically into the left intrahepatic system or transduodenally into the common bile duct, and a 0.018" or 0.035" guidewire is passed through the needle antegrade and through the papilla into the duodenum. The echoendoscope is withdrawn leaving the guidewire in place. A standard duodenoscope is then passed into the duodenum to grasp the wire and perform standard retrograde ERCP.

In patients with native anatomy, an alternative to rendezvous is creation of a choledochoduodenostomy, especially when access to the papilla is not possible due to duodenal obstruction [41]. This is a consideration for elderly patients with a bile duct ≥12 mm in diameter, since there are long-term concerns about development of sump syndrome in this cohort.

Endoscopic Ultrasound-Guided Therapy of Common Bile Duct Stones in Patients with Surgically Altered Gastrointestinal Anatomy

While there are a variety of postsurgical anatomies that face the endoscopist, the most commonly seen in which CBDS occur are those with Roux-en-Y gastric bypass (RYGB). In patients with an intact gallbladder who will undergo cholecystectomy, the primary approach is laparoscopic-assisted ERCP at the time of laparoscopic cholecystectomy. In this situation, the excluded stomach is accessed intraoperatively to allow antegrade ERCP.

In RYGB patients who are post-cholecystectomy or poor operative candidates for cholecystectomy, intraoperative laparoscopic-assisted ERCP is still an option. An alternative approach that can be performed in the endoscopy suite is EUS-directed therapy.

There are two main approaches to RYGB patients with CBDS. The approach taken depends on the urgency of decompression. In patients with nonurgent CBDS (hemodynamically stable, minimal or resolved symptoms, lack of cholangitis), EUS-guided gastrostomy using recently developed and commercially available lumen-apposing metal stents (LAMS) allows endoscopic access to the excluded stomach to accomplish conventional ERCP [42].

Using a linear echoendoscope positioned in the gastric pouch, the excluded stomach can be seen ultrasonographically and a 19G needle used to puncture into it (Fig. 13.4a, b). A 0.035" wire is advanced into the excluded stomach. The LAMS is deployed to create a gastrogastric anastomosis (GGA). The largest-diameter LAMS currently available is 15 mm, and attempts to pass a standard adult duodenoscope immediately after GGA often result in stent dislodgement and free perforation due to the resistance in the stent (even in spite of 15 mm balloon dilation after deployment) and the angulation of entry into the LAMS. Therefore, a waiting period of 2–4 weeks is necessary prior to ERCP. It is possible to perform immediate ERCP through the LAMS using a pediatric duodenoscope or standard upper gastroscope. However, the former is not readily available in most units and accessories are limited; the latter is possible but fraught with difficulties due to the

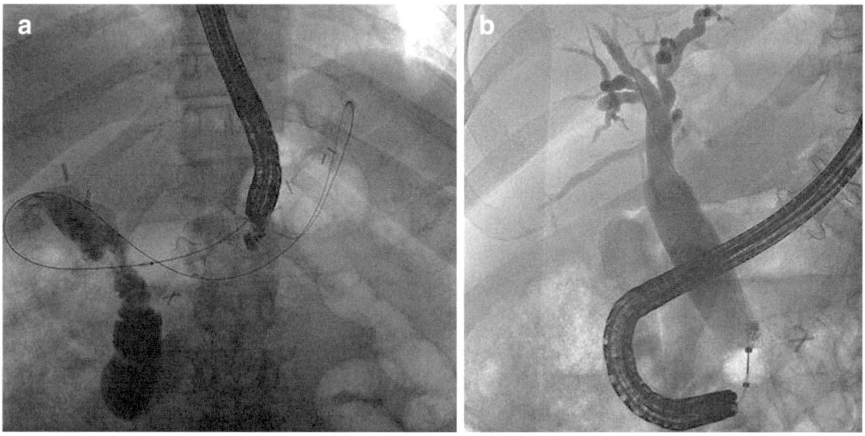

Fig. 13.4 Removal of stones following EUS-guided gastrogastric anastomosis (GGA) in a Roux-en-Y gastric bypass patient. (**a**) Creation of a GGA. Fluoroscopic image shows oblique linear echoendoscope positioned in gastric pouch. There are contrast and guidewire across into the excluded stomach. A 15-mm-diameter lumen-apposing stent can be seen immediately after deployment across the GGA. (**b**) Fluoroscopic image of ERCP and sweeping of the duct for stone removal. ERCP was done at the same session using a standard gastroscope after dilation of the stent to 15 mm

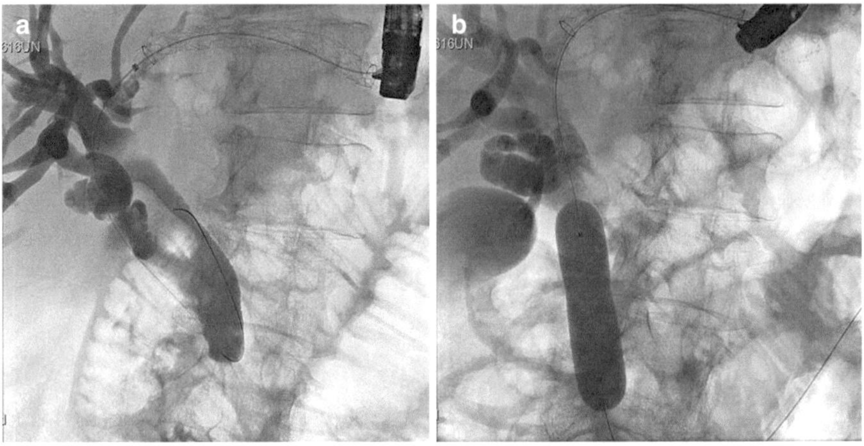

Fig. 13.5 Removal of stones following EUS-guided hepaticogastrostomy (HG) in a Roux-en-Y gastric bypass patient. (**a**) A standard duodenoscope is positioned in the stomach, and the bile duct has been accessed antegrade through the HG self-expanding stent. A large stone is seen. (**b**) Large-diameter balloon dilation of the distal bile duct and biliary sphincter is performed to facilitate stone passage. The bile duct was eventually cleared and the HG stent removed

forward-viewing optics. The GG stent is removed when access to the excluded stomach is no longer necessary and should be delayed for at least 4 weeks after LAMS placement to allow an established fistula. A 20 mm LAMS has just recently become approved by the US Food and Drug Administration (FDA) (but not yet commercially available) and may allow immediate ERCP to be performed.

In patients who need immediate decompression and in the presence of even mild ductal dilation, we prefer to perform EUS-guided hepaticogastrostomy (HG) (Fig. 13.5a, b) [43]. The initial puncture and wire placement are described earlier for rendezvous using a transgastric- transhepatic approach through the left lobe. It is not necessary to pass the wire across the papilla. After guidewire placement into the biliary tree, the tract is balloon dilated to 4–6 mm, and a 6–8 cm, fully covered, self-expanding biliary stent is deployed. This provides both immediate decompression and immediate access to the biliary tree, if desired. Stone removal is then accomplished by antegrade maneuvers through the HG stent. This entails antegrade balloon dilation of the biliary sphincter and distal bile duct and advancement of stone retrieval balloons from proximal to distal to push stones into the duodenum, as is done by interventional radiologists. If needed, cholangioscopy with intraductal lithotripsy can also be performed to facilitate stone clearance. The HG stent is removed after stone clearance is assured and should not be done before 4 weeks so as to allow an established fistula and to avoid bile leak.

The aforementioned techniques are currently offered only in selected tertiary centers. Adverse events associated with the GG approach are perforation, usually due to stent misdeployment or dislodgement (prior to anastomotic maturation). In addition, there remains a concern for persistent GGA after stent removal and bypass "reversal" leading to weight regain. Fortunately, this may be managed endoscopically with endoluminal suturing devices or large over-the-scope clips. Adverse events related to the HG approach are bile peritonitis, which usually only occurs with puncture and dilation of the tract, and loss of access or stent misdeployment.

Endoscopic Ultrasound-Guided Gallbladder Drainage

EUS-guided gallbladder drainage (EUSGBD) was first described in 2007 [44]. It entails transgastric or transduodenal puncture of the gallbladder and transmural placement of stents [45]. Because the gallbladder is not adherent to the gastrointestinal lumen, 10-mm-diameter covered self-expanding stents are used, either short biliary (4 cm long) or LAMS [46], which are 1 cm long. EUSGBD is primarily performed for treatment of clinically severe acute cholecystitis. It is reserved for patients who are nonoperative candidates, since creation of an anastomosis can interfere with or preclude subsequent cholecystectomy. EUSGBD can also allow for internalization of percutaneous gallbladder catheters in patients who are deemed nonoperative candidates and are catheter dependent [47].

EUSGBD can also be utilized in patients with CBDS when ERCP fails and the cystic duct is patent, since it allows for decompression of the biliary tree.

Endoscopic Ultrasound-Guided Drainage of Pancreatic Fluid Collections Following Complicated Gallstone Pancreatitis

Pancreatic fluid collections can occur as a complication of acute gallstone pancreatitis. In such patients, the pancreatitis is usually clinically severe. Collections that arise and that require drainage are most often pancreatic pseudocysts and walled-off pancreatic necrosis (WOPN) (Fig. 13.6a–c). EUS-guided transmural drainage has been shown to be superior to non-EUS-guided drainage of pancreatic pseudocysts [48] and at least equivalent to surgical cystgastrostomy [49]. With the advent of large-diameter (15 mm) LAMS, as described previously, endoscopic drainage of WOPN has been simplified [50, 51].

The large diameter allows egress of fluid and debris while permitting influx of gastric acid to facilitate resolution without the absolute requirement for direct endoscopic necrosectomy (DEN). If DEN is needed, a standard or therapeutic gastroscope is advanced into the necrotic cavity, and grasping devices are used to remove necrotic debris.

Summary

EUS-guided rendezvous for treatment of bile duct stones is becoming commonplace as EUS is being integrated into community settings. This approach is useful for patients with native gastrointestinal anatomy and who have accessible papillae but have failed

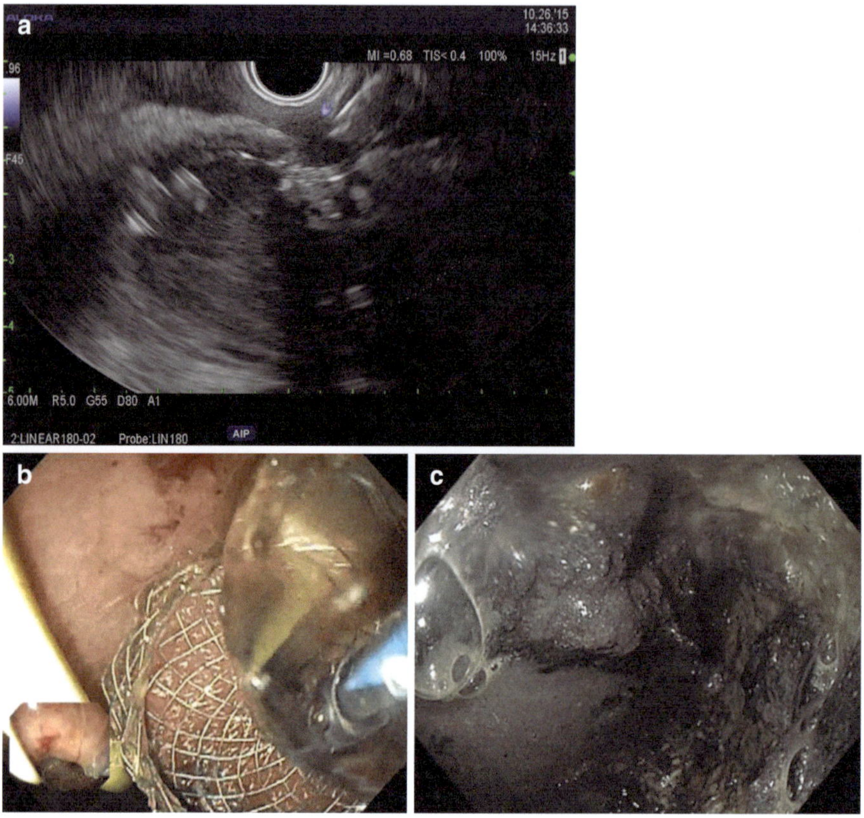

Fig. 13.6 EUS-guided transgastric drainage of walled-off pancreatic necrosis that developed after gallstone pancreatitis. (**a**) EUS showing necrotic pancreatic collection. (**b**) Endoscopic view of balloon dilation performed immediately after deployment of lumen-apposing self-expanding stent to facilitate direct necrosectomy. (**c**) Endoscopic view of necrotic cavity after passage of gastroscope into collection

ERCP cannulation. More advanced therapeutic techniques using transmural access to the excluded stomach and biliary tree are limited to tertiary care centers. Drainage of pancreatic fluid collections is now widely available. All of these therapeutic EUS therapeutic techniques are used to avoid percutaneous and more invasive surgical approaches.

References

1. ASGE Standards of Practice Committee, Maple JT, Ben-Menachem T, Anderson MA, Appalaneni V, Banerjee S, et al. The role of endoscopy in the evaluation of suspected choledocholithiasis. Gastrointest Endosc. 2010;71(1):1–9.
2. Nebiker CA, Baierlein SA, Beck S, von Flue M, Ackermann C, Peterli R. Is routine mr cholangiopancreatography (mrcp) justified prior to cholecystectomy? Langenbeck's Arch Surg. 2009;394(6):1005–10.

3. Desai R, Shokouhi BN. Common bile duct stones–their presentation, diagnosis and management. Indian J Surg. 2009;71(5):229–37.
4. Fanelli RD, Andrew BD. Making the diagnosis: surgery, a rational approach to the patient with suspected CBD stones. In: Hazey JW, Conwell DL, Guy GE, editors. Multidisciplinary management of common bile duct stones: an interdisciplinary textbook. New York: Springer; 2016. p. 37–48.
5. Schmidt S, Chevallier P, Novellas S, Gelsi E, Vanbiervliet G, Tran A, et al. Choledocholithiasis: repetitive thick-slab single-shot projection magnetic resonance cholangiopancreaticography versus endoscopic ultrasonography. Eur Radiol. 2007;17(1):241–50.
6. Aljebreen A, Azzam N, Eloubeidi MA. Prospective study of endoscopic ultrasound performance in suspected choledocholithiasis. J Gastroenterol Hepatol. 2008;23(5):741–5.
7. Petrov MS, Savides TJ. Systematic review of endoscopic ultrasonography versus endoscopic retrograde cholangiopancreatography for suspected choledocholithiasis. Br J Surg. 2009;96(9):967–74.
8. Ang TL, Teo EK, Fock KM. Endosonography- vs. endoscopic retrograde cholangiopancreatography-based strategies in the evaluation of suspected common bile duct stones in patients with normal transabdominal imaging. Aliment Pharmacol Ther. 2007;26(8):1163–70.
9. Lee YT, Chan FKL, Leung WK, Chan HLY, Wu JCY, Yung MY, et al. Comparison of eus and ercp in the investigation with suspected biliary obstruction caused by choledocholithiasis: A randomized study. Gastrointest Endosc. 2008;67(4):660–8.
10. Borie F, Fingerhut A, Millat B. Acute biliary pancreatitis, endoscopy, and laparoscopy. Surg Endosc. 2003;17(8):1175–80.
11. Videhult P, Sandblom G, Rudberg C, Rasmussen IC. Are liver function tests, pancreatitis and cholecystitis predictors of common bile duct stones? Results of a prospective, population-based, cohort study of 1171 patients undergoing cholecystectomy. HPB (Oxford). 2011;13(8):519–27.
12. Sheen AJ, Asthana S, Al-Mukhtar A, Attia M, Toogood GJ. Preoperative determinants of common bile duct stones during laparoscopic cholecystectomy. Int J Clin Pract. 2008;62(11):1715–9.
13. Suarez AL, LaBarre NT, Cotton PB, Payne KM, Cote GA, Elmunzer BJ. An assessment of existing risk stratification guidelines for evaluation of patients with suspected choledocholithiasis. Surg Endosc. 2016;30(10):4613–8.
14. Einstein DM, Lapin SA, Ralls PW, Halls JM. The insensitivity of sonography in the detection of choledocholithiasis. AJR Am J Roentgenol. 1984;142(4):725–8.
15. Almadi MA, Barkun JS, Barkun AN. Management of suspected stones in the common bile duct. CMAJ. 2012;184(8):884–92.
16. Sakai Y, Tsuyuguchi T, Yukisawa S, Tsuchiya S, Sugiyama H, Miyakawa K, et al. Diagnostic value of magnetic resonance cholangiopancreatography for clinically suspicious spontaneous passage of bile duct stones. J Gastroenterol Hepatol. 2008;23(5):736–40.
17. Peng WK, Sheikh Z, Paterson-Brown S, Nixon SJ. Role of liver function tests in predicting common bile duct stones in acute calculous cholecystitis. Br J Surg. 2005;92(10):1241–7.
18. Yang MH, Chen TH, Wang SE, Tsai YF, Su CH, Wu CW, et al. Biochemical predictors for absence of common bile duct stones in patients undergoing laparoscopic cholecystectomy. Surg Endosc. 2008;22(7):1620–4.
19. Rickes S, Treiber G, Monkemuller K, Peitz U, Csepregi A, Kahl S, et al. Impact of the operator's experience on value of high-resolution transabdominal ultrasound in the diagnosis of choledocholithiasis: a prospective comparison using endoscopic retrograde cholangiography as the gold standard. Scand J Gastroenterol. 2006;41(7):838–43.
20. Grönroos JM, Haapamäki MM, Gullichsen R. Effect of the diameter of the common bile duct on the incidence of bile duct stones in patients with recurrent attacks of right epigastric pain after cholecystectomy. Eur J Surg. 2001;167(10):767–9.
21. Al-Jiffry BO, Elfateh A, Chundrigar T, Othman B, Almalki O, Rayza F, et al. Non-invasive assessment of choledocholithiasis in patients with gallstones and abnormal liver function. World J Gastroenterol: WJG. 2013;19(35):5877–82.

22. Tseng CW, Chen CC, Chen TS, Chang FY, Lin HC, Lee SD. Can computed tomography with coronal reconstruction improve the diagnosis of choledocholithiasis? J Gastroenterol Hepatol. 2008;23(10):1586–9.
23. Lee JK, Kim TK, Byun JH, Kim AY, Ha HK, Kim PN, et al. Diagnosis of intrahepatic and common duct stones: combined unenhanced and contrast-enhanced helical CT in 1090 patients. Abdom Imaging. 2006;31(4):425–32.
24. Soto JA, Alvarez O, Múnera F, Velez SM, Valencia J, Ramírez N. Diagnosing bile duct stones. Am J Roentgenol. 2000;175(4):1127–34.
25. Topal B, Van de Moortel M, Fieuws S, Vanbeckevoort D, Van Steenbergen W, Aerts R, et al. The value of magnetic resonance cholangiopancreatography in predicting common bile duct stones in patients with gallstone disease. Br J Surg. 2003;90(1):42–7.
26. Boraschi P, Gigoni R, Braccini G, Lamacchia M, Rossi M, Falaschi F. Detection of common bile duct stones before laparoscopic cholecystectomy. Evaluation with ME cholangiography. Acta Radiol. 2002;43(6):593–8.
27. Raval B, Kramer LA. Advances in the imaging of common duct stones using magnetic resonance cholangiography, endoscopic ultrasonography, and laparoscopic ultrasonography. Semin Laparosc Surg. 2000;7(4):232–6.
28. Stiris MG, Tennøe B, Aadland E, Lunde OC. MR cholangiopancreaticography and endoscopic retrograde cholangiopancreaticography in patients with suspected common bile duct stones. Acta Radiol. 2000;41(3):269–72.
29. Kejriwal R, Liang J, Andrewson G, Hill A. Magnetic resonance imaging of the common bile duct to exclude choledocholithiasis. ANZ J Surg. 2004;74(8):619–21.
30. Mendler MH, Bouillet P, Sautereau D, Chaumerliac P, Cessot F, Le Sidaner A, et al. Value of mr cholangiography in the diagnosis of obstructive diseases of the biliary tree: a study of 58 cases. Am J Gastroenterol. 1998;93(12):2482–90.
31. Sharma SK, Larson KA, Adler Z, Goldfarb MA. Role of endoscopic retrograde cholangiopancreatography in the management of suspected choledocholithiasis. Surg Endosc. 2003;17(6):868–71.
32. Kubota Y, Takaoka M, Yamamoto S, Shibatani N, Shimatani M, Takamido S, et al. Diagnosis of common bile duct calculi with intraductal ultrasonography during endoscopic biliary cannulation. J Gastroenterol Hepatol. 2002;17(6):708–12.
33. Urbach DR, Khajanchee YS, Jobe BA, Standage BA, Hansen PD, Swanstrom LL. Cost-effective management of common bile duct stones: a decision analysis of the use of endoscopic retrograde cholangiopancreatography (ERCP), intraoperative cholangiography, and laparoscopic bile duct exploration. Surg Endosc. 2001;15(1):4–13.
34. Mukai S, Itoi T, Tsuchiya T, Tanaka R, Tonozuka R. Eus-guided intrahepatic bile duct stone extraction via choledochoduodenostomy created by a lumen-apposing metal stent. Gastrointest Endosc. 2016;83(4):832–3.
35. Overby DW, Richardson W, Fanelli R. Choledocholithiasis after gastric bypass: a growing problem. Surg Obes Relat Dis. 2014;10(4):652–3.
36. Menon S. Eus in biliary stone disease. Gastrointest Endosc. 2008;68(4):810.
37. Alper E, Arabul M, Aslan F, Cekic C, Celik M, Ipek S, et al. Radial eus examination can be helpful in predicting the severity of acute biliary pancreatitis. Medicine (Baltimore). 2016;95(3):e2321.
38. Sharma M, Shoukat A, Kirnake V, Bennett A. Idiopathic acute pancreatitis: role of EUS with reference to biliary and pancreatic ascariasis. Am J Gastroenterol. 2015;110(9):1367–9.
39. Zhan X, Guo X, Chen Y, Dong Y, Yu Q, Wang K, et al. Eus in exploring the etiology of mild acute biliary pancreatitis with a negative finding of biliary origin by conventional radiological methods. J Gastroenterol Hepatol. 2011;26(10):1500–3.
40. Tsuchiya T, Itoi T, Sofuni A, Tonozuka R, Mukai S. Endoscopic ultrasonography-guided rendezvous technique. Dig Endosc. 2016;28(Suppl 1):96–101.
41. Tyberg A, Desai AP, Kumta NA, Brown E, Gaidhane M, Sharaiha RZ, Kahaleh M. EUS-guided biliary drainage after failed ERCP: a novel algorithm individualized based on patient anatomy. Gastrointest Endosc. 2016;84(6):941–6.

42. Tyberg A, Nieto J, Salgado S, Weaver K, Kedia P, Sharaiha RZ, Gaidhane M, Kahaleh M. Endoscopic ultrasound (EUS)-directed transgastric endoscopic retrograde cholangiopancreatography or EUS: mid-term analysis of an emerging procedure. Clin Endosc. 2017;50(2):185–90.
43. Siripun A, Sripongpun P, Ovartlarnporn B. Endoscopic ultrasound-guided biliary intervention in patients with surgically altered anatomy. World J Gastrointest Endosc. 2015;7(3):283–9.
44. Baron TH, Topazian MD. Endoscopic transduodenal drainage of the gallbladder: implications for endoluminal treatment of gallbladder disease. Gastrointest Endosc. 2007;65(4):735–7.
45. Baron TH, Grimm IS, Swanstrom LL. Interventional approaches to gallbladder disease. N Engl J Med. 2015;373(4):357–65.
46. Irani S, Baron TH, Grimm IS, Khashab MA. EUS-guided gallbladder drainage with a lumen-apposing metal stent (with video). Gastrointest Endosc. 2015;82(6):1110–5.
47. Law R, Grimm IS, Stavas JM, Baron TH. Conversion of percutaneous cholecystostomy to internal transmural gallbladder drainage using an endoscopic ultrasound-guided, lumen-apposing metal stent. Clin Gastroenterol Hepatol. 2016;14(3):476–80.
48. Varadarajulu S, Christein JD, Tamhane A, Drelichman ER, Wilcox CM. Prospective randomized trial comparing EUS and EGD for transmural drainage of pancreatic pseudocysts (with videos). Gastrointest Endosc. 2008;68(6):1102–11.
49. Varadarajulu S, Bang JY, Sutton BS, Trevino JM, Christein JD, Wilcox CM. Equal efficacy of endoscopic and surgical cystogastrostomy for pancreatic pseudocyst drainage in a randomized trial. Gastroenterology. 2013;145(3):583–90.e1.
50. Siddiqui AA, Kowalski TE, Loren DE, Khalid A, Soomro A, Mazhar SM, et al. Fully covered self-expanding metal stents versus lumen-apposing fully covered self-expanding metal stent versus plastic stents for endoscopic drainage of pancreatic walled-off necrosis: clinical outcomes and success. Gastrointest Endosc. 2017;85(4):758–65.
51. Sharaiha RZ, Tyberg A, Khashab MA, Kumta NA, Karia K, Nieto J, et al. Endoscopic therapy with lumen-apposing metal stents is safe and effective for patients with pancreatic walled-off necrosis. Clin Gastroenterol Hepatol. 2016;14(12):1797–803.

Chapter 14
Laparoscopic-Assisted Endoscopic Retrograde Cholangiopancreatography

Thadeus L. Trus and B. Fernando Santos

Introduction

Patients with altered anatomy who require endoscopic retrograde cholangiopancreatography (ERCP) present a challenge to the surgeon and require a specialized approach. In the past, most patients had altered anatomy secondary to duodenal ulcer operations, specifically a Billroth II reconstruction with afferent and efferent limbs. More common in the current era are patients with altered anatomy secondary to bariatric surgery, specifically laparoscopic Roux-en-Y gastric bypass (RYGB), which has become one of the most commonly performed general surgery operations over the last decade. Traditionally, cholecystectomy was performed concurrently on all patients undergoing open bariatric surgery due to the risk of gallstone development with rapid postoperative weight loss and to avoid the difficulty of cholecystectomy in the re-operative upper abdomen [1]. This practice has fallen out of favor particularly with data supporting the use of ursodiol to prevent biliary complications after bariatric surgery and with the ease of laparoscopic cholecystectomy after laparoscopic bariatric surgery due to decreased adhesion formation with laparoscopy [2]. Our experience indicates that approximately 14% of patients eventually develop

Electronic supplementary material The online version of this chapter (doi: 10.1007/978-3-319-74503-9_14) contains supplementary material, which is available to authorized users.

T. L. Trus, MD (✉)
Department of Surgery, Geisel School of Medicine, Dartmouth-Hitchcock Medical Center, Lebanon, NH, USA
e-mail: Thadeus.trus@hitchcock.org

B. F. Santos, MD
Department of Surgery, Geisel School of Medicine, Dartmouth College, Hanover, NH, USA

Veterans Affairs Medical Center, White River Junction, Hartford, VT, USA
e-mail: byron.santos-aleman@va.gov

© Springer International Publishing AG, part of Springer Nature 2018

B. F. Santos, N. Soper (eds.), *Choledocholithiasis*,
https://doi.org/10.1007/978-3-319-74503-9_14

symptomatic biliary colic and require cholecystectomy after bariatric surgery, with some of these patients also having concurrent choledocholithiasis.

Cholecystectomy in patients with altered anatomy can usually be performed laparoscopically, but access to the duodenum and the major papilla via transoral ERCP may be extremely difficult and frequently impossible. Even if one is able to access the duodenum using a transoral approach, impaired visualization of the papilla and scope instability can reduce the likelihood of deep biliary cannulation and technical success. Given the difficulty and poor success rate of transoral ERCP in RYGB patients, laparoscopic-assisted ERCP has developed as a safe and reliable way to allow ERCP.

Indications

Indications for ERCP (besides choledocholithiasis) in patients with altered anatomy include biliary leak or injury postcholecystectomy, biliary and/or pancreatic lesions such as strictures, and progressive common bile duct dilation after RYGB thought to be secondary to tonic sphincter of Oddi contraction, that is, ampullary achalasia [3]. In a recent review by Banerjee et al., the most common indications for laparoscopically assisted ERCP were sphincter of Oddi dysfunction/suspected papillary stenosis and choledocholithiasis accounting for 51% and 20% of all reported cases, respectively [4].

Preoperative Evaluation

For patients undergoing cholecystectomy who have altered anatomy, it is important that the surgeon preoperatively risk-stratify them for choledocholithiasis. In addition to the usual laboratory studies and right upper quadrant ultrasound, magnetic resonance cholangiopancreatography (MRCP) should be considered, especially if the surgeon does not perform intraoperative imaging and does not have the capability to perform common duct exploration (see Chap. 3 for further discussion of recommended evaluation for these patients). In general, we recommend routine intraoperative cholangiography in all of these patients given that a missed stone will require another trip back to the operating room for clearance. Identifying in advance which patients will definitely need or have a good chance of needing ERCP allows for coordination of ERCP ahead of time, leads to a smoother and more expeditious operation, and reduces the possibility that the patient will require a second operation.

Choice of Approach

In patients with an intact distal stomach, one can perform either a single- or two-stage procedure. In a two-stage procedure, the surgeon places a laparoscopic gastrostomy tube and then uses the mature tract as an access point at a later date for antegrade ERCP [5]. Alternatively, access and ERCP can be performed as a single-stage procedure, which is our preferred method. Patients without an intact distal stomach require access through the afferent limb (in the case of a prior Billroth II reconstruction) or the biliopancreatic limb (in the case of prior gastric bypass) for retrograde ERCP. These procedures through the small bowel are performed in a single stage since it is not possible to place a tube for interval access (as in the case of a gastrostomy tube placed into the gastric remnant). Most published single-stage procedures describe access to the excluded stomach by creating a laparoscopic gastrostomy and then placing a trocar, usually 15 or 18 mm in size, through which a duodenoscope is introduced into the distal stomach and duodenum for ERCP [6–9]. Once access is achieved, transgastric ERCP success rates are greater than 98% [4]. Adverse events are relatively infrequent and can be gastrostomy related (83%) or

Table 14.1 Gastrostomy-related and ERCP-related complications

Categorizable adverse events		
Adverse events $N = 63$	Gastrostomy related $N = 52$	ERCP related $N = 11$
Wound infection	19	0
Perforation	3	3
Bleeding	5	1
Pulmonary embolism	1	0
Persistent gastrocutaneous fistula after PEG tube removal	2	0
Pneumoperitoneum	1	0
False tract creation	1	0
Pneumothorax	1	0
Enterocutaneous fistula	1	0
Abdominal wall hematoma	3	0
Gastrostomy tube dislodgement/leak	4	0
Post-ERCP pancreatitis	0	7
Enterotomy in Roux limb	2	0
Incisional hernia	1	0
Wound dehiscence	1	0
Bile staining from LOA between gastric remnant/liver	1	0
Intra-abdominal leak	2	0
Injury to posterior gastric wall	3	0
Gastric outlet obstruction	1	0

Reprinted with permission from Banerjee N, Parepally M, Byrne TK, Pullatt RC, Coté GA, Elmunzer BJ. Systemic review of transgastric ERCP in Roux-en-Y gastric bypass patients. Surg Obes Relat Dis. 2017;13(7):1236–42

ERCP endoscopic retrograde cholangiopancreatography, *LOA* lysis of adhesions, *PEG* percutaneous endoscopic gastrostomy tube

ERCP related (17%). Wound infection is by far the most common complication (Table 14.1) [4].

Operative Considerations

Equipment

The operating table should be compatible with any radiographic equipment used for cholangiography, usually a portable C-arm.

Two monitors should be positioned on either side of the bed, at the level of the patient's upper body.

ERCP equipment is usually brought on a portable cart along with appropriate guidewires, balloon catheters, and separate cautery unit. A trained endoscopy technician familiar with ERCP should accompany the endoscopist to function as an assistant.

Patient Preparation

Typically the patient is positioned supine on the operating room table, with both arms tucked to allow for positioning the C-arm for cholangiography. The surgeon stands on the patient's right side, and the endoscopist eventually stands on the patient's left. The C-arm is positioned to the right side of the patient and off to the side of the room until ERCP is performed (Fig. 14.1).

An orogastric tube is not usually necessary in patients with gastric bypass since the gastric pouch is extremely small.

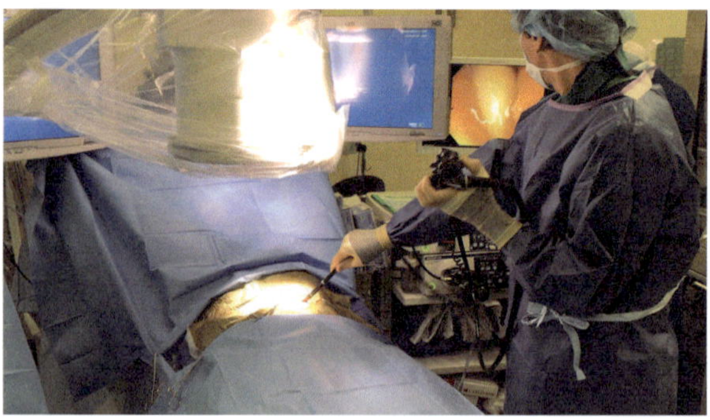

Fig. 14.1 Patient and room setup for laparoscopic-assisted ERCP. The C-arm is positioned on the right side of the patient, and the endoscopist stands at the left side of the patient. Additional drapes are placed during the ERCP procedure to maintain sterility

Surgical Technique

1. Laparoscopy is typically performed with three trocars:

   a. A 5 or 10 mm trocar is placed at the umbilicus. A Veress needle or open technique can be used to enter the abdomen. Alternatively, we prefer an optical trocar placement just to the left of the midline, approximately 18 to 20 cm below the xiphoid process (this allows placement through the rectus muscle, which minimizes the risk of subsequent trocar site hernia). After insufflating the abdomen to 15 mmHg, the 30° or 45° laparoscope is inserted and the abdomen explored.
   b. Under direct vision, two additional 5 mm trocars are placed: one in the right upper quadrant and one in the mid-abdomen to the right of the midline. A liver retractor is rarely necessary.

2. Adhesions, if present in the upper abdomen, should be divided and the Roux limb identified at the level of the gastrojejunostomy. This is then followed down to the jejunojejunostomy to ensure there is no internal hernia either under the Roux limb mesentery or at the jejunojejunostomy site. If an internal hernia is found, it is recommended that one runs the bowel from the terminal ileum proximally as this makes reduction far easier. Any potential internal hernia defects should be closed with suture.
3. Patients with an intact gastric remnant:

   a. The distal stomach remnant is usually easily identified, and the lateral anterior wall is grasped and elevated toward the anterior abdominal wall in the left upper quadrant to ensure it will reach (Fig. 14.2, Video 14.1).
   b. A stay stitch is then placed through the anterior wall of the stomach. A small (15 mm) incision is then made in the left upper quadrant. We prefer to then place a small Alexis™ wound protector (Applied Medical Resources Corp, Rancho Santa Margarita, CA) through this wound and deliver the stay suture and exteriorize a small portion of the anterior stomach.

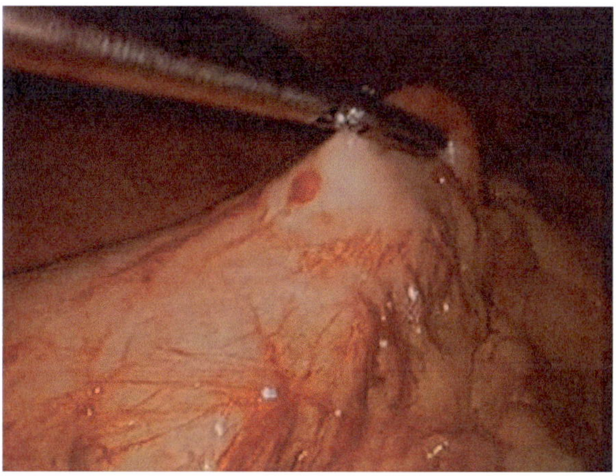

Fig. 14.2 A suitable site on the greater curvature of the gastric remnant that will reach the abdominal wall is identified

c. Most will place a purse-string suture on the anterior stomach wall and/or place a 15 mm trocar or 15 mm balloon tip trocar through a gastrostomy at this site. Alternatively, we prefer creating the gastrostomy and suturing the gastrostomy wall circumferentially to the wound protector ring on the skin surface. Usually four points of fixation are enough. This gastrostomy provides direct access to the stomach and removes the stiffness of the port that makes scope manipulation more difficult.

4. Patients without a gastric remnant:

   a. Access will need to be through the small bowel. The biliopancreatic limb (RYGB anatomy) or proximal afferent limb (Billroth II anatomy) will provide the most direct route for retrograde ERCP and will be less likely to develop a symptomatic stricture after closure (compared to the Roux limb or common channel). A point approximately 30 cm from the ligament of Treitz that will easily reach the left upper quadrant is chosen (Video 14.2).
   b. A window is made on the mesenteric side of the chosen small bowel site to pass a cotton umbilical tape (or Penrose drain). The proximal side of this loop

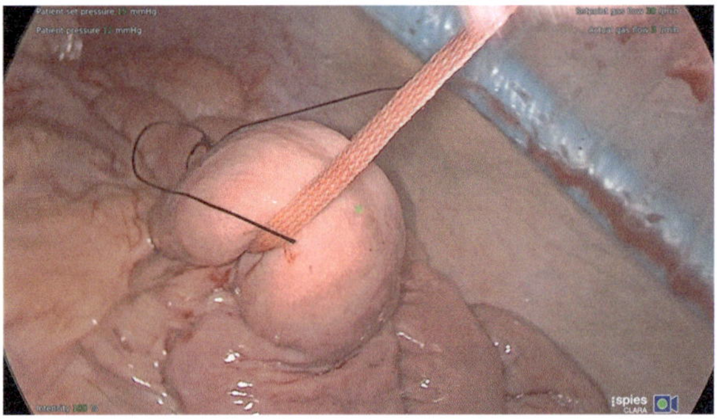

Fig. 14.3 The biliopancreatic limb has been encircled with an umbilical tape and marked with a stay suture to identify the proximal direction. The bowel is then exteriorized through a wound protector

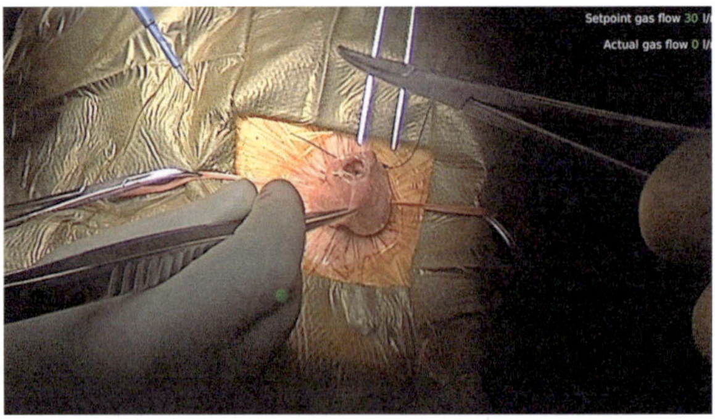

Fig. 14.4 Additional drapes are placed to maintain a sterile barrier during the ERCP. The small bowel is secured externally by securing the umbilical tape with hemostats. An enterotomy is made to allow retrograde ERCP access

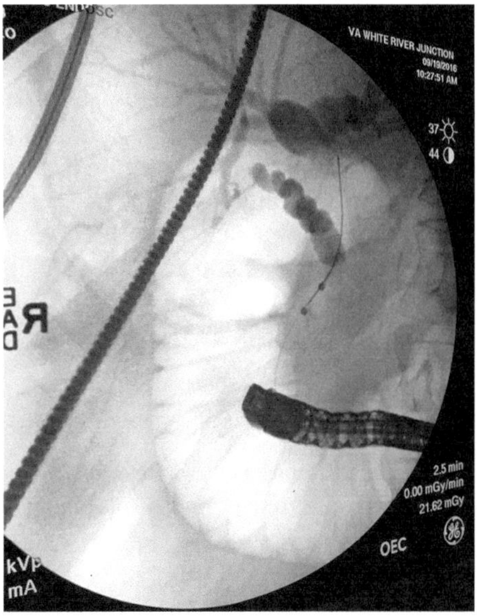

Fig. 14.5 Fluoroscopic view of retrograde ERCP through biliopancreatic limb. Note the position of the duodenoscope in the distal duodenum

of bowel can be marked with a suture or clip to facilitate orientation (Fig. 14.3, Video 14.2).

c. The small bowel loop is exteriorized by grasping the umbilical tape through a small left upper quadrant incision (through a wound protector, as for gastric access). Blue towels are placed around the wound protector, and the site is covered with a sheet of Ioban (this, along with drapes, will provide a barrier to the sterile field during ERCP). A small hole is cut in the Ioban to allow the bowel to be exposed. The umbilical tape is secured on either side to the blue towels to fix the small bowel in place in the proper orientation (proximal limb cephalad). Securing the bowel with the umbilical tape instead of stay sutures allows for less traumatic fixation during scope manipulation. A linear enterotomy is made, large enough to accommodate the ERCP scope (Fig. 14.4, Video 14.2).

5. The C-arm is brought in from the patient's right side to provide fluoro-imaging for ERCP performance (Fig. 14.5). The endoscopist then performs the ERCP.
6. After completion of the ERCP, the scope is withdrawn and the gastrostomy closed in two layers of permanent suture. The stomach is then released into the abdominal cavity and the fascia closed to allow for re-insufflation and reinspection of the abdominal cavity to assure hemostasis. Closure of the small bowel (if small bowel access was required for retrograde ERCP) is performed in a transverse fashion in two layers.

Postoperative Care

Patients are recovered in the postanesthesia care unit (PACU) and usually admitted for observation. If stable in the morning after procedure, they are discharged on a regular diet. We have successfully discharged about 20% of patients on the same day as the operation.

Patients whose ERCP was difficult or those with persistent or increasing pain undergo laboratory studies and/or imaging to rule out pancreatitis or perforation.

Conclusion

In summary, laparoscopic-assisted ERCP is generally safe and effective. It is imperative that general or bariatric surgeons become familiar with this procedure given the frequency of gastric bypass in the current environment.

References

1. Grover BT, Kothari SN. Biliary issues in the bariatric population. Surg Clin North Am. 2014;94:413–25.
2. Sugerman HJ, Brewer WH, Shiffman ML, Brolin RE, Fobi MA, Linner JH, et al. A multicenter, placebo-controlled, randomized, double-blind, prospective trial of prophylactic ursodiol for the prevention of gallstone formation following gastric-bypass-induced rapid weight loss. Am J Surg. 1995;169:91–6.
3. Ponsky JL, Jones N, Rodriguez JH, Kroh MD, Strong AT. Massive biliary dilation after Roux-en-Y gastric bypass: is it ampullary achalasia? J Am Coll Surg. 2017;224(6):1097–103.
4. Banerjee N, Parepally M, Byrne TK, Pullatt RC, Coté GA, Elmunzer BJ. Systemic review of transgastric ERCP in Roux-en-Y gastric bypass patients. Surg Obes Relat Dis. 2017;13(7):1236–42.
5. Choi EK, Chiorean MV, Coté GA, El Hajj II, Ballard D, Fogel EL, et al. ERCP via gastrostomy vs. double balloon enteroscopy in patients with prior bariatric Roux-en-Y gastric bypass surgery. Surg Endosc. 2013;27(8):2894–9.
6. Chavalitdhamrong D, Wagh M, Lara L, Ben-David K, Draganov P. Prospective evaluation of the clinical utility of laparoscopy-assisted ERCP in patients with Roux-en-Y gastric bypass. Am J Gastroenterol. 2014;109:S590–1.
7. Snauwaert C, Laukens P, Dillemans B, Himpens J, De Looze D, Deprez PH, et al. Laparoscopy-assisted transgastric endoscopic retrograde cholangiopancreatography in bariatric Roux-en-Y gastric bypass patients. Endosc Int Open. 2015;3(5):E458–63.
8. Neto MG, Falcao M, Campos JM, Bandeira Ferrax AA. Laparoscopy-assisted transgastric ERCP and papillotomy in gastric bypass bariatric patients. Initial series of 16 cases. Obes Surg. 2010;20(8):1000.
9. Lin C, Aragon RJ, Carr AD, Ali MR. Direct access ERCP: a novel and reliable surgical technique for patients with Roux-en-Y anatomy. Surg Endosc. 2014;28:422.

Chapter 15
Percutaneous Treatment of Biliary Stone Disease

Frank J. Brennan

Introduction

A variety of percutaneous approaches to the biliary system for a variety of interventions including treatment of biliary stones are possible. The options for percutaneous access to the biliary system include direct puncture of the gallbladder or transhepatic puncture of the intrahepatic biliary ducts. In patients with prior biliary surgery, access can be through an indwelling catheter or T-tube placed at time of operation. In cases of more complex biliary surgery, such as hepaticojejunostomy, access can be obtained by puncture of the surgically created limb or loop of bowel. The percutaneous route can be successful in cases where surgical approaches are felt to be high risk due to medical comorbidities or when conventional routes such as transoral endoscopic retrograde cholangiopancreatography (ERCP) are not feasible for anatomic reasons.

The tools and techniques currently available for the percutaneous treatment of biliary stones have developed over time through the work of many individuals, building on the work of prior investigators. This chapter gives a short history of the techniques developed for percutaneous treatment of biliary conditions. Although not an exhaustive recitation of works in the field, these selected works serve to indicate the directions that the field of percutaneous treatment of biliary stone disease has taken over the past several decades.

Electronic supplementary material The online version of this chapter (doi: 10.1007/978-3-319-74503-9_15) contains supplementary material, which is available to authorized users.

F. J. Brennan, MD (✉)
Department of Radiology, Veteran Affairs Medical Center, White River Junction, VT, USA

Department of Radiology, Geisel School of Medicine, Dartmouth College, Hanover, NH, USA
e-mail: frank.brennan@va.gov; frank.j.brennan@dartmouth.edu

© Springer International Publishing AG, part of Springer Nature 2018

B. F. Santos, N. Soper (eds.), *Choledocholithiasis*,
https://doi.org/10.1007/978-3-319-74503-9_15

Percutaneous Cholecystostomy

Elyaderani and Gabriele [1] first reported a case of gallbladder puncture and drainage in a 72-year-old woman with obstructive jaundice in 1979. Bacteremia and fevers made surgery unfeasible. The gallbladder was localized by ultrasound (US) and puncture performed with a 20 ga (gauge) sheathed needle, and a 6.3 Fr (French) straight catheter with end and side holes was used for drainage. The gallbladder was aspirated, demonstrating pus that grew *Escherichia coli* and *Klebsiella* in culture. The patient improved clinically and eventually had a choledochojejunostomy for a malignant distal common bile duct obstruction.

Shaver et al. [2] reported the technique and clinical follow-up in a series of 13 patients treated with percutaneous cholecystostomy, 5 for acute cholecystitis and 8 for common duct obstruction. The acute cholecystostomy patients were deemed poor surgical candidates, and the biliary obstruction patients had failed transhepatic drainage. Their technique was to puncture using a needle system with a preloaded 5 Fr Teflon sheath to enter the gallbladder in either the anterior abdominal wall or the right midaxillary line. Either 6 Fr or 8.3 Fr drainage catheters were then placed over a guidewire with successful catheter placement achieved in all 13 patients.

Percutaneous cholecystostomy has now become widely used for patients with acute cholecystitis who are deemed too high risk for emergency cholecystectomy, most often as a bridge to interval cholecystectomy once the acute illness has resolved. Although many patients eventually go on to have cholecystectomy, up to 50% of patients experience mortality from their underlying comorbidities in the first 2 years after drain placement—for these patients percutaneous cholecystostomy may serve as the only intervention for their biliary symptoms. Percutaneous cholecystostomy also has utility in certain cases where there may be uncertainty between the diagnoses of acute cholecystitis versus acute cholangitis, as it can temporize acute cholecystitis and in the case of cholangitis may decompress the biliary tree as long as the cystic duct is patent.

Percutaneous Treatment of Biliary Stone Disease: Access via T-Tubes

Lamis et al. [3] in 1969 presented a series of three patients with retained common duct stones after cholecystectomy. They described a process of exchanging the T-tube for a coude tip rubber catheter and using saline irrigation and tube manipulation to clear the intrahepatic ducts and common duct of stones. The technique was successful in two of three patients.

Fennessy and You [4] in 1970 addressed retained stones demonstrated on a postoperative T-tube cholangiogram by exchanging the T-tube for a 14 Fr soft rubber urinary catheter, which was then used to push the stones through the sphincter of Oddi and into the duodenum.

Burhenne [5] in 1973 described a novel technique to extract retained stones using a Dormia basket designed for retrieval of ureteral stones. Via a T-tube tract, they inserted a 14 Fr curved tip polyethylene catheter with side port for the injection of contrast. The curved tip allowed them to steer the catheter such that they could reach stones in the hepatic or common ducts. To engage stones that were too large to fit in the Dormia basket, they fashioned custom guidewire loop snares.

Even though now in the current "laparoscopic" surgical era T-tubes have become rare, the techniques and instruments that allow intervention through percutaneous tube tracts have continued to evolve. There are now myriad access sheaths, dilation systems, stents, balloons, baskets, and guidewires to allow access to biliary tree and facilitate interventions through percutaneous tube tracts. Strictly percutaneous techniques such as papillary balloon dilation followed by flushing of stone out of the common duct are effective options (discussed in Chap. 9) in situations in which access to the biliary tree via ERCP is otherwise difficult (as in patients with altered anatomy). In parallel with the evolution of percutaneous techniques, there have been tremendous advances in flexible endoscope technology, taking advantage of the miniaturization and wide availability of cheaper, higher definition camera technology in the digital age. For biliary interventions, ultrathin (2.8 mm diameter), ultra-flexible (270-degree bi-directional flexion) choledochoscopes with "chip-on-the-tip" video technology have recently become available (Karl Storz, Tuttlingen, Germany) and will replace previous generations of flexible scopes that relied on fragile fiber-optic bundles (resulting in a "honey-combed" image) and had limited flexion capabilities. These new video scopes can be used through percutaneous access to retrieve stones, pass wires, biopsy suspicious ductal lesions, and perform lithotripsy using technologies such as a holmium laser.

Transhepatic Access

Perez [6], in 1979, reported a case of fever and hyperbilirubinemia in a patient after cholecystectomy. Transhepatic cholangiography demonstrated a radiolucent stone in the distal common bile duct. Due to the patient's poor clinical condition from cholangitis, the risk of reoperation was judged to be high. Transhepatic access into the biliary system was obtained with a 5 Fr sheath over a 16 ga needle. The stone was captured in a Dormia basket. After attempts to crush the stone within the basket were unsuccessful, the stone and basket were successfully pushed through the ampulla, and the stone was released in the duodenum.

Mueller et al. [7] in 1980 discussed refinements in the percutaneous transhepatic cholangiography (PTC) technique and reported a large experience of 450 cases. Success rates for opacification of the biliary system were 99% in patients with a dilated system and 74% in patients with non-dilated ducts. Most procedures were done purely with fluoroscopic guidance, but they described the supplemental use of ultrasound (US) and computed tomography (CT), especially in biliary obstruction cases requiring selective puncture of the right or left lobe from stones, inflammation, or tumor. They also advocated the use of positional maneuvers during the filling of the biliary system to avoid the misinterpretation of layering in the posterior ducts as an obstruction at the level of the hilum. This "periportal pseudo obstruction" can be resolved by tilting the patient to reverse Trendelenburg and turning the patient toward left lateral decubitus or both to allow the heavier contrast to spill into the common bile duct. This is a good example of a potential interpretative pitfall in determining both level and underlying cause of obstruction. The use of positional maneuvers can "spill" contrast from one part of the duct system into another to yield more complete opacification and avoid the danger of overpressuring the ductal system that could lead to increased risk of post-procedural sepsis.

Ferrucci et al. [7] described the technique of percutaneous transhepatic biliary internal/external drainage as an effective alternative to surgical treatment of biliary obstruction. Their discussion of new options for the nonoperative care of biliary disorders also included biliary stone extraction.

Currently, PTC is a mature technique that allows the placement of external or internal/external biliary drains when the biliary tree is unable to be accessed using conventional transoral ERCP (Fig. 15.1 and Video 15.1), as well as percutaneous therapy to address biliary stone disease that has otherwise failed or is not accessible via endoscopic therapy.

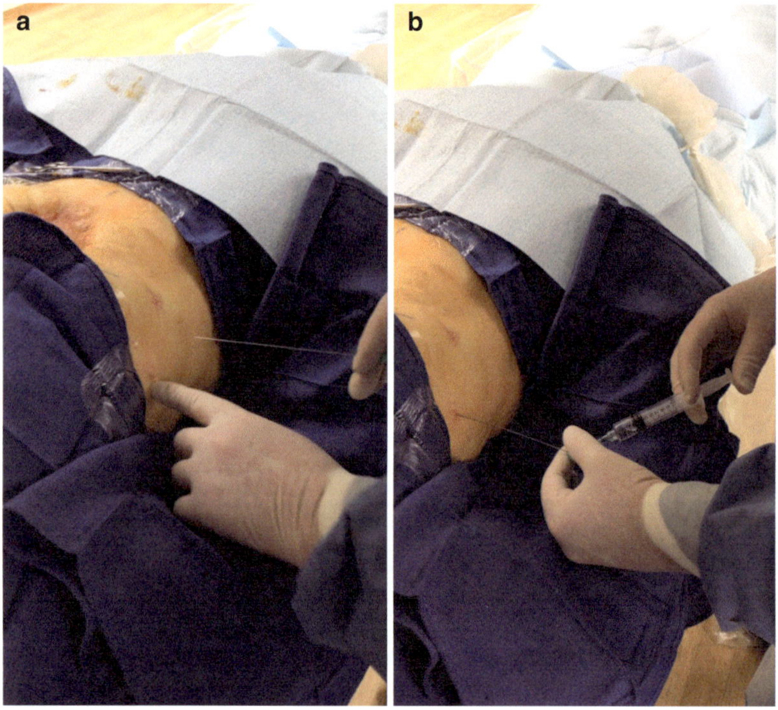

Fig. 15.1 Percutaneous transhepatic cholangiography and internal-external biliary catheter placement. (**a**) A suitable intercostal space is chosen for needle insertion. (**b**) Needle advancement is monitored under fluoroscopy with injection to opacify the intrahepatic structures. (**c**) Contrast injection reveals position in a hepatic vein branch. Note contrast draining in the direction of the inferior vena cava. (**d**) Repositioning of needle and repeat injection opacifies the biliary tree. (**e**) Wire is advanced into distal common bile duct. (**f**) Catheter access to the duodenum is obtained, with wire exchange for a stiff guidewire over which the internal-external biliary drain is advanced, with distal pigtail end in the duodenum

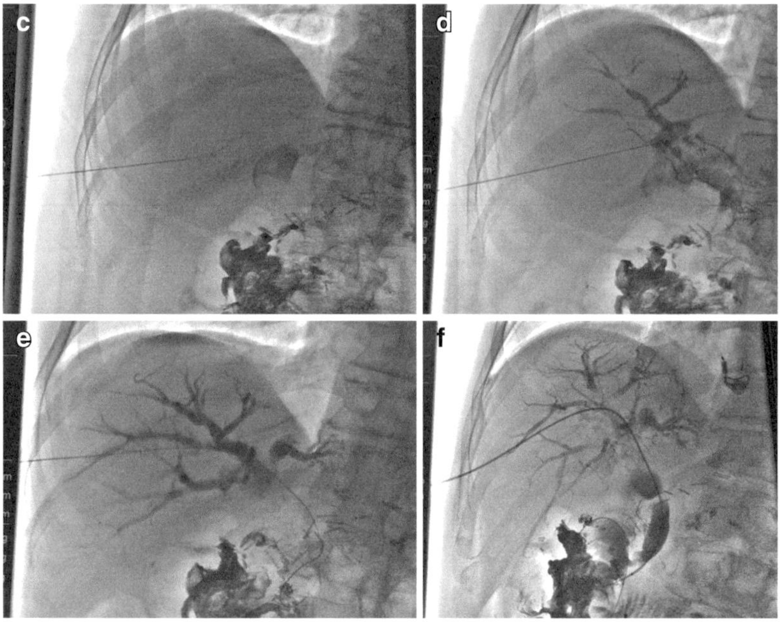

Fig. 15.1 (continued)

PTC is also sometimes used to perform rendezvous procedures, wherein the radiologist accesses the biliary tree and passes a wire into the common bile duct, past the papilla, and into the duodenum. The wire can then be snared by the ERCP operator and used to achieve deep biliary cannulation over the wire. These rendezvous procedures are most frequently necessary when there is an inability to cannulate the papilla via ERCP due to obstructing periampullary malignancies or distal strictures.

Direct Puncture of Small Bowel to Access Bilioenteric Anastomoses

Russell [8] described percutaneous access through surgically created jejunal access in which the distal end of the Roux limb (known as a "Hutson loop") was marked with metal clips and tacked to the anterior abdominal wall, fashioned to allow linear access to the bile ducts in anticipation of percutaneous intervention in the future. These patients required repeated access for balloon dilation of benign disease including sclerosing cholangitis and post-traumatic strictures.

Using Chiba needles directed through the anterior abdominal wall, Martin [9] punctured jejunal limbs on 13 occasions in 10 different patients. In two of the patients, a surgically created chimney had been brought up to the peritoneum and marked with clips for identification under fluoroscopy. In the remaining patients, passes with the Chiba needle were based on anatomic landmarks aiming for the porta hepatis. Successful needle entry into the jejunal loop was then verified with contrast injection. The indications for these procedures were recurrent cholangitis or hyperbilirubinemia. Two of the patients underwent stone retrieval using baskets.

Perry [10] reported direct puncture of antegrade jejunal loop for access to the postoperative biliary system in patients. Patients had undergone antegrade Roux-en-Y loops with choledochojejunostomy or hepaticojejunostomy but without surgical techniques such as fixation to the abdominal wall to facilitate subsequent percutaneous access.

Transcholecystic Access

Mazzariello [11] in 1978 reported the nonoperative extraction of residual postoperative biliary stones in 1086 patients over a period of 14 years. The majority of patients were treated by dilation of a T-tube tract. However, he also described transcholecystic techniques for the extraction of both gallbladder and choledochal stones. He described accessing the common bile duct via the gallbladder and cystic duct used in 48 patients as giving great satisfaction in patients with high operative risk. He noted that the success rate was not as high as with transcholedochal access and that the procedure required more time and dedication. He intubated the cystic duct with curved catheters and sounds. Once access to the common bile duct was established, he used sequential dilation with open-ended sounds, sizing up to progressively larger gauges every several days.

Long-term results of percutaneous cholecystostomy involving high-risk or debilitated patients with subsequent tract dilation and stone removal as an alternative to surgical cholecystectomy indicate that mean survival is around 33 months; although 40% of patients develop recurrent gallstones on ultrasound, only 12% of patients overall develop recurrent symptoms of stone recurrence [12]. These results support the role of this procedure as an effective and safe palliative procedure in nonoperative patients.

Cholangioscopy and Lithotripsy

Nimura et al. [13] discussed the value of transhepatic cholangioscopy for both malignant and benign disease. They began performing transhepatic cholangioscopy in 1977, treating 82 patients with common bile duct stones and 70 patients with intrahepatic stones. Beginning in 1982, they treated gallbladder stones with percutaneous transhepatic cholecystoscopy. Mechanical lithotripters, Nd-YAG laser, and electrohydraulic shock wave were used to break up large gallstones with cholecystoscope visualization. Since then, there have been numerous series describing hybrid approaches utilizing PTC to access the biliary tree and serving as a channel for flexible, small-diameter endoscopes to perform therapy. These procedures sometimes use a combination of approaches, such as percutaneous papillary balloon dilation to open the sphincter, lithotripsy to break up large stones, and pushing of stones into the duodenum using biliary balloon extractors through the access sheath. Large series have been reported for percutaneous transhepatic cholangioscopy for the treatment of hepatolithiasis, a disease common in Asia but rare in the West, as well as treatment of common duct stones [14, 15]. Clearance of biliary stones in a large series of 916 patients in Japan was performed using papillary balloon dilation followed by pushing or flushing the stones through the dilated papilla [16]. The technique of dilation was described as using an 8–10 mm for non-dilated ducts, and larger (according to the size of the largest stone) for dilated bile ducts, but never larger than the size of the bile duct. The duration of inflation was 10–20 s, with no episodes of pancreatitis experienced. Success rates greater than 95% have been reported with these techniques, with incidence of complications of around 7–9%. Minor complications included nausea, vomiting, abdominal pain, and hemobilia managed nonoperatively, and major complications included cholangitis, subcapsular biloma or hematoma, bile peritonitis, duodenal perforation, gastroduodenal artery pseudoaneurysm, and right hepatic artery transection. PTC procedures naturally lend themselves to innovation, as illustrated by two reports of sphincterotomy using cholangioscopy, the first as early as 1982 [17, 18]. These reports describe using a "push-type" sphincterotome taped to the outside of a flexible cystoscope that is passed through the papilla and retroflexed. The sphincterotome is then used under retroflexed visualization by the cystoscope to create a sphincterotomy. The efficacy and safety of these procedures remains to be determined. Nevertheless, these reports serve as examples of the multidisciplinary teamwork that is often required for these interesting and challenging cases.

Safety and Complications of Percutaneous Biliary Intervention

A thorough review of possible complications of percutaneous biliary intervention was published in 2017 by Venkatanarasimha et al. [19]. They note an overall complication rate of 3–10%. Potential complications vary from relatively minor, such as pain at the tube insertion site, to major or life-threatening, such as major hemorrhage and sepsis. Access-related complications include pain, pleural space transgression, inadvertent access into the extrahepatic biliary tree with bile leak and peritonitis, and bowel perforation when the colon is interposed between the diaphragm and surface of the liver. Nonvascular complications include bile leakage, acute pancreatitis, biloma, and cholangitis. Vascular complications include pseudoaneurysm, bilioarterial fistula, and bilioportal vein fistula. Many of these conditions can be managed by percutaneous techniques. They also describe preventative measures based on lessons learned by root cause analysis of the complications.

Case Studies

The following cases illustrate variations on the theme of percutaneous cholecystostomy followed by biliary stone extraction. The multidisciplinary nature of these cases is emphasized by cooperative work between the general surgeon, interventional radiologist, gastroenterologist, and even urologist to aid in laser lithotripsy of stones. Each case is followed by a list of technical tips, including the utilization of certain catheters, wires, and access kits that are currently commercially available and that the author has found to be useful.

Case 1

A 61-year-old man presented with abdominal pain and elevated alkaline phosphatase. CT scan demonstrated findings of acute cholecystitis and a 1.2 cm gallstone located in the gallbladder neck. Multiple medical comorbidities including obesity, chronic obstructive pulmonary disease (COPD) requiring 4–6 L oxygen by nasal cannula at home, severe pulmonary hypertension, and atrial fibrillation treated with anticoagulation made the patient a high risk for surgery or anesthesia.

Percutaneous cholecystostomy was performed with CT guidance due to the proximity of the colon to the gallbladder fundus seen on the diagnostic CT. Puncture was performed using a transhepatic route into the gallbladder using a 5 Fr Yueh (Cook, Bloomington, IN) sheathed needle/catheter (Fig. 15.2). After sequential dilation over an 80 cm Amplatz Ultra Stiff wire (Cook, Bloomington, IN), a 12 Fr locking pigtail catheter (Cook, Bloomington, IN) was placed (Fig. 15.3). The catheter was attached to a gravity bag for external drainage.

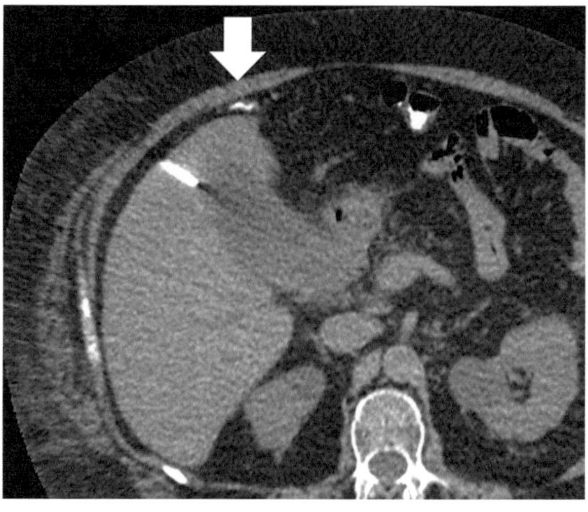

Fig. 15.2 Needle placement during CT-guided percutaneous cholecystostomy. Note: Transhepatic tract and portion of colon anterior to liver (white arrow)

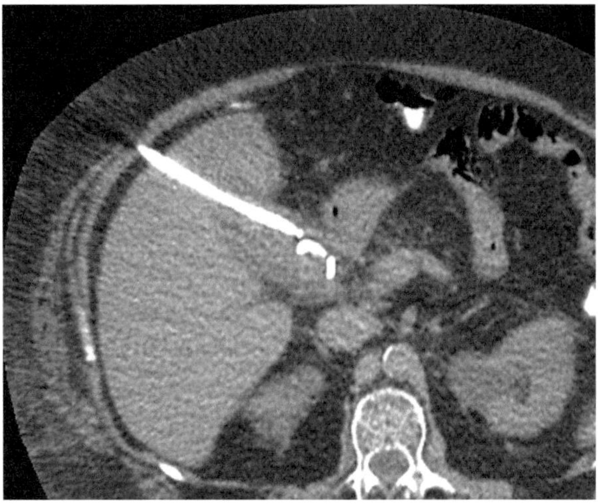

Fig. 15.3 Drainage catheter in gallbladder. Note position of locking loop in region of gallbladder neck, a longer length of catheter within the gallbladder lumen can reduce chance of inadvertent removal

A cholangiogram performed through the tube 5 days after placement demonstrated interval decompression of the gallbladder distension, continued intraluminal filling defects consistent with stones and debris, and a patent common bile duct with free flow of contrast into the duodenum. As there were no filling defects within the common bile duct to suggest choledocholithiasis, the tube was capped for a trial of internal drainage. However, recurrent right upper quadrant pain necessitated reestablishing external drainage the following day.

The patient was followed in outpatient interventional radiology (IR) clinic with the tube draining externally awaiting improvement of his medical condition. Even after he had recovered 4 weeks later, he was deemed not a candidate for cholecystectomy given his severe comorbidities and risk of mortality. Given his recurrent symptoms whenever the tube was capped, and the inconvenience and discomfort of living with a cholecystostomy tube indefinitely, a plan for percutaneous stone extraction was agreed upon. A plan was developed with anesthesia, surgery, and interventional radiology to attempt stone extraction under monitored anesthesia care using a flexible endoscope through the percutaneous cholecystostomy tract.

At the time of the procedure, the patient received prophylactic antibiotics and sedation by the anesthesia service. An initial cholangiogram was performed via the existing pigtail catheter. This demonstrated good position of the pigtail portion of the catheter within a contracted, lobulated appearing gallbladder lumen felt to represent post-inflammatory scarring. The existing catheter was removed over an Amplatz Ultra Stiff guidewire, 0.035″ diameter with 80 cm length. A series of dilators from a gastrostomy insertion kit (Cook, Bloomington, IN) was used to sequentially dilate the tract (Fig. 15.4). This allowed placement of the 20 Fr peel-away sheath from the same kit through the percutaneous tract into the gallbladder lumen. A 2.8 mm flexible choledochoscope could then be inserted through the sheath for direct visualization of the gallbladder stones. Debris from the gallbladder lumen was flushed out by irrigation. At this time, the patient's respiratory status declined

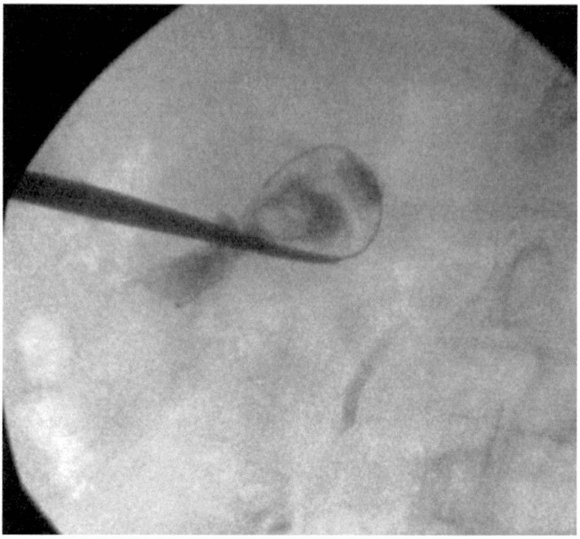

Fig. 15.4 Fluoroscopic-guided tract dilation in preparation for placing sheath for cholecystoscopy. Note loop of guidewire beyond tip of dilator protecting gallbladder wall from inadvertent puncture by dilator tip

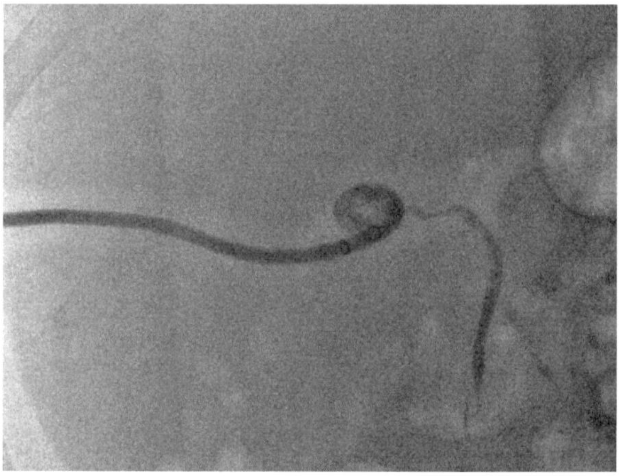

Fig. 15.5 Tube cholangiogram at time of tube removal demonstrating patent cystic and common bile ducts. Note that the gallbladder lumen has contracted down around the catheter loop

to the extent that anesthesia recommended aborting any further attempts at stone extraction. The peel-away sheath was removed over a guidewire and a 14 Fr locking pigtail catheter used to maintain access into the gallbladder. External drainage continued for another month with multiple discussions with the patient about management choices. The patient expressed a strong desire to be rid of the tube and decided to proceed with another capping trial. The tube was capped for 1 week without recurrent symptoms and the tube removed uneventfully after another cholangiogram confirmed patency of the cystic duct and common bile duct (Fig. 15.5).

At the time of writing, the patient has been tube-free and symptom-free for 7 months without the need for further intervention. Subsequent imaging, both US and CT, has described a small, contracted gallbladder with a thickened wall. This case suggests that patients who have undergone prolonged external drainage can have a thickened wall due to scarring, and this finding alone does not necessarily imply acute cholecystitis. Therefore, caution must be exercised in the interpretation of such studies to avoid the mistaken impression of an acute process that could lead to unnecessary re-intervention.

Technical Tips:

- CT for percutaneous access is helpful to avoid possible transgression of the colon when the colon is interposed between the diaphragm and anterolateral liver.
- Shorter guidewires 80 cm long are sufficient for catheter placement and exchanges and avoid the cumbersome length of standard guidewire lengths, 145 cm and 180 cm.
- To dilate a tract using a stiff guidewire, make sure to keep the dilator oriented along the axis of the wire to avoid kinking the wire and possible damage to surrounding structures.
- Dilate in steps, increasing the size of the dilators 2–4 Fr at a time.
- When advancing a dilator over a guidewire, use a rotational twisting instead of a straight push; this helps dissipate the friction and the dilator will track easier through tissue.
- Dilators have different tapers. Generally, the longer the taper the easier the dilation. However, small structures such as the gallbladder may not be large enough to accommodate the entire taper. A shorter, more bullet-shaped taper is useful, especially when placing a peel-away sheath.

Case 2

A 69-year-old male was admitted to the intensive care unit (ICU). His multiple medical problems included diabetes, cirrhosis, coronary artery disease, and recent stroke. Presenting symptoms were hypotension, fever, and mental status changes. An abdominal ultrasound was consistent with acute cholecystitis. Due to high surgical and anesthesia risk, interventional radiology was consulted for percutaneous cholecystectomy (Fig. 15.6).

Anticoagulation because of the recent stroke reversed with fresh frozen plasma. Sedation was administered by the anesthesia service. Using a subcostal, transhepatic approach, a 21 gauge percutaneous thin-walled entry needle (Cook, Bloomington, IN) advanced under direct ultrasound visualization into the gallbladder lumen. An 0.018″ wire coiled in the lumen under fluoroscopic control. The tract was dilated with an Accustick system (Boston Scientific, Natick, MA) to allow passage of a 0.035″ working wire. An 8.5 Fr pigtail multipurpose drainage catheter was placed over the working wire with extra length of catheter looped in the gallbladder lumen (Fig. 15.7).

Cholangiogram after medical stabilization demonstrated free flow of contrast through the common bile duct into the duodenum. However, nonobstructing filling defects in the cystic dust and gallbladder were consistent with numerous small stones.

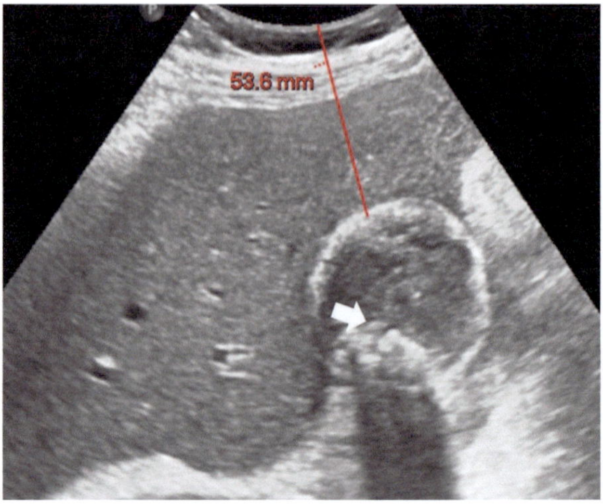

Fig. 15.6 Ultrasound demonstrating planned needle trajectory for percutaneous cholecystostomy using a transhepatic approach. Note gallbladder lumen filled with debris/sludge and dependent stones. The stones are evident by posterior acoustical shadowing (*white arrow*)

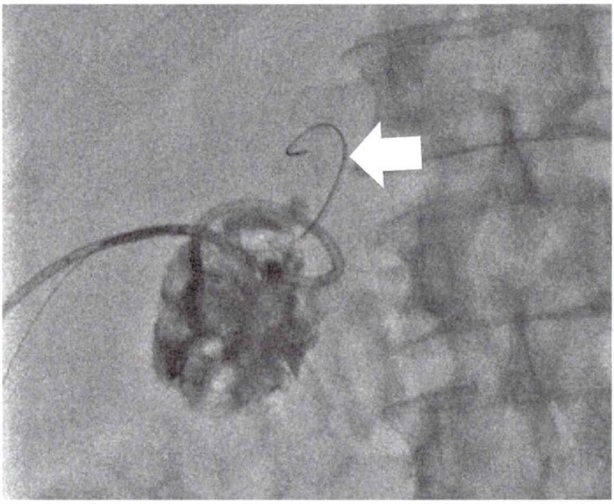

Fig. 15.7 Fluoroscopic verification of catheter location following ultrasound-guided puncture. A redundant loop of catheter has been coiled in the gallbladder lumen to reduce chance of inadvertent removal. Note the microwire from initial puncture (*white arrow*) has been left as a "safety" wire to be removed once drainage catheter position is confirmed

The patient was seen in an outpatient IR clinic every couple of weeks for tube exchanges, with sizing up of the tube to 10.2 Fr and then 12 Fr in anticipation of placing a larger intraoperative access at the time of planned stone extraction (Fig. 15.8). At each tube exchange, copious irrigation with normal saline yielded quantities of grit and gravel, which helped decrease the overall load of material within the gallbladder lumen.

An inadvertent removal of the catheter occurred even with the cautionary redundancy of catheter in the lumen and frequent dressing checks (Fig. 15.9). As the tract was well established, access was reestablished by opacification of the tract by gentle injection of contrast into the tract by means of a Christmas tree adaptor. Use of a directional catheter with an angled tip (Kumpe catheter, Angiodynamics, Latham, NY) and a combination of flexible, hydrophilic guidewires (Advantage wire, Terumo and Roadrunner wire, Cook) allowed a new 12 Fr drainage catheter to be placed.

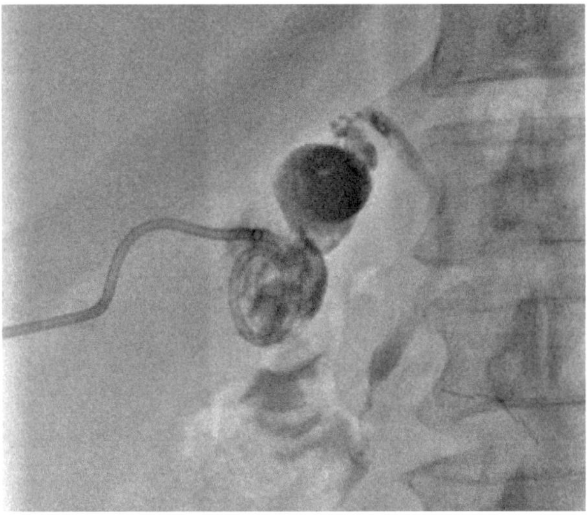

Fig. 15.8 Tube cholangiogram 6 weeks after original placement showing stones in the gallbladder fundus and cystic duct. The cystic duct and common bile ducts are patent. Note: the redundant loop of catheter at time of placement has partially pulled out due to patient activity, but the locking loop remains in the gallbladder fundus

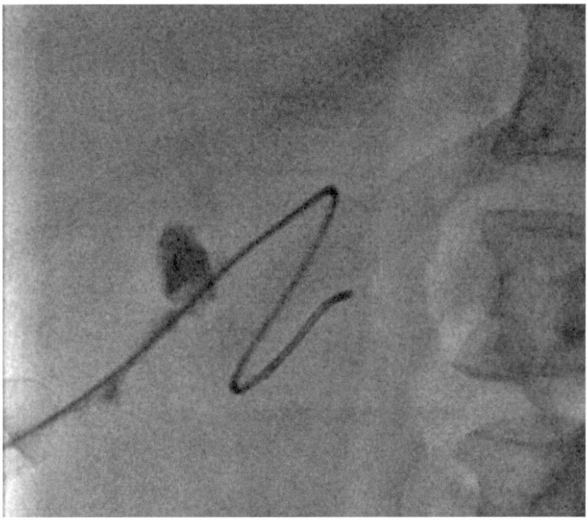

Fig. 15.9 Inadvertent removal of drainage catheter. Tract opacified with contrast injected through "Christmas tree" adaptor. Tract then re-cannulated by use of directional Kumpe catheter and glidewire

Biliary stone extraction was performed in operating room. Percutaneous tract was dilated to 16 French for placement of sheath for endoscope insertion (Fig. 15.9). Multiple stones, 52 by count, were removed by snare under direct endoscopic visualization (Figs. 15.10, 15.11, and 15.12, Video 15.2). Urology service is assisted with laser fragmentation of larger stones.

Cholangiography before and after stone extraction demonstrated free flow through the common bile duct into the duodenum. A 14 Fr pigtail catheter was replaced at the end of the case to maintain access.

ERCP with sphincterotomy and balloon sweeping of duct by gastroenterology was performed 4 days later to assess for any stones that might have migrated into the CBD during instrumentation (Fig. 15.13).

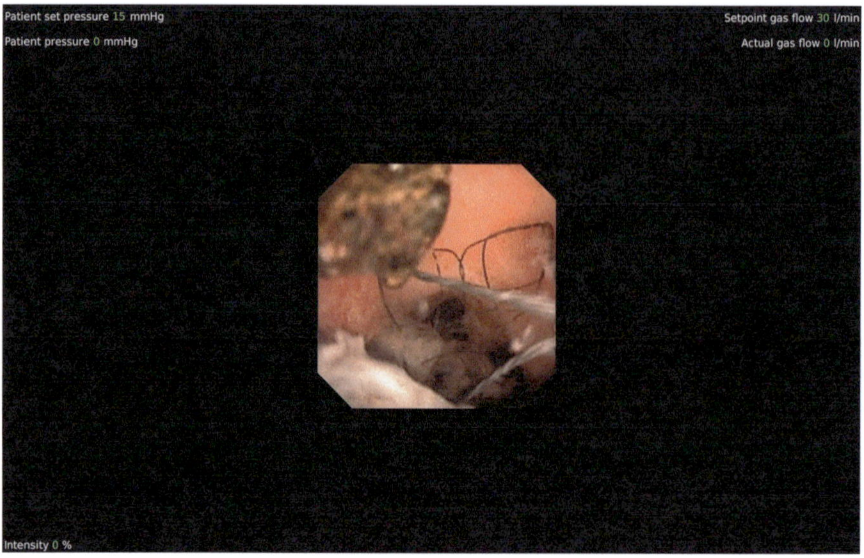

Fig. 15.10 Flexible choledochoscope visualizing the inside of the gallbladder. Stone basket used to entrap stones for removal

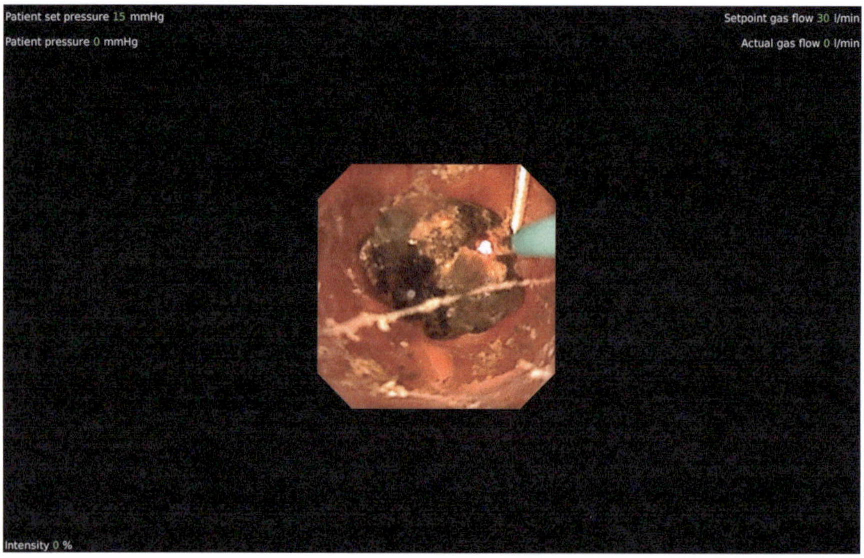

Fig. 15.11 Flexible choledochoscope with use of holmium laser for lithotripsy of residual large gallstones

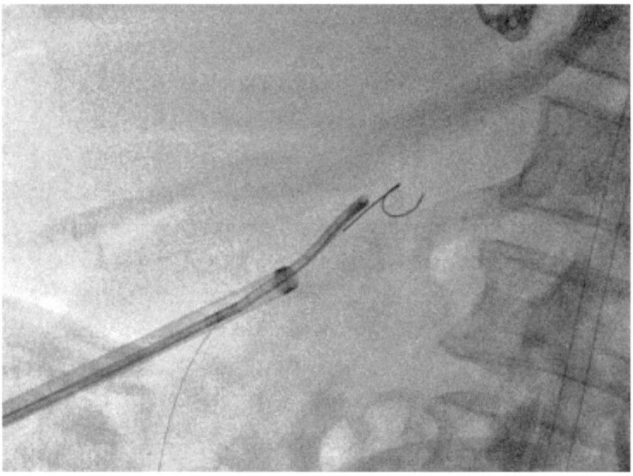

Fig. 15.12 Endoscope via sheath for cholecystoscopy and choledochoscopy. Note safety wire adjacent to sheath and scope; this will maintain access if sheath is backed out of the gallbladder

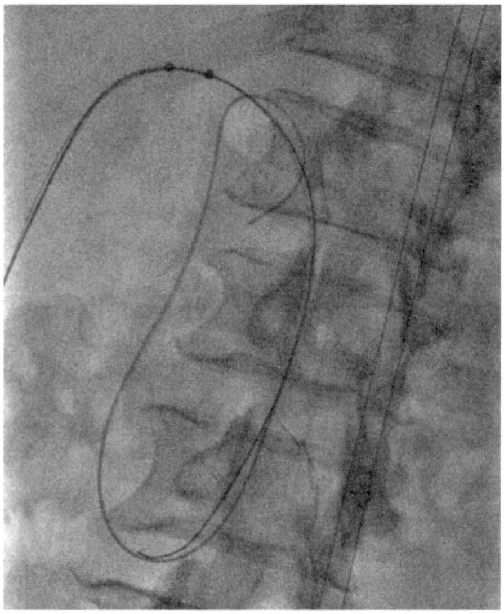

Fig. 15.13 Balloon clearing of cystic duct and common bile duct pushing balloon over stiff guidewire. Note diameter difference between 0.018″ safety wires adjacent to 0.035″ working wire

The patient returned to the operating room for second look and endoscopic removal of several residual stones. Attempted canalization of the cystic duct was unsuccessful. The lack of success was attributable to poor visualization of fine anatomic detail in the patient with large body habitus using mobile C-arm fluoroscopy.

The procedure was rescheduled for the fixed angiographic unit (General Electric) in the interventional radiology suite. This resulted in a successful cannulation of the cystic duct. This allowed visualization of the entire common bile duct and cystic duct by endoscope. The technique used for traversing the tortuous cystic duct included the use of a double curve 0.018″ glidewire (Terumo, Somerset, NJ) and a Quickcross microcatheter (Spectranetics, Colorado Springs, CO). Once the microwire traversed the cystic duct, this was followed by a Greb set (Vascular Solutions, Minneapolis, MN), which was used to maneuver through the ampulla into the duodenum. The hydrophilic glidewire was then exchanged for a pair of Nitinol 0.018″ wires (Nitrex, ev3/Covidien, Plymouth, MN) into the duodenum. Reinsertion of the Greb introducer allowed placement of a 0.035" Coons wire (Cook, Bloomington, IN) into the duodenum over which a biliary balloon was used to sweep the CBD and cystic duct back into the gallbladder. An endoscope could then be used for direct visualization of the biliary system from the ampulla back into the gallbladder. As no further stones could be seen with endoscopy and no further filling defects could be appreciated by fluoroscopy, we had a high degree of certainty that the patient was now rendered stone free. A capped pigtail catheter was left in the gallbladder to maintain access. This was removed 2 days later as the patient was asymptomatic, a cholangiogram showed patency of the biliary system, and a tractogram during removal demonstrated a well-formed tract without intra-abdominal leakage.

At follow-up 12 months after tube removal, the patient remained asymptomatic and an ultrasound demonstrated a contracted gallbladder with expected mild thickening of the gallbladder wall without pericholecystic fluid, recurrent stones, sonographic Murphy's sign, or biliary ductal dilation. The patient is now greater than 12 months out from the procedure without need for further intervention.

Technical Tips:

- Society of Interventional Radiology (SIR) Guidelines classify percutaneous cholecystostomy as a procedure with moderate risk of bleeding and recommend that international normalized ratio (INR) be corrected to ≤1.5 and platelets >50,000.
- The triaxial Accustick (Boston Scientific) system allows placement of a 0.035″ working wire alongside the original microwire. The microwire can be left in situ as a safety wire.
- Microwires will often have a radio-opaque platinum tip to aid in visibility under fluoroscopy.
- Stainless steel microwires are stiffer than Nitinol and less likely to flex sideways during initial dilator advancement. However, if they kink, the bend is permanent and will make subsequent use difficult.
- Nitinol microwires offer superior kink resistance compared with standard stainless steel wires. Additionally, their increased flexibility will allow them to track through tortuous structures more easily than stainless steel wires.
- Redundant coiling of catheter within the gallbladder lumen may lessen the chance of inadvertent removal.
- In case of inadvertent removal, a combination of a directional catheter and hydrophilic guidewire can salvage the access if the tract is sufficiently mature, generally 2–4 weeks.
- Nitinol microwires make good safety wires at time of stone extraction to aid in reentry to the gallbladder if the sheath for the endoscope backs out.

- Flexible microwires in combination with directional catheters and low-profile crossing catheters can traverse valves within the cystic duct in an atraumatic fashion.
- The coaxial Greb set allows placement of a short directional catheter over a microwire, which gives the system good steerability. The lumen is large enough to fit a second microwire alongside the original as safety wire. The Greb set coaxial introducer is then removed and reinserted over a single 0.018″ wire to allow placement of an 0.035″ wire.

References

1. Elyaderani M, Gabriele OF. Percutaneous cholecystostomy and cholangiography in patients with obstructive jaundice. Radiology. 1979;130(3):601–2.
2. Shaver RW, Hawkins IF, Soong J. Percutaneous cholecystostomy. Am J Roentgenol Radium Therapy, Nucl Med. 1982;138(6):1133–6.
3. Lamis PA, Letton AH, Wilson JP. Retained common duct stones: a new nonoperative technique for treatment. Surgery. 1969;66(2):291–6.
4. Fennessy JJ, You K-D. A method for the expulsion of stones retained in the common bile duct. Am J Roentgenol Radium Therapy, Nucl Med. 1970;110(2):256–9.
5. Burhenne HJ. Nonoperative retained biliary tract stone extraction: a new roentgenologic technique. Am J Roentgenol Radium Therapy, Nucl Med. 1973;117(2):388–99.
6. Perez MR, Oleaga JA, Freiman DB, McLean GL, Ring EJ. Removal of a distal common bile duct stone through percutaneous transhepatic catheterization. Arch Surg. 1979;114(1):107–9.
7. Ferrucci JT Jr, Mueller PR, Harbin WP. Percutaneous transhepatic biliary drainage: technique, results, and applications. Radiology. 1980;135(1):1–13.
8. Russell E, Yrizarry JM, Huber JS, Nunez D Jr, Hutson DG, Schiff E, et al. Percutaneous transjejunal biliary dilatation: alternate management for benign strictures. Radiology. 1986;159(1):209–14.
9. Martin EC, Laffey KJ, Bixon R. Percutaneous transjejunal approaches to the biliary system. Radiology. 1989;172(3):1031–4.
10. Perry LJ, Stokes KR, Lewis WD, Jenkins RL, Clouse ME. Biliary intervention by means of percutaneous puncture of the antecolic jejunal loop. Radiology. 1995;195(1):163–7.
11. Mazzariello RM. A fourteen-year experience with nonoperative instrument extraction of retained bile duct stones. World J Surg. 1978;2(4):447–54.
12. Courtois CS, Picus DD, Hicks ME, Darcy MD, Aliperti G, Edmundowicz S, Hovsepian DM. Percutaneous gallstone removal: long-term follow-up. J Vasc Interv Radiol. 1996;7(2):229–34.
13. Nimura Y, Shionoya S, Hayakawa N, Kamiya J, Kondo S, Yasui A. Value of percutaneous transhepatic cholangioscopy (ptcs). Surg Endosc. 1988;2(4):213–9.
14. Cannavale A, Bezzi M, Cereatti F, Lucatelli P, Fanello G, Salvatori FM, et al. Combined radiological-endoscopic management of difficult bile duct stones: 18-year single center experience. Therap Adv Gastroenterol. 2015;8(6):340–51.
15. Ozcan N, Kahriman G, Mavili E. Percutaneous transhepatic removal of bile duct stones: results of 261 patients. Cardiovasc Intervent Radiol. 2012;35(3):621–7.
16. Shin JS, Shim HJ, Kwak BK, Yoon HK. Biliary stone removal through the percutaneous transhepatic biliary drainage route, focusing on the balloon sphincteroplasty flushing technique: a single center study with 916 patients. Jpn J Radiol. 2017;35(8):440–7.
17. Nimura Y, Hayakawa N, Suzuki T, Iyomasa Y. Counterplan to remunant stone-technique and application of endoscopic sphincterotomy. Jpn J Gastroenterol Surg. 1982;15:570–5.

18. Itoi T, Shinohara Y, Takeda K, Nakamura K, Sofuni A, Itokawa F, et al. A novel technique for endoscopic sphincterotomy when using a percutaneous transhepatic cholangioscope in patients with an endoscopically inaccessible papilla. Gastrointest Endosc. 2004;59(6):708–11.
19. Venkatanarasimha N, Damodharan K, Gogna A, Leong S, Too CW, Patel A, et al. Diagnosis and management of complications from percutaneous biliary tract interventions. Radiographics. 2017;37(2):665–80.

Part IV
Institutional Adoption of Laparoscopic Common Bile Duct Exploration Techniques and Training

Chapter 16
Training in Laparoscopic Common Bile Duct Exploration: Role of Simulation and Its Impact on Clinical Outcomes

Ben Schwab, Ryan Albert Campagna, and Eric S. Hungness

Introduction

Surgical education in the United States has long been influenced by the ideology of William Halsted, MD, FACS, and William Osler, MD, in which the role of graduated responsibility under the close supervision of an experienced surgeon was paramount [1, 2]. This "apprenticeship model" would go on to form the foundation of surgical training for years to come. Surgeons who trained during this era were often exposed to a broad range of surgical disease and pathology since there were no viable alternatives at the time. This allowed them to become experts in the management of a large number of conditions. A number of factors in the current era of surgery and graduate medical education (GME) have contributed to limit the utility of apprenticeship education. Numerous technological and educational advancements have resulted in the development and proliferation of alternative treatments that have lessened the dependence on surgical intervention to treat human disease. In addition, restrictions placed on resident training in addition to the expansion of specialized postgraduate fellowships have served to limit exposure to a wide range of procedures for general surgical trainees in the modern era when compared to their predecessors [3].

Electronic supplementary material The online version of this chapter (doi: 10.1007/978-3-319-74503-9_16) contains supplementary material, which is available to authorized users.

B. Schwab, MD · E. S. Hungness, MD (✉)
Department of Surgery, Northwestern Memorial Hospital, Chicago, IL, USA
e-mail: ben.schwab@northwestern.edu; Eric.Hungness@nm.org

R. A. Campagna, MD
Department of Surgery, Northwestern University Feinberg School of Medicine, Chicago, IL, USA
e-mail: ryan.campagna@northwestern.edu

© Springer International Publishing AG, part of Springer Nature 2018

B. F. Santos, N. Soper (eds.), *Choledocholithiasis*,
https://doi.org/10.1007/978-3-319-74503-9_16

Numerous examples of this evolution can be found in the field of hepatopancreatobiliary (HPB) surgery, which has traditionally fallen under the scope of general surgery. Various developments have served to fundamentally alter the approach to managing hepatobiliary pathology in a way that has had profound implications for the training of general surgeons. Management of biliary disease in particular is one area that has seen a major evolution in the surgical approach to managing these conditions. For example, the introduction of the laparoscopic cholecystectomy caused an almost overnight revolution in the management of gallbladder disease, resulting in a precipitous drop in the number of open cholecystectomies being performed by general surgeons [4]. While this development had obvious benefits for patients in the form of reduced postoperative pain and a shorter length of stay, the near universal incorporation of the technique had a number of implications for the practice of general surgery, and for the training of general surgery residents in particular. While the widespread use of laparoscopic cholecystectomy encouraged surgeons to become comfortable with general laparoscopic techniques, it also served to significantly limit their exposure to the principles of open hepatobiliary surgery.

The approach to the management of common bile duct stones provides another example of how surgical practice and education has been profoundly influenced by the introduction and widespread adoption of an alternative treatment. The first use of endoscopic retrograde cholangiopancreatography (ERCP) for the management of biliary disease occurred in the 1970s [5]. While ERCP allows patients to avoid surgery in many cases, the procedure is not without risk. Post-procedural pancreatitis and hemorrhage are two feared complications of ERCP that can result in significant morbidity and mortality. Despite these considerations, ERCP rapidly replaced common duct exploration (CDE) as a primary treatment for choledocholithiasis. A 2005 study analyzing the effect of decreased utilization of surgical CDE on complication rates estimated that approximately 47,000 CDEs were performed per year in the late 1970s prior to the widespread introduction of ERCP. This number would fall to less than 10,000 cases per year by 2001 and has continued to decrease [6, 7]. While it is tempting to accept that surgical exploration of the common bile duct (CBD) has been rendered obsolete by ERCP, it should be remembered that the use of LCBDE offers distinct advantages over endoscopy. A single-stage operation with LCBDE at the time of laparoscopic cholecystectomy (LC) obviates the need for patients to undergo a two-stage procedure with ERCP either before or after LC, thereby avoiding a second anesthetic in addition to adding the previously described risks of ERCP. Multiple studies have demonstrated that LCBDE is equivalent to ERCP for achieving clearance of ductal stones [8, 9].

The declining utilization of LCBDE has serious implications for training of general surgeons (Fig. 16.1). A recent study examining the operative case logs of graduating chief general surgery residents showed that residents only participated in an average of 1.7 open CDEs and 0.7 LCBDEs over the course of their training [10]. These findings have raised concerns that the next generation of general surgeons is receiving inadequate exposure to the surgical management of biliary disease. While ERCP provides an attractive alternative for patients hoping to avoid surgery, sur-

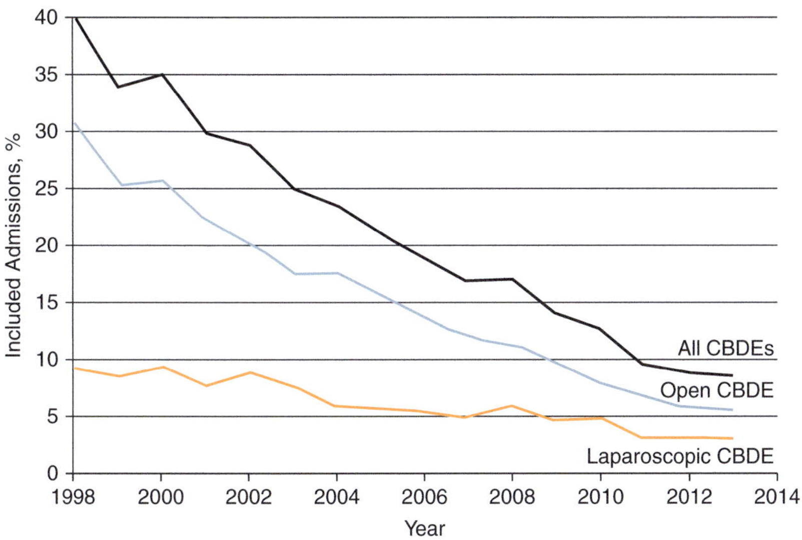

Fig. 16.1 Utilization trends of surgical common bile duct exploration from 1998 to 2013. Reprinted with permission from Wandling et al. [7]

geons need to be proficient in the general principles of CDE as surgical intervention is now generally the last resort for patients with choledocholithiasis not resolved after endoscopic intervention.

Simulation and Laparoscopic Common Bile Duct Exploration

One of the commonly cited reasons for the lack of utilization of the LCBDE procedure is that it requires advanced laparoscopic skills in order to successfully obtain clearance of the CBD. While it is true that a transcholedochal exploration requires the surgeon to be familiar with advanced laparoscopic maneuvers including intracorporeal suturing in order to repair the choledochotomy, the transcystic approach can be safely attempted by any surgeon with basic laparoscopic training. There are a series of operative steps that must be followed in order to increase the likelihood of successfully clearing any CBD obstruction via the laparoscopic approach. However, as is the case with any procedure that is done infrequently, many surgeons are unfamiliar with the procedural steps of LCBDE. Most also lack knowledge regarding strategies that can be employed when dealing with a variety of intraoperative scenarios, including obtaining and maintaining guidewire access, accessing the CBD with the choledochoscope, manipulation of the choledochoscope during stone retrieval, and appropriate management of the cystic duct stump (see Video 16.1). Surgical simulation has emerged as a viable option for training of novice physicians in a multitude of procedures and is not limited only to those in procedural fields.

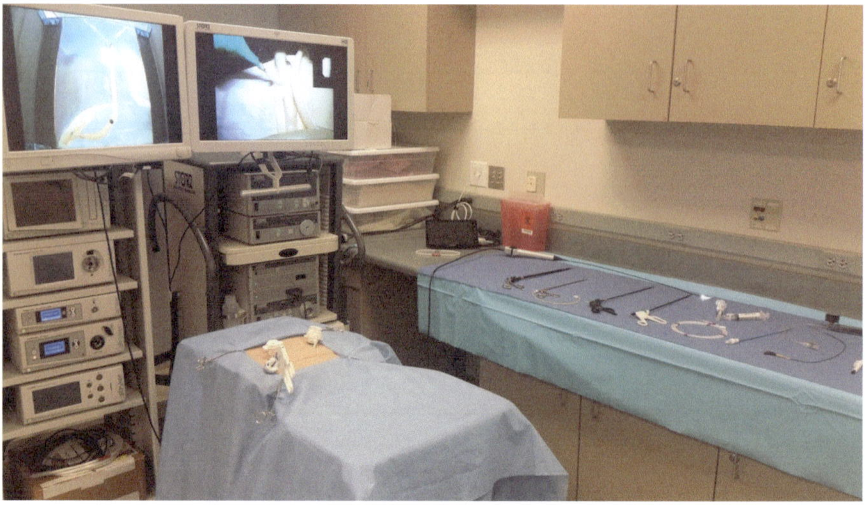

Fig. 16.2 External view of LCBDE simulator and equipment

The scope of these simulators ranges widely, including various low-cost inanimate task trainers aimed primarily at practicing a single skill, up to live animal models that afford trainees the opportunity to practice skills in an environment that closely approximates that found in the operating room—but these models are limited by issues of cost and ethical concerns.

In an attempt to improve upon previous LCBDE simulation models, Santos and colleagues at Northwestern University Feinberg School of Medicine developed a low-cost LCBDE simulation program aimed at teaching learners a stepwise approach to performance of an LCBDE (Fig. 16.2) [11]. The development of the simulator began by defining a comprehensive algorithm covering the cognitive and technical considerations necessary for successfully performing an LCBDE (Fig. 16.3).

The physical simulator was then developed and incorporated multiple modalities utilized during a clinical LCBDE case, including a laparoscopic image utilizing the static camera of a Fundamentals of Laparoscopic Surgery™ trainer box, a simulated fluoroscopic view by using a second camera and mirror in addition to the endoscopic image provided by a flexible choledochoscope for retrieving the CBD "stone" (Fig. 16.4).

Performance on a simulated task is improved when learners are provided with targeted assessment and feedback at the conclusion of the training session. Therefore, in addition to development of the multimodality LCBDE simulator, procedure-specific rating scales based on the objective structured assessment of technical skills (OSATS) principles were developed for the purpose of evaluating a participant's performance on the simulator. Rather than using a generic rating scale based solely on technical skill, the rating scale was based on the previously developed algorithm and assessed learners on their cognitive understanding of the

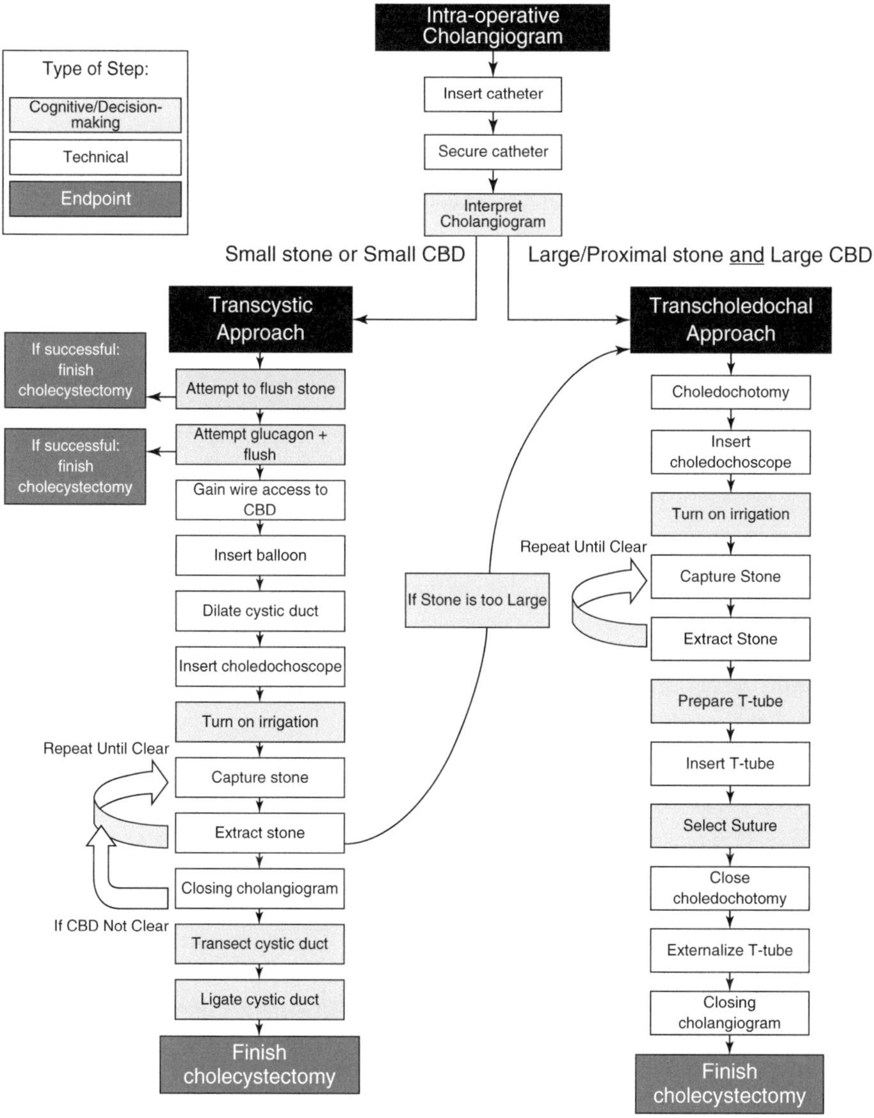

Fig. 16.3 Algorithm outlining key cognitive and technical steps of LCBDE. Reprinted with permission from Santos et al. [11]

LCBDE procedure in addition to their technical skill. Examples of these components included assessing the understanding of the available adjuncts available for clearing the CBD prior to embarking on a laparoscopic exploration, in addition to managing the cystic duct stump at the conclusion of the procedure. Learners were also asked to provide justification for their choice of operative approach, as the simulator was

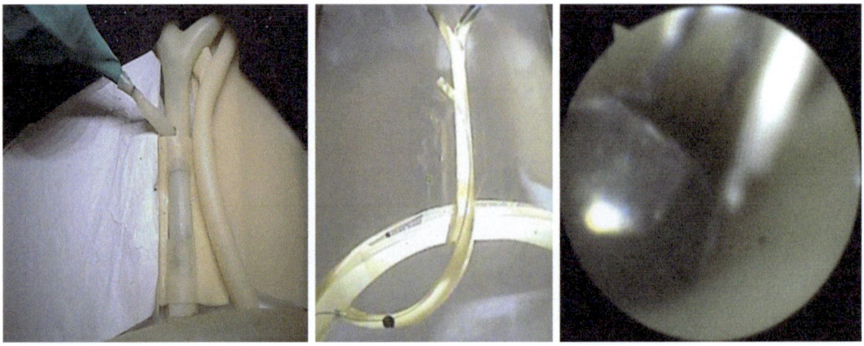

Fig. 16.4 LCBDE simulated views. (**a**) Laparoscopic view demonstrating liver (black), gallbladder (green), cystic duct, and common bile duct (CBD). (**b**) Fluoroscopic view demonstrating distal filling defect (black) after establishment of guidewire access. (**c**) Endoscopic view demonstrating CBD stone (black) trapped in endoscopic basket retrieval device

originally designed to permit either a transcholedochal or a transcystic laparoscopic exploration. Given the complex nature of the decision-making process necessary for performing LCBDE, utilizing this approach allows raters to better assess a participant's overall understanding of the various considerations that must be accounted for during the performance of an LCBDE procedure.

Mastery Learning

While simulation certainly provides advantages for learners, isolated performance of a simulated procedure is not adequate preparation for optimal performance in a real-world situation. Rather, simulation should function as one part of a comprehensive, goal-directed curriculum designed to provide learners with a global understanding of the subject material. Mastery learning (ML) is an educational strategy that has undergone a resurgence, particularly in the field of medical education and simulation. ML is founded on the principle that any motivated learner has the capacity to reach a predefined competency level, otherwise known as the "mastery" standard, provided they are given the necessary time and resources in order to attain a particular educational goal. This approach is in contrast to the contemporary model, whereby learners are given a discrete unit of time in which to accomplish the educational task. This has traditionally resulted in variable educational outcomes given that a proportion of learners will be unable to achieve the defined educational standard within the allotted time. In contrast, mastery learning is focused on universal achievement at the expense of variable learning time and requires a paradigm shift in medical education, and particularly surgical education, given the time constraints placed on residents. The concept of mastery learning has traditionally been broken down into seven core features (Table 16.1) [12].

Table 16.1 Seven core principles of the mastery learning bundle

1. Baseline or diagnostic testing
2. Clear learning objectives, sequenced as units usually in increasing difficulty
3. Engagement in educational activities (e.g., skills practice, data interpretation, reading) focused on reaching the objectives
4. A set minimum passing standard (e.g., test score) for each educational unit
5. Formative testing to gauge unit completion at the preset minimum passing standard for mastery
6. Advancement to the next educational unit given measured achievement at or above the mastery standard
7. Continued practice or study on an educational unit until the mastery standard is reached

Reprinted with permission from McGaghie et al. [12]

One of the key tenets of ML is the concept of "deliberate practice" [13]. Deliberate practice describes a process of immersive, goal-directed practice and involves targeted and immediate feedback for the learner. The timely provision of this feedback provides learners with an opportunity to quickly correct mistakes and increases the likelihood of reaching the defined mastery standard within the allotted time. This process fosters a high level of achievement among learners while simultaneously reducing variation in educational outcomes, the keystone of the mastery learning approach. ML concepts are widely applicable and have found fertile ground in the field of medical simulation [14–17].

Simulation-based mastery learning (SBML) has emerged as a unique opportunity in the field of surgical education as a strategy to address training deficiencies while promoting graduated responsibility among surgical residents. There are a variety of applications for well-designed SBML curricula. SBML can be used to provide novices with exposure to various surgical techniques prior to applying those techniques in the operating room. Another benefit of SBML is the ability to provide residents with exposure to surgical procedures not commonly encountered during the normal course of their clinical training. As described earlier, one of the commonly cited reasons for the low utilization of LCBDE is lack of exposure to the procedure during clinical training.

Using the previously described simulator, Teitelbaum and colleagues designed an SBML educational curriculum aimed at teaching senior surgical residents the essential steps for performing both a transcystic and a transcholedochal LCBDE [18]. The curriculum consisted of a pretest, where resident surgeons were asked to perform a simulated LCBDE without any preparation. They were then provided with didactic materials and given opportunities for deliberate practice followed by a posttest assessment on the simulator. The minimum passing score, or "mastery standard," was previously defined by two senior surgeons with prior LCBDE experience utilizing the previously described OSATS assessment tool. The SBML curriculum was then evaluated among a group of ten senior surgical residents with no prior LCBDE experience. None of the original ten residents who participated in the study achieved the mastery standard during the initial pretest. However, all residents were able to achieve the mastery standard on their posttest after a period of deliberate practice using the LCBDE simulator. In addition to achieving the mastery standard, pre- and post-surveys completed by the participating residents demonstrated a significant improvement in their perceived ability to perform an LCBDE independently. Importantly, steps were taken to include operating room (OR) nurses and staff in the training sessions. This served two primary functions: It improved OR staff awareness of the equipment needed when the decision is made to proceed to LCBDE and also acquainted them with the key procedural steps. Senior residents rotating on the minimally invasive surgery service are now required to demonstrate successful completion of the LCBDE mastery curriculum as a core requirement of the rotation.

Preliminary work examining the clinical impact of the LCBDE curriculum demonstrates a number of trends that have significant implications, both for patients presenting with choledocholithiasis and for the training of surgical residents. First, an analysis of LCBDE utilization before and after implementation of the SBML curriculum demonstrated a statistically significant increase in the clinical use of LCBDE, both in terms of the absolute number of cases being performed per year and the overall percentage of patients presenting with choledocholithiasis who underwent single-stage management with LC/LCBDE compared to two-stage management with LC + ERCP. In addition to the overall increase in the use of LCBDE, the analysis demonstrated that the majority of cases done after curriculum implementation were performed by surgical faculty who had no prior LCBDE experience with the assistance of a resident who had successfully completed the LCBDE curriculum. This is an example of an educational intervention aimed solely at residents that resulted in a change in the pattern of surgical practice within an institution and represents a profound deviation from the traditional structure of surgical education. Additionally, when compared to ERCP + LC, the use of LCBDE among similarly matched patients resulted in significant cost savings and a reduced length of stay. These unpublished results (in press) provide an example of the potential benefits of implementing a targeted intervention designed to address a deficiency in current surgical practice and suggest that a well-designed SBML curriculum can effectively supplement the traditional apprenticeship model for the benefit of trainee surgeons while also resulting in significantly improved patient-level outcomes.

Conclusion

The use of LCBDE remains a clearly underutilized modality for managing patients who present with uncomplicated choledocholithiasis, despite continued evidence of its efficacy and cost-effectiveness when compared to the use of ERCP. While there is clearly a role for endoscopic management of these patients, it must be remembered that the procedure is not without its attendant risks, some of which can result in major morbidity or mortality. In addition, the use of single-stage LCBDE and laparoscopic cholecystectomy has obvious benefits to patients by avoiding multiple procedures, limiting anesthetic interventions, and shortening hospital stay. We believe that LCBDE should be the first choice for appropriately selected patients who present with choledocholithiasis.

Given the current clinical environment where ERCP is often the first step in management, opportunities for surgical residents to gain experience with the techniques necessary to perform a safe and therapeutic LCBDE are limited. Performing LCBDE does require surgeons to follow a series of cognitive and technical steps that will increase the likelihood of success and is not necessarily intuitive to those unfamiliar with the procedure. In an attempt to address the decline of LCBDE in surgical training and clinical use, researchers at Northwestern University designed, built, and evaluated a low-cost, multimodality LCBDE simulator and developed an SBML curriculum aimed at teaching novices the necessary skills to perform the procedure. Analysis of utilization trends and clinical outcomes demonstrated a significant increase in the use of LCBDE in addition to significant decreases in hospital length of stay and cost for patients who underwent LCBDE after implementation of the curriculum.

The success of this intervention represents an example of translational science in action, namely, a comprehensive SBML program designed to address a specific clinical deficiency in surgical training resulted in clinically significant high-level outcomes in the form of reduced cost, length of stay, and a high return of investment for the home institution. SBML will continue to serve as a powerful tool for surgical educators as they strive to prepare the next generation of surgeons for practice in an era of increasing technological advances and evolving patient care management strategies.

References

1. Halsted WS. The training of the surgeon. Bull Johns Hopkins Hosp. 1904;15(162):267–75.
2. Osler W. The hospital as a college. In: Osler W, editor. Aequanimitas. Philadelphia: P. Blakiston's Son & Co.; [1903] 1932.
3. Bell RH Jr, Biester TW, Tabuenca A, Rhodes RS, Cofer JB, Britt LD, Lewis FR Jr. Operative experience of residents in U.S. general surgery programs: a gap between expectation and experience. Ann Surg. 2009;249:719–24.
4. Begos DG, Modlin IM. Laparoscopic cholecystectomy: from gimmick to gold standard. J Clin Gastroenterol. 1994;19(4):325–30.
5. Katon RM, Lee TG, Parent JA, Bilbao MK, Smith FW. Endoscopic retrograde cholangiopancreatography (ERCP). Experience with 100 cases. Am J Dig Dis. 1974;19(4):295–306.
6. Livingston EH, Rege RV. Technical complications are rising as common duct exploration is becoming rare. J Am Coll Surg. 2005;201(3):426–33.
7. Wandling MW, Hungness ES, Pavey ES, Stulberg JJ, Schwab B, Yang AD, et al. Nationwide assessment of trends in choledocholithiasis management in the United States from 1998 to 2013. JAMA Surg. 2016;151(12):1125–30.
8. Dasari BV, Tan CJ, Gurusamy KS, Martin DJ, Kirk G, McKie L, et al. Surgical versus endoscopic treatment of bile duct stones. Cochrane Database Syst Rev. 2013;12:CD003327.
9. Rogers SJ, Cello JP, Horn JK, Siperstein AE, Schecter WP, Campbell AR, et al. Prospective randomized trial of LC+LCBDE vs ERCP/S+LC for common bile duct stone disease. Arch Surg. 2010;145(1):28–33.

10. Helling TS, Khandelwal A. The challenges of resident training in complex hepatic, pancreatic, and biliary procedures. J Gastrointest Surg. 2008;12(1):153–8.
11. Santos BF, Reif TJ, Soper NJ, Nagle AP, Rooney DM, Hungness ES. Development and evaluation of a laparoscopic common bile duct exploration simulator and procedural rating scale. Surg Endosc. 2012;26(9):2403–15.
12. McGaghie WC, Siddall VJ, Mazmanian PE, Myers J. Lessons for continuing medical education from simulation research in undergraduate and graduate medical education: effectiveness of continuing medical education: American college of chest physicians evidence-based educational guidelines. Chest. 2009;135(3, Suppl):62S–8S.
13. Ericsson KA, Krampe RT, Tesch-Römer C. The role of deliberate practice in the acquisition of expert performance. Psychol Rev. 1993;100:363–406.
14. Barsuk JH, Cohen ER, Vozenilek JA, et al. Simulation-based education with mastery learning improves paracentesis skills. J Grad Med Educ. 2012;4:23–7.
15. Wayne DB, Barsuk JH, O'Leary KJ, Fudala MJ, McGaghie WC. Mastery learning of thoracentesis skills by internal medicine residents using simulation technology and deliberate practice. J Hosp Med. 2008;3(1):48–54.
16. Barsuk JH, McGaghie WC, Cohen ER, O'Leary KJ, Wayne DB. Simulation-based mastery learning reduces complications during central venous catheter insertion in a medical intensive care unit. Crit Care Med. 2009;37:2697–701.
17. Zendejas B, Cook DA, Hernández-Irizarry R, Huebner M, Farley DR. Mastery learning simulation-based curriculum for laparoscopic TEP inguinal hernia repair. J Surg Educ. 2012;69:208–14.
18. Teitelbaum EN, Soper NJ, Santos BF, Rooney DM, Patel P, Nagle AP, et al. A simulator-based resident curriculum for laparoscopic common bile duct exploration. Surgery. 2014;156(4):880–7.

Chapter 17
Economic Aspects of the Management of Choledocholithiasis

Harry C. Sax and Brian Weinberg

Introduction

With significant pressures to optimize care and control costs, surgical procedures are under scrutiny. New programs, such as the Medicare Comprehensive Joint Replacement program, are shifting risk to the hospital and practitioners by limiting total payment for an episode of care to a specified amount including technical and professional components [1]. Even in those situations where a bundle is not created, the responsibility to care for larger populations of patients in a risk-sharing environment will increase. As the healthcare environment evolves to a population health model rather than a fee-for-service model, medical centers are increasingly accepting up-front capitation payments for a given patient population; and as patients utilize services, the costs of those services are not additionally reimbursed beyond the initial capitation payment. In other chapters, we have discussed methods to address the patient with common bile duct (CBD) stones. This chapter will examine the economics involved and attempt to quantify the differences between two-stage and single-stage management of CBD stones.

Clearly identifying costs and revenues is quite difficult. There is little correlation between charges and true cost or clear understanding of how incentive alignment drives practitioner behaviors. The procedures required to care for CBD stone patients can be a two-stage or single-stage intervention and may be accomplished as inpatient, outpatient, or some combination of the two. Reimbursements vary depending on individual carriers, geography, and delivery system integration.

H. C. Sax, MD (✉)
Department of Surgery, Cedars-Sinai Medical Center, Los Angeles, CA, USA
e-mail: Harry.Sax@cshs.org

B. Weinberg, BA, BS, MBA
Department of Clinical Care Finance, Cedars-Sinai Health System, Los Angeles, CA, USA
e-mail: brian.weinberg@cshs.org

© Springer International Publishing AG, part of Springer Nature 2018

B. F. Santos, N. Soper (eds.), *Choledocholithiasis*,
https://doi.org/10.1007/978-3-319-74503-9_17

Nonetheless an attempt must be made to examine the true costs of laparoscopic common bile duct exploration in comparison to staged procedures of laparoscopic cholecystectomy followed or preceded by ERCP with stone extraction.

Accounting Terminology

To better understand the issues involved, some basic definitions are necessary.

Revenue is the actual amount of money reimbursed by a carrier for services rendered. It includes a *professional* component, paid to the physician, and a *technical* component or *facility fee* paid to the organization where the service took place. *Charges* are created for each of these components. However, the actual payment is usually much less due to contractual adjustments and fee schedules. Revenue is further complicated because different medical centers will have different payer mixes for their patients, and additionally each institution will have a fee schedule or a contracted reimbursement rate that may be different than the rates that other institutions receive.

Of greater importance is an understanding of true cost structure. Most healthcare institutions use a form of differential financial accounting that separates various costs into direct or indirect buckets. A *direct cost* is one that can be fairly assigned to the services rendered. For example, the sutures during a hernia repair are directly related to that repair, and the cost would not have been accrued if the procedure was not done. In the case of management of CBD stones, direct costs would include disposable laparoscopic trocars, baskets, and dilating balloons and various endoscopic instruments used for ERCP. In addition, many organizations will include the labor involved in the care of the patient. The postoperative care of a patient who is on the ward with one nurse assigned to four patients will include the equivalent of 0.25 FTE (full-time equivalent). Other direct costs are patient medications, meals, and laboratory tests. Direct costs are important because they are the one area that is potentially controllable through negotiations with suppliers as well as improvements in clinical efficiency and appropriateness.

Indirect costs are also an important component of the overall delivery of care. These include such items as heating and cooling of the building, salaries for administrative and support personnel, and other expenses such as maintenance, laundry services, housekeeping, and depreciation. These costs are allocated to each encounter using various formulas including square footage, budgets, or volumes. It is important to remember that indirect costs do not go away even if the procedure is not done.

Total cost reflects both direct and indirect costs. In academic institutions, it may also include an allocation for the teaching mission.

All institutions must generate a *positive margin* on their total book of business if they are to have long-term viability. Margins take several forms:

Contribution margin is defined as revenue less direct costs. For an institution, it is the most basic reflection of the financial implications of providing a service. You cannot have a negative margin and “make it up on volume.” Contribution margin is a bit more esoteric for a physician. *Opportunity cost* to the physician is the difference in income received in choosing to do one procedure in lieu of another.

For example, if it takes an extra 2 h to do a LCBDE and this generates an additional $100, the surgeon will weigh that against doing another simple laparoscopic cholecystectomy instead in those 2 h that pays $600. This may begin to shift as more physicians move to employed models, and gain-sharing arrangements are created for efficiency in the overall cost of care.

Total margin is revenue less total costs. It is not uncommon for an episode of care to have a positive contribution margin but negative total margin after allocation of indirect costs.

Costs Associated with the Treatment of Common Bile Duct Stones

This chapter will focus on the actual costs in the care of CBD stones. The costs are born by the institution for the technical component and by the insurance carrier who pays both the physician and the institution. We identified patients at Cedars-Sinai Medical Center (CSMC) who underwent laparoscopic cholecystectomy with or without cholangiogram (CPT 47562 or 47563) for our fiscal year 2016, ending June 30, 2016. This large cohort was then narrowed to those who also had a LCBDE (CPT 47564) or ERCP with stone extraction (CPT 43260, 43262, or 43264). For a measure of professional costs, we used the published Medicare CPT reimbursements, rounded to the nearest dollar. These include 91 different geographic locations [2]. From our internal financial database, we also quantified direct and total costs, excluding the academic component, as well as length of stay (LOS). Data provided include median, minimum, and maximum values and expressed as US dollars.

Results

We identified 14 patients who underwent cholecystectomy and LCBDE as a single procedure and compared them to 23 whose common duct stones were handled in a staged manner—either before or after cholecystectomy. Tables 17.1, 17.2, 17.3, and 17.4 represent only those patients who had both procedures done at CSMC. It is entirely possible that one of the procedures was carried out in a private, non-Cedars environment.

Table 17.1 Medicare professional fees for cholecystectomy

CPT	Median	Minimum	Maximum
47562—LC	680	555	868
47563—LC/IOC	739	604	944
47564—LCBDE	1150	942	1472

LC laparoscopic cholecystectomy, *LC/IOC* laparoscopic cholecystectomy with cholangiogram, *LCBDE* laparoscopic common bile duct exploration, *ERCP* endoscopic retrograde cholangiopancreatography, *LOS* hospital length of stay, *CPT* current procedural terminology

Table 17.2 Medicare professional fees for ERCP with stone extraction

CPT	Median	Minimum	Maximum
43260—Diagnostic ERCP	343	295	455
43262—ERCP with sphincterotomy	380	326	504
43264—ERCP with CBD stone removal	388	333	513

CPT current procedural terminology, *ERCP* endoscopic retrograde cholangiopancreatography, *CBD* common bile duct

Table 17.3 Costs

Procedure type	Median direct	Direct range	Median total	Total range
LCBDE	7905	5784–10,752	15,114	10,892–20,455
ERCP/LC	13,865	6723–78,488	26,926	12,745–153,092

LCBDE laparoscopic common bile duct exploration, *ERCP* endoscopic retrograde cholangiopancreatography, *LC* laparoscopic cholecystectomy

Table 17.4 Hospital length of stay

Procedure type	Median LOS	Range	Outpatient (%)
LCBDE	1.0	1.0–2.0	36
ERCP/LC	3.0	1.0–29.0	0

LCBDE laparoscopic common bile duct exploration, *ERCP* endoscopic retrograde cholangiopancreatography, *LC* laparoscopic cholecystectomy

Discussion

It is not surprising that staging the management of CBD stones is more expensive from a facility point of view. Of interest, the profession fees for a single-stage LCBDE are similar to the additive costs of a laparoscopic cholecystectomy and separate ERCP with stone extraction. However, the current dynamics of fee-for-service practice come into play. Surgeons are dependent on referrals from gastroenterologists, especially for other high-value procedures, such as colectomies. These factors may make a surgeon less willing to do a single-stage procedure, depending on the additional time and effort required. This is less of an issue in closed staff models, where clinicians share in gains for clinical efficiency. As more clinical conditions move to bundled payments, and Stark laws are modified to allow risk and gain sharing between doctors and hospitals, these incentives may change.

We choose not to discuss margins in the various scenarios, as reimbursement is highly variable based on payer mix, local geography, and hospital negotiations. Maximizing reimbursement by staging procedures may have been appropriate in the previous payment paradigm, but not with the move to population health.

There are also implications directly related to patient care. Staged procedures require separate anesthetics and an additive risk of complication to the patient. Pancreatitis or perforation after ERCP occurs in up to 5% of patients and leads to prolonged hospitalizations and increased costs [3]. LCBDE also carries risk, primarily related to the dilation needed to place the choledochoscope as well as bile leaks [4]. There are various scenarios that can be generated including the costs for treating each complication and the likelihood of that occurring. Further, neither procedure is 100% successful on the first attempt, requiring subsequent interventions [5, 6]. For this study, we chose to focus on an "apples to apples" comparison, assuming no complications and optimal success rates.

Reduction in length of stay is beneficial for both the patient and the institution. LCBDE patients are discharged to family and activity earlier and have a lower risk of nosocomial infection related to ERCP disinfection issues [7]. Institutions free up bed capacity to improve patient throughput. In our institution, more than one-third of the LCBDE patients were treated as outpatients, with no bed required.

Finally, there are other costs related to the purchase and maintenance of the choledochoscopes and duodenoscopes. These have finite life expectancies that must be amortized over the number of procedures performed, as well as the need for cleaning and repairs. There has been increased scrutiny of ERCP after recent clustered outbreaks of drug-resistant colonization [8]. We also did not include professional fees related to multiple anesthetics or additional radiology studies (e.g., magnetic resonance imaging or endoscopic ultrasound) that would be seen in the staged situation.

There are limitations to our analysis. Every hospital has its own cost structure, physician alignment, and patient demographics. CSMC's costs for labor and supplies are higher, as it must compete in the Los Angeles market. The advanced laparoscopic and endoscopic cases tend to cluster to a few physicians, which optimizes outcomes from both a success and procedural time perspective. We also have a pluralistic model of physician employment and do not have direct access to professional charges or reimbursement to our individual staff members. Nonetheless, the differential in costs being related to the facility costs seems intuitive.

Conclusion

Single-stage LCBDE offers significant opportunities to reduce cost, reduce length of stay, and improve the patient experience. For these goals to be reached, expansion in the training of surgical residents in the management of CBD stones and a shift in incentive alignment are vital.

References

1. Comprehensive care for joint replacement model. https://innovation.cms.gov/initiatives/cjr. Accessed 15 Nov 2016.
2. Medicare physician fee schedule search tool. https://www.cms.gov/apps/physician-fee-schedule/overview.aspx. Accessed 1 Nov 2016.

3. Mann K, Belgaumkar AP, Singh S. Post-endoscopic retrograde cholangiography after laparoscopic cholecystectomy: challenging but safe. JSLS. 2013;17(3):371–5.
4. Dasari BV, Tan CJ, Gurusamy KS, Martin DJ, Kirk G, McKie L, Diamond T, Taylor MA. Surgical versus endoscopic treatment of bile duct stones. Cochrane Database Syst Rev. 2013;9:CD003327.
5. Rogers SJ, Cello JP, Horn JK, Siperstein AE, Schecter WP, Campbell AR, et al. Prospective randomized trial of LC+LCBDE vs ERCP/S+LC for common bile duct stone disease. Arch Surg. 2010;145(1):28–33.
6. Chan DS, Jain PA, Khalifa A, Hughes R, Baker AL. Laparoscopic common bile duct exploration. Br J Surg. 2014;101(11):1448–52.
7. Keswani RN, Soper NJ. Endoscopes and the "Superbug" outbreak. JAMA Surg. 2015;150(9):831–2.
8. Supplemental measures to enhance duodenoscope reprocessing: FDA safety communication. http://www.fda.gov/MedicalDevices/Safety/AlertsandNotices/ucm454766.htm. Accessed 15 Nov 2016.

Index

© Springer International Publishing AG, part of Springer Nature 2018

B. F. Santos, N. Soper (eds.), *Choledocholithiasis*,
https://doi.org/10.1007/978-3-319-74503-9

MIX
Papier aus verantwortungsvollen Quellen
Paper from responsible sources
FSC® C105338

If you have any concerns about our products,
you can contact us on
ProductSafety@springernature.com

In case Publisher is established outside the EU,
the EU authorized representative is:
Springer Nature Customer Service Center GmbH
Europaplatz 3, 69115 Heidelberg, Germany

Printed by Libri Plureos GmbH
in Hamburg, Germany